T0202206

THE CDC FIELD EPIDEMIOLOGY MANUAL

THE CDC FIELD EPIDEMIOLOGY MANUAL

Edited by
Sonja A. Rasmussen and Richard A. Goodman

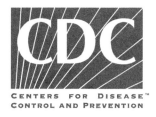

US Department of Health and Human Services
Centers for Disease Control and Prevention
Atlanta, Georgia

OXFORD
UNIVERSITY PRESS

OXFORD
UNIVERSITY PRESS

Oxford University Press is a department of the University of Oxford. It furthers
the University's objective of excellence in research, scholarship, and education
by publishing worldwide. Oxford is a registered trade mark of Oxford University
Press in the UK and certain other countries.

Published in the United States of America by Oxford University Press
198 Madison Avenue, New York, NY 10016, United States of America.

Library of Congress Cataloging-in-Publication Data
Names: Rasmussen, Sonja A., editor. | Goodman, Richard A. (Richard Alan), 1949– editor. |
Centers for Disease Control and Prevention (U.S.)
Title: The CDC field epidemiology manual / edited by Sonja A. Rasmussen, Richard A. Goodman.
Other titles: Field epidemiology. | Centers for Disease Control and Prevention field epidemiology manual |
Field epidemiology manual
Description: Fourth edition. | Oxford ; New York : Oxford University Press, [2019] |
Preceded by Field epidemiology / edited by Michael B. Gregg. 3rd ed. c2008. |
Includes bibliographical references and index.
Identifiers: LCCN 2018025581 | ISBN 9780190624248 (pbk. : alk. paper) |
ISBN 9780190933692 (hardcover : alk. paper)
Subjects: | MESH: Epidemiologic Methods
Classification: LCC RA651 | NLM WA 950 | DDC 614.4—dc23
LC record available at https://lccn.loc.gov/2018025581

9 8 7

Paperback printed by Sheridan Books, Inc., United States of America
Hardback printed by Bridgeport National Bindery, Inc., United States of America

The mark "CDC" is owned by the US Dept. of Health and Human Services (HHS) and is used with permission. Use of
this logo is not an endorsement by HHS or CDC of any particular product, service, or enterprise.

SUGGESTED CITATION

Rasmussen SA and Goodman RA. *The CDC Field Epidemiology Manual*. New York: Oxford University Press, 2019.

>

DISCLAIMERS

The findings and conclusion in this report are those of the authors and do not necessarily represent the official position of the Centers for Disease Control and Prevention or the authors' institutions.

References to non-CDC Internet sites are provided as a service to readers and do not constitute or imply endorsement of these organizations or their programs by the US Department of Health and Human Services, the Public Health Service, or CDC. CDC is not responsible for the content of these sites. URL addresses were current as of the date of publication.

NOTICE

This material is not intended to be, and should not be considered, a substitute for medical or other professional advice. Treatment for the conditions described in this material is highly dependent on the individual circumstances. While this material is designed to offer accurate information with respect to the subject matter covered and to be current as of the time it was written, research and knowledge about medical and health issues are constantly evolving, and dose schedules for medications and vaccines are being revised continually, with new side effects recognized and accounted for regularly. Readers must, therefore, always check the product information and clinical procedures with the most up-to-date published product information and data sheets provided by the manufacturers and the most recent codes of conduct and safety regulation. Oxford University Press and the authors make no representations or warranties to readers, express or implied, as to the accuracy or completeness of this material, including without limitation that they make no representations or warranties as to the accuracy or efficacy of the drug dosages mentioned in the material. The authors and the publishers do not accept, and expressly disclaim, any responsibility for any liability, loss, or risk that may be claimed or incurred as a consequence of the use and/or application of any of the contents of this material.

The Publisher is responsible for author selection and the Publisher and the Author(s) make all editorial decisions, including decisions regarding content. The Publisher and the Author(s) are not responsible for any product information added to this publication by companies purchasing copies of it for distribution to clinicians.

For additional copies, please contact Oxford University Press, or order online at www.oup.com/us.

This book is dedicated to the thousands of public health professionals globally who work tirelessly to protect the public's health by responding rapidly to acute disease outbreaks and other emerging public health issues.

CONTENTS

PREFACE

Field epidemiology, defined as "epidemiology with the goal of immediate action to address a public health problem of concern" (see Chapter 1), is a primary function in US public health practice and has been integral to the mission of CDC since the creation of the agency's Epidemic Intelligence Service (EIS) Program in 1951. After several years in development, the first edition of *Field Epidemiology*, edited by Michael B. Gregg, MD, was published in 1996. In the preface to that edition, Carl W. Tyler, Jr., MD—who had helped conceive the need for the initial text during his tenure as Director of CDC's Epidemiology Program Office during the mid-1980s—wrote, "There is a need for a clearly written, highly usable book devoted to field epidemiology—the timely use of epidemiology in solving public health problems. This process involves the application of basic epidemiologic principles as in real time, place, and person to solve health problems of an urgent or emergency nature." The uptake, use, and success of that first edition led to second and third editions, the latter published in 2008. The decade after the 2008 edition has been marked by the continuing emergence of public health challenges that require epidemiologic field investigative responses as well as innovations in the science and art of the methods of field epidemiology. For these reasons, CDC recognized the need to update the volume's scope and contents. The result of this renewal is this fourth edition, now under a new title, the *CDC Field Epidemiology Manual*, to reflect the evolution in scope, methods, venues, and other aspects of the application of field epidemiology.

The preface to the first edition stated, "This book takes its roots from the experience of the Centers for Disease Control and Prevention (CDC) over more than 40 years of training health professionals in the science and art of field epidemiology." This new, fourth edition sustains that tradition: the principles of field epidemiology in this manual continue to draw from and reflect the foundation of the curriculum used each year in training newly arriving EIS officers. However, this focus on principles central to CDC's training of EIS officers should not be interpreted as limiting the book's utility only to epidemiologic field investigations conducted by CDC. As was the case for the previous editions, one of the new edition's main goals is for public health professionals and many other allied health workers to be able to use all the chapters in addressing a broad spectrum of problems in multiple field settings.

Another major goal we pursued in developing this new edition was to make the book more usable to epidemiologists in the planning and implementation phases of field investigations. Also as noted in the first edition's preface, "Copies of this book should be more often in the briefcases of field epidemiologists than on the shelves of libraries." However, the page length of previous editions had expanded dramatically, from 267 pages in the first edition, to 411 in the second, and 523 in the third. To enable this new edition to have greater utility in the field, we pursued a more readable format, including boxes and bulleted points, as are sometimes used in portable clinical manuals. We hope public health practitioners and other readers will find the tighter chapters and easier-to-read format helpful when using this manual in epidemiologic field investigations.

In this edition, we also removed the background chapters on principles of epidemiology and surveillance because we expect that most users already have a basic fund of knowledge of these areas and because other sources cover these topics in great depth. For similar reasons, we also removed other chapters, including the chapters on communicating epidemiologic findings, which focused on how to write a scientific paper, and immunization practices. Because this new edition is designed to be used in planning and implementing investigations in a greater spectrum of field settings, we also removed the chapter on field investigations from the state and local health department perspective.

This fourth edition of CDC's compendium on field epidemiology has preserved the core elements in approaching field investigations of public health problems that require prompt action and solutions. Meanwhile, this edition has augmented the core elements by incorporating a broad set of innovations, including design changes that impart portability, increased utilities, and enhanced readability, and an expansion in scope that accommodates major evolutionary changes in methods for epidemiologic field investigations that have emerged since the last edition's publication in 2008. To undertake such substantial change and to ensure that this new edition is responsive to the needs of persons who actively perform field investigations, we established a steering committee made up of members with broad experiences in field epidemiology in local, state, national, and international settings. We then charged those committee members with proposing new chapter topics and authors for the fourth edition as well as making recommendations for maximizing the manual's usefulness across wide-ranging field settings. We are grateful to the committee members (listed in the Acknowledgments) who provided this expert guidance early in this edition's development.

Since the inception of *Field Epidemiology* as CDC's first dedicated edition on field epidemiology, this domain's core principles have remained unchanged, and the representation of those principles has remained consistent across all of the editions. In contrast, however, substantial changes have occurred in certain approaches, methods, and types of settings in which field investigations are conducted. Accordingly, in this fourth edition, all chapters have been updated to include the latest advances in field epidemiology wherever possible. As in the previous editions, chapters in this edition's first section on "The Field Investigation" remain organized according to the progression of the basic steps in an outbreak investigation, including, for example, the sequencing from "Defining Field Epidemiology" and "Initiating Operations," to "Developing Interventions" and "Communicating During an Outbreak or Public Health Investigation." Each chapter in this first section focuses on an activity, as evidenced by their action-oriented titles.

This edition also places an increased emphasis on the importance of collaborations during field investigations. Accordingly, the chapter on laboratory science now is included in the first section on Field Investigations but has been strengthened and retitled ("Optimizing Epidemiology–Laboratory Collaborations") to give greater attention to the importance of these collaborations, beginning at the earliest phase of planning an investigation. The importance of collaborations in multistate and international settings is now highlighted by the addition of new chapters addressing these concerns in the section on Special Considerations ("Coordination of Multiple States and Federal Agencies" and "Multinational Outbreak Investigations"). Finally, to address the need for collaboration in investigating public health problems that might be associated with malicious use of biologic or toxic agents, a new chapter ("Suspected Intentional Use of Biologic and Toxic Agents") covers collaborations between public health, law enforcement, and other non-traditional partners.

The new edition has recognized substantive advances in some of the key tools used during field investigations through the addition of new chapters and updates to others. For example, because portable computers are now a standard, fully integrated component in field investigations, the chapter on this topic from the previous edition has been supplanted by a new chapter ("Using Technologies for Data Collection and Management") that discusses an expanding array of technologies—from mobile devices to environmental sensors—that can improve the efficiency and effectiveness of field responses. Other additions covering advances in tools are a new chapter on the use of geographic information system data and, to encompass the increasing use of qualitative data in epidemiology, a new chapter on "Collecting and Analyzing Qualitative Data."

Finally, because of a progression in the types of scenarios that might prompt epidemiologic field investigations, this edition includes new chapters reflecting these scenarios. For example, a chapter in the third edition on the scenario of investigations in out-of-home child care settings has been supplanted in this edition by a new chapter ("Community Congregate Settings") that covers such situations as educational institutions, workplaces, mass gatherings, and detention facilities. A new chapter on "Acute Enteric Disease Outbreaks" provides information on methods for detecting, investigating, and controlling foodborne, waterborne, and other enteric pathogen–associated outbreaks, with a particular focus on multijurisdictional investigations of foodborne illness. Finally, to address the epidemiologic phenomenon of the spread of violent injury in patterns that echo the transmission of certain infectious conditions, this fourth edition includes a new chapter on field investigations of "Suicide, Violence, and Other Forms of Injury."

Although this new edition features many changes, we have retained historically important principles and traditions of field epidemiology to preserve the spirit of CDC's earlier progenitors of this branch of epidemiology. Foremost among these leaders were Alexander Langmuir, MD, originator of the EIS Program and powerful advocate for broader uses of epidemiology in public health practice; Philip Brachman, MD, long-time director of CDC's Bureau of Epidemiology, who promoted the EIS Program and led in the creation of the globe-spanning Field Epidemiology Training Program based on the EIS; Carl Tyler, MD, former director of CDC's Epidemiology Program Office who had a vision for continually modernizing field epidemiology and who championed creation of the first edition of *Field Epidemiology*; and Michael B. Gregg, MD, editor of the first three editions, who also served as editor of CDC's *Morbidity and Mortality Weekly Report* (*MMWR*) for 21 years and as CDC's dean of training in field epidemiology.

We hope investigators will find the chapters in this fourth edition useful as they seek to address public health challenges and identify interventions to decrease disease and disability and save lives.

—Sonja A. Rasmussen
Atlanta, Georgia

—Richard A. Goodman
(Associate Editor, *Field Epidemiology*, First Edition, 1996)
Atlanta, Georgia

ACKNOWLEDGMENTS

We acknowledge the *CDC Field Epidemiology Manual* Steering Committee members who provided crucial guidance early in the planning of the book, including input regarding potential chapter topics and authors and on ways to make the book more useful across the array of field settings. Members of the steering committee were Guthrie Birkhead, Megan Davies, Kate Glynn, Patricia M. Griffin, Marci Layton, Frank Mahoney, Josephine Malilay, Joshua Mott, and Robert V. Tauxe.

We also acknowledge the experts who provided their guidance through their review of individual chapters: Katherine Lyon Daniel, Chad Heilig, and Michael Iademarco. We are also grateful to CDC experts who reviewed all chapters as part of the CDC clearance process. In particular, we would like to highlight the outstanding work of Paul Z. Siegel who reviewed nearly all book chapters as a reviewer for CDC's Center for Surveillance, Epidemiology, and Laboratory Services.

We also acknowledge Todd Goldfarb, Charmika Placide, Samantha Riemer, and John Vagas who helped with organizational and logistical aspects of the book, including arranging steering committee conference calls, monitoring the status of all book chapters, and assisting with completion of the contents and list of contributors.

We are especially grateful for the dedicated efforts of the managing editors of the book, Karen L. Foster and C. Kay Smith, who edited all chapters for style and clarity and prepared chapters for final submission to the publisher. We believe their hard work has substantially improved the readability and usefulness of the book for future field investigators.

ABOUT THE EDITORS

Sonja A. Rasmussen, MD, MS, was the Director of CDC's Division of Public Health Information Dissemination in the Center for Surveillance, Epidemiology, and Laboratory Services (CSELS) and Editor-in-Chief of the *Morbidity and Mortality Weekly Report* (*MMWR*) Series while serving as the editor of this book. She is currently Professor of Pediatrics and Epidemiology at the University of Florida College of Medicine and College of Public Health and Health Professions. She has held leadership positions in several CDC emergency responses, including 2009 H1N1 influenza, Middle East respiratory syndrome (MERS) coronavirus, and Ebola and Zika viruses.

Richard A. Goodman, MD, JD, MPH, is Professor of Medicine at Emory University's School of Medicine and Rollins School of Public Health. Dr. Goodman held leadership and senior staff positions at the Centers for Disease Control and Prevention from 1978 to 2015, serving as Editor-in-Chief of CDC's *Morbidity and Mortality Weekly Report* (*MMWR*) Series for a decade, Co-Director CDC's Public Health Law Program, and Associate Director of CDC's Epidemiology Program Office.

About the Centers for Disease Control and Prevention:
The Centers for Disease Control and Prevention (CDC), headquartered in Atlanta, Georgia, is a United States federal agency under the Department of Health and Human Services.

CONTRIBUTORS

Erica Adams, MS, MPH
Contract Spatial Epidemiologist
Booz Allen Hamilton
Assigned to the Geospatial Research
    Analysis and Services Program
National Center for Environmental
    Health/Agency for Toxic Substances
    and Disease Registry
Centers for Disease Control and
    Prevention
Atlanta, Georgia

Diana M. Bensyl, PhD, MA, FACE
CAPT, US Public Health Service
Lead, Global Emergency Alert and
    Response Service
Division of Global Health Protection
Center for Global Health
Centers for Disease Control and
    Prevention
Atlanta, Georgia

Jennifer R. Black, JD
Contract Public Health Analyst
Cherokee Nation Assurance
Assigned to the Public Health Law
    Program
Center for State, Tribal, Local, and
    Territorial Support (Proposed)
Centers for Disease Control and
    Prevention
Atlanta, Georgia

Jeffrey L. Bryant, MS, MSS
Director
Division of Emergency Operations
Office of Public Health Preparedness and
    Response
Centers for Disease Control and
    Prevention
Atlanta, Georgia

James W. Buehler, MD
Clinical Professor, Health Management
    and Policy
Dornsife School of Public Health
Drexel University
Philadelphia, Pennsylvania

Bryan E. Christensen, PhD, MEPC
CDR, US Public Health Service
Environmental Health Officer
Division of Healthcare Quality Promotion
National Center for Emerging and
    Zoonotic Infectious Diseases
Centers for Disease Control and
    Prevention
Atlanta, Georgia

Melissa Corkum, MA
Chief of Polio
United Nations International Children's
    Emergency Fund
Kabul, Afghanistan

Kristin J. Cummings, MD, MPH
Visiting Scientist
Chief (Former)
Field Studies Branch
Respiratory Health Division
National Institute for Occupational Safety
    and Health
Centers for Disease Control and
    Prevention
Morgantown, West Virginia

David Daigle, MA
Lead
Strategic Partnerships and Media
    Relations
Division of Healthcare Quality Promotion
National Center for Emerging and
    Zoonotic Infectious Diseases
Centers for Disease Control and
    Prevention
Atlanta, Georgia

Andrew Dent, MBA, MA
Director
Geospatial Research Analysis and Services
    Program
National Center for Environmental
    Health/Agency for Toxic Substances
    and Disease Registry
Centers for Disease Control and
    Prevention
Atlanta, Georgia

Richard C. Dicker, MD, MS
Lead
Curriculum Development Unit
Workforce and Institute
    Development Branch
Division of Global Health Protection
Center for Global Health
Centers for Disease Control and
    Prevention
Atlanta, Georgia

Ian Dunn, MPH, GISP
Contract Geographic Information System
    Analyst
DRT Strategies
Assigned to the Geospatial Research,
    Analysis, and Services Program
National Center for Environmental
    Health/Agency for Toxic Substances
    and Disease Registry
Centers for Disease Control and
    Prevention
Atlanta, Georgia

Danice K. Eaton, PhD, MPH

CAPT, US Public Health Service

Lead, Epidemiology Workforce Branch

Division of Scientific Education and
 Professional Development

Center for Surveillance, Epidemiology,
 and Laboratory Services

Centers for Disease Control and
 Prevention

Atlanta, Georgia

Ryan P. Fagan, MD, MPH&TM

CAPT, US Public Health Service

Medical Officer, Division of Healthcare
 Quality Promotion

National Center for Emerging and
 Zoonotic Infectious Diseases

Centers for Disease Control and
 Prevention

Atlanta, Georgia

Jerry Fagliano, PhD, MPH

Associate Clinical Professor and Chair

Department of Environmental and
 Occupational Health

Dornsife School of Public Health

Drexel University

Philadelphia, Pennsylvania

Robert E. Fontaine, MD, MSc

Senior Advisor

Workforce and Institute
 Development Branch

Division of Global Health Protection

Center for Global Health

Centers for Disease Control and
 Prevention

Atlanta, Georgia

Stephanie Foster, MPH, MA

Lead

Geospatial Epidemiology and Applied
 Research Unit

Geospatial Research, Analysis, and
 Services Program

National Center for Environmental
 Health/Agency for Toxic Substances
 and Disease Registry

Centers for Disease Control and
 Prevention

Atlanta, Georgia

Joanna Gaines, PhD, MPH, CHES

CDR, US Public Health Service

Senior Epidemiologist, Travelers'
 Health Branch

Division of Global Migration and
 Quarantine

National Center for Emerging and
 Zoonotic Infectious Diseases

Centers for Disease Control and
 Prevention

Atlanta, Georgia

Sudevi Navalkar Ghosh, JD, MPH

Senior Attorney

US Department of Health and Human
 Services

Office of the General Counsel

Public Health Division

Centers for Disease Control and
 Prevention Branch

Atlanta, Georgia

Richard A. Goodman, MD, JD, MPH
Professor of Medicine
Department of Family and Preventive
    Medicine
Emory University School of Medicine
and
Department of Epidemiology
Emory University Rollins School of
    Public Health
Atlanta, Georgia

Patricia M. Griffin, MD
Chief
Enteric Diseases Epidemiology Branch
Division of Foodborne, Waterborne, and
    Environmental Diseases
National Center for Emerging and
    Zoonotic Infectious Diseases
Centers for Disease Control and
    Prevention
Atlanta, Georgia

James L. Hadler, MD, MPH
Clinical Professor of Epidemiology and
    Public Health
Emerging Infections Program
Yale School of Public Health
New Haven, Connecticut
and
Public Health Consultant
New York City Department of Health and
    Mental Hygiene
New York City, New York

Janet J. Hamilton, MPH
Senior Manager
Surveillance and Surveillance Systems
Bureau of Epidemiology
Florida Department of Health
Tallahassee, Florida

Craig Hedberg, PhD
Professor
Environmental Health Sciences
School of Public Health
University of Minnesota
Minneapolis, Minnesota

Katrina Hedberg, MD, MPH
Health Officer and State Epidemiologist
Oregon Health Authority
Public Health Division
Portland, Oregon

James D. Holt, JD, LLM
Senior Attorney
US Department of Health and Human
    Services
Office of the General Counsel
Public Health Division
Centers for Disease Control and
    Prevention Branch
Washington, District of Columbia

Richard S. Hopkins, MD, MSPH
Courtesy Professor
Department of Epidemiology
University of Florida
Gainesville, Florida

Brendan R. Jackson, MD, MPH
CDR, US Public Health Service
Lead, Epidemiology Team
Mycotic Diseases Branch
Division of Foodborne, Waterborne, and
    Environmental Diseases
Centers for Disease Control and
    Prevention
Atlanta, Georgia

Timothy Jones, MD
State Epidemiologist
Tennessee Department of Health
Nashville, Tennessee

M. Shannon Keckler, PhD, MS, MPH
Laboratory Leadership Service Fellow
Clinical and Environmental
    Microbiology Branch
Division of Healthcare Quality Promotion
National Center for Emerging and
    Zoonotic Infectious Diseases
Centers for Disease Control and
    Prevention
Atlanta, Georgia

Michael E. King, PhD, MSW
CAPT, US Public Health Service
Senior Epidemiologist, Epidemiology
    Workforce Branch
Division of Scientific Education and
    Professional Development
Center for Surveillance, Epidemiology,
    and Laboratory Services
Centers for Disease Control and
    Prevention
Atlanta, Georgia

Kathleen Kreiss, MD
Chief (Retired)
Field Studies Branch
Respiratory Health Division
National Institute for Occupational Safety
    and Health
Centers for Disease Control and
    Prevention
Sitka, Alaska

James W. Le Duc, PhD
Director
Galveston National Laboratory
Professor, Department of Microbiology
    and Immunology
John Sealy Distinguished University Chair
    in Tropical and Emerging Virology
University of Texas Medical Branch
Galveston, Texas

Joseph E. Logan, PhD
Behavioral Scientist and Epidemiologist
Division of Violence Prevention
National Center for Injury Prevention and
    Control
Centers for Disease Control and
    Prevention
Atlanta, Georgia

Anna Leena Lohiniva, MSc, MA
Cultural Anthropologist
World Health Organization
Eastern Mediterranean Office
Cairo, Egypt

Julie Maher, PhD, MS
Director
Program Design and Evaluation Services
Oregon Health Authority and Multnomah
    County Health Department
Portland, Oregon

Frank Mahoney, MD
Senior Immunization Officer
International Federation of Red Cross
Red Crescent National Societies
Geneva, Switzerland

James A. Mercy, PhD
Director
Division of Violence Prevention
National Center for Injury Prevention and
    Control
Centers for Disease Control and
    Prevention
Atlanta, Georgia

Joshua A. Mott, PhD
CAPT, US Public Health Service
Chief, Epidemiology Workforce Branch
    and Epidemic Intelligence Service
Division of Scientific Education and
    Professional Development
Center for Surveillance, Epidemiology,
    and Laboratory Services
Centers for Disease Control and
    Prevention
Atlanta, Georgia

Glen Nowak, PhD
Director
Center for Health and Risk
    Communication
and
Professor
Department of Advertising and Public
    Relations
Grady College of Journalism and Mass
    Communication
University of Georgia
Athens, Georgia

Stephen Papagiotas, MPH
Public Health Advisor
Emergency Preparedness and
    Response Branch
Division of Preparedness and Emerging
    Infections
National Center for Emerging and
    Zoonotic Infectious Diseases
Centers for Disease Control and
    Prevention
Atlanta, Georgia

Sonja A. Rasmussen, MD, MS
Director
Division of Public Health Information
    Dissemination
and
Editor-in-Chief
Morbidity and Mortality Weekly
    Report Series
Center for Surveillance, Epidemiology,
    and Laboratory Services
Centers for Disease Control and
    Prevention
Atlanta, Georgia

Stephen C. Redd, MD
RADM and Assistant Surgeon General,
    US Public Health Service
Director, Office of Public Health
    Preparedness and Response
Centers for Disease Control and
    Prevention
Atlanta, Georgia

Reynolds M. Salerno, PhD
Director
Division of Laboratory Systems
Center for Surveillance, Epidemiology,
    and Laboratory Services
Centers for Disease Control and
    Prevention
Atlanta, Georgia

Kelly Shannon, MPH
Unit Chief
Weapons of Mass Destruction Directorate
Federal Bureau of Investigation
Washington, District of Columbia

Michael W. Shaw, PhD
Senior Advisor for Laboratory Science
Office of Infectious Diseases
Centers for Disease Control and
    Prevention
Atlanta, Georgia

Daniel M. Sosin, MD, MPH, FACP
Deputy Director and Chief Medical
    Officer
Office of Public Health Preparedness and
    Response
Centers for Disease Control and
    Prevention
Atlanta, Georgia

Abbigail J. Tumpey, MPH, CHES
Associate Director for Communication
    Science
Center for Surveillance, Epidemiology,
    and Laboratory Services
Centers for Disease Control and
    Prevention
Atlanta, Georgia

Amra Uzicanin, MD, MPH
Lead
Community Interventions for Infection
    Control Unit
Division of Global Migration and
    Quarantine
National Center for Emerging and
    Zoonotic Infectious Diseases
Centers for Disease Control and
    Prevention
Atlanta, Georgia

Jay K. Varma, MD
Senior Advisor
Africa Centers for Disease Control and
    Prevention
Addis Ababa, Ethiopia

Duc J. Vugia, MD, MPH
Chief
Infectious Diseases Branch
California Department of Public Health
Richmond, California
and
Clinical Professor
Department of Epidemiology and
    Biostatistics
University of California, San Francisco
San Francisco, California

Ronald Waldman, MD, MPH
Professor of Global Health
Milken Institute School of Public Health
George Washington University
Washington, District of Columbia

Sharon M. Watkins, PhD
State Epidemiologist and Director
Bureau of Epidemiology
Pennsylvania Department of Health
Harrisburg, Pennsylvania

Laura Whitlock, MPH
Communication Lead
Outbreak Response and
    Prevention Branch
Division of Foodborne, Waterborne, and
    Environmental Diseases
National Center for Emerging and
    Zoonotic Infectious Diseases
Centers for Disease Control and
    Prevention
Atlanta, Georgia

Tim W. Wiedrich, MS
Chief
Emergency Preparedness and Response
    Section
North Dakota Department of Health
Bismarck, North Dakota

Ian T. Williams, PhD, MS
Chief
Outbreak Response and
    Prevention Branch
Division of Foodborne, Waterborne, and
    Environmental Diseases
National Center for Emerging and
    Zoonotic Infectious Diseases
Centers for Disease Control and
    Prevention
Atlanta, Georgia

Matthew E. Wise, PhD, MPH
CDR, US Public Health Service
Deputy Branch Chief for Response
Outbreak Response and
    Prevention Branch
Division of Foodborne, Waterborne, and
    Environmental Diseases
National Center for Emerging and
    Zoonotic Infectious Diseases
Centers for Disease Control and
    Prevention
Atlanta, Georgia

Brent Wolff, PhD, MHS
Team Lead
Demand Policy & Communication
Immunization Systems Branch
Global Immunization Division
Centers for Disease Control and
    Prevention
Atlanta, Georgia

The Field Investigation

/// 1 /// DEFINING FIELD EPIDEMIOLOGY

RICHARD A. GOODMAN, JAMES W. BUEHLER, AND JOSHUA A. MOTT

INTRODUCTION

Although epidemiologists work in field settings in different contexts, the term *field epidemiology* as used in this manual describes investigations initiated in response to urgent public health problems. A primary goal of field epidemiology is to guide, as quickly as possible, the processes of selecting and implementing interventions to lessen or prevent illness or death when such problems arise. Despite continuing changes in the contexts within which epidemiologists operate, as well as the types and quantity of information that epidemiologists have at their disposal, the core principles of field epidemiology remain largely constant.

The constellation of problems faced by epidemiologists who investigate urgent public health problems shapes the definition of field epidemiology. For example, consider the following scenario: At 8:30 AM on Monday, August 2, 1976, Dr. Robert B. Craven, an Epidemic Intelligence Service (EIS) officer assigned to the Center for Disease Control's (CDC) Viral Diseases Division, received a telephone call from a nurse at a veterans' hospital in Philadelphia, Pennsylvania. The nurse reported two cases of severe respiratory illness (including one death) in persons who had attended the recent American Legion Convention in Philadelphia. Subsequent conversations with local and state public health officials revealed that 18 persons who had attended the convention during July 21–24 had died during July 26–August 2, primarily from pneumonia. By the evening of August 2, an additional 71 cases had been identified among Legionnaires. As a consequence of this information, a massive epidemiologic investigation was immediately initiated that involved local, state, and federal public health agencies. This problem became known as the outbreak of Legionnaires' disease, and the investigation of the problem led directly to discovery of the bacterial pathogen, *Legionella pneumophila* (1,2), enabling further studies of the nature and modes of transmission of this organism, the epidemiology, and natural history of *Legionella* infections, as well as more precise recommendations for prevention and treatment.

The Legionnaires' disease outbreak and the public health response it triggered illustrate the raison d'être for field epidemiology. Using this epidemic as an example, we can define *field epidemiology* as the application of epidemiology under the following general conditions:

- The timing of the problem is unexpected.
- A timely response is demanded.
- Public health epidemiologists must travel to and work in the field to solve the problem.
- The extent of the investigation is likely to be limited because of the imperative for timely intervention and by other situational constraints on study designs or methods.

Although field investigations of acute problems share many characteristics with prospectively planned epidemiologic studies, they differ in at least three important aspects.

- Because field investigations often start without specific hypotheses about the cause or source of disease, they require the use of descriptive studies to generate hypotheses before analytic studies can be designed and conducted to test these hypotheses.
- As noted previously, when acute problems occur, an immediate need exists to protect the community's health and address its concerns. These responsibilities drive the epidemiologic field investigation beyond the confines of data collection and analysis and into the realm of public health policy and action.
- Field epidemiology forces the epidemiologist to consider when the findings are sufficient to take action rather than to ask what additional questions might be answered by additional data collection or analyses or, alternatively, to take initial actions that might be modified as additional information is obtained through further investigation.

Although the timing of acute public health problems that prompt field investigations is typically unexpected, emergencies often unmask latent threats to health that had gone unrecognized or had been "waiting to happen." For example, sporadic or epidemic illness might be inevitable if restaurants fail to adhere to food management guidelines, if hospitals fail to properly sterilize instruments, if employers fail to maintain workplace safety standards, or if members of social networks engage in unsafe sexual behaviors. As a result, field investigations can prompt both immediate interventions and longer term recommendations, or they can identify problems that require further study after the immediate problem has been addressed.

Experiences during 2014–2016 with the Ebola virus disease (EVD) outbreak in West Africa underscore how networks of professionals trained in the basics of field epidemiology can play key roles in mitigating the health and economic effects of emerging disease threats, such as EVD. When left unchecked in many locations in West Africa, the EVD outbreak resulted in more than 28,000 cases and 11,000 deaths (3,4). However, in July 2014, when a case of EVD was introduced into Nigeria, epidemiologists, in close partnership with the Ministry of Health, nongovernmental organizations, and other community members, conducted rapid field investigations to prevent further transmission (5). Given the population size of Nigeria, timely epidemiologic response might have helped to avert a considerably larger disaster.

The concepts and methods used in field investigations derive from clinical medicine, epidemiology, laboratory and behavioral sciences, decision theory, an expanding array of other scientific disciplines, skill in communications, and common sense. In this manual, the guidelines and approaches for conducting epidemiologic field investigations reflect the urgency of discovering causative factors, use of evolving multifaceted methods, and need to make timely practical recommendations.

DETERMINANTS FOR FIELD INVESTIGATIONS

Health departments become aware of possible disease outbreaks or other acute public health problems in different ways. Situations might gain attention because astute clinicians recognize unusual patterns of disease among their patients and alert health departments, surveillance systems for monitoring disease or hazard trends detect increases, the diagnosis of a single case of a rare disease heralds a broader problem or potential threat, or members of the public are concerned and contact authorities.

After such alerts, the first step is to decide whether to conduct a field investigation. Initial assessments might dispel concerns or affirm that further investigation is warranted. After initiated, decisions must be made at successive stages about how far to pursue an investigation. These decisions are necessary to make the most effective use of public health resources, including capacities to conduct field investigations and optimize opportunities for disease prevention.

In addition to the need to develop and implement control measures to end threats to the public's health, such as the Legionnaires' disease and EVD outbreaks, other determinants that shape field investigations include (1) epidemiologic, programmatic, and resource considerations; (2) public and political considerations; (3) research and learning opportunities; (4) legal obligations; and (5) training needs.

Epidemiologic, Programmatic, and Resource Considerations

Certain disease control programs at national, state, and local levels have specific and extensive requirements for epidemiologic investigation. For example, as part of the measles elimination effort in the United States, a measles outbreak is defined as a chain of transmission including three or more cases linked in time and space (6). Accordingly, every case of measles might be investigated to identify and vaccinate susceptible persons and to evaluate other control strategies, such as the exclusion from school of children who cannot provide proof of vaccination. This recommendation reflects the epidemiology of measles in the United States, where most cases result from travel-related introduction of measles into the country and where vaccination programs have dramatically reduced the incidence of measles although pockets of vulnerability to transmission remain.

Additional situations in which investigations are likely to be initiated after the diagnoses of individual cases include the emergence of highly pathogenic infections, such as influenza A(H5N1) and A(H7N9) in Asia and Middle East respiratory syndrome coronavirus. Given past experiences with influenza pandemics and severe acute respiratory syndrome (SARS), detection of such events have prompted multiple field investigations. The diagnoses of individual illnesses that might be associated with bioterrorism also should prompt investigations, at least to the point of dismissing concerns that exposure resulted from an intentional act. For example, diagnosis of a case of inhalation anthrax in a photo editor for a national media company in 2001, an occupation not associated with exposure to naturally occurring anthrax, was the first of 22 cases of terrorism-related anthrax and five associated deaths that were exhaustively investigated (7) and led to massive increases in investments in public health emergency preparedness in the United States. The anthrax attacks and other bioterrorism-related concerns brought about a lowering of the threshold of suspicion necessary for triggering a full field investigation (8,9).

Different clinical, laboratory, and surveillance technologies have the potential to enhance recognition of situations that merit investigation, including detection of individual cases of disease that might signal a larger threat to public health, early detection of disease outbreaks, or detection of environmental hazards that can result in widespread disease. Conversely, the potential benefits of these technologies might be offset by increasing the likelihood of detecting situations that do not represent public health threats yet require time and resources to draw that conclusion. At the individual level, the advent of multipathogen detection platforms also enables the simultaneous detection of multiple viruses and bacteria in a single clinical specimen. Although this technology can provide important clinical health benefits, it can challenge efforts to distinguish pathogens that are potentially related to disease outbreaks versus organisms that are merely commensal (10). At the outbreak level, the advent of highly automated public health surveillance systems that incorporate statistical algorithms to detect unusual trends can provide an early warning for the onset of outbreaks as well as statistical aberrations that do not herald substantial threats (11). At the level of environmental monitoring, debates surrounding proposed enhancements in the pathogen monitoring capacities of the US BioWatch system for detecting airborne biological hazards included consideration of the potential for more frequent alerts resulting from the detection of naturally occurring microbes that do not represent substantial public health threats (12).

Global disease elimination and eradication programs, international preparedness and coordination for emerging threats, and advances in surveillance and laboratory technologies have helped to strengthen public health. However, these developments also place new pressures on epidemiology program managers to prioritize resources. Any expenditure of public resources should be judicious. Field investigations can be costly in personnel time and other resources and can incur opportunity costs by detracting from other public health activities. In addition, field investigations consume the time and effort of persons investigated and of persons whose collaboration is often essential. Thus, the capacity to conduct field work can be limited not only by the resources or capacity of individual public health agencies, but also by competing demands of other programs within an agency or by other situational demands. Resource constraints also might shape the extent to which investigations are conducted. In the United States, state health departments might help local governments when needed, and state or local health departments might request assistance from the CDC when their capacities are exceeded by the demands of an event. Globally, the World Health Organization and its network of regional offices serve as resources to national governments.

Public and Political Considerations

Scrutiny from the public, political leaders, and the media can occur at all stages of field investigations, including the stage when initial assessments are conducted to determine whether a field investigation is warranted. This scrutiny can affect the perceived urgency of a situation or the perceived need for investigations. The importance that others attach to problems and the conclusions that others draw from initial knowledge of situations might differ from or align with the positions of epidemiologists responsible for conducting field investigations or those of more senior public health officials responsible for determining when field investigations should be started.

In certain instances, a citizen's alert can lead to recognition of a major public health problem, such as with Lyme disease in Lyme, Connecticut, in 1976 (13). In other cases, however, public concerns and attendant pressures might lead to investigations that otherwise are premature or unlikely to be fruitful from a scientific perspective but are critical in terms of community relations. Small clusters of disease (e.g., leukemia or adverse fetal outcomes) are an example of problems that frequently generate substantial public concern. Perceived clusters of disease might prove to represent unrelated events after formal scrutiny; small clusters of disease might occur by chance alone, and field investigations are often inconclusive and only occasionally yield new information about etiologic links to putative exposures (14). However, because community members might perceive a health threat, and certain clusters do represent specific preventable risks, some public health agencies have developed standard procedures for investigating such clusters even though the likelihood of identifying a remediable cause is low (15).

Determining how long an investigation should be continued can become a matter of public controversy. A decision to postpone interventions pending completion of thorough epidemiologic investigations might be perceived as community experimentation or bureaucratic delay. For example, in a large *Escherichia coli* enteric disease outbreak at Crater Lake National Park, Oregon, in 1975, a 1-day delay in implementing control measures to obtain more definitive epidemiologic data resulted in a Congressional hearing and charges of a cover-up (16).

Research and Learning Opportunities

Because almost all outbreaks are "natural experiments," they present opportunities to address questions of importance both to basic scientists and to persons in the applied science of public health practice. Even when a clear policy exists for control of a specific problem, investigation can still provide opportunities to identify new agents and risk factors for infection or disease, define the clinical spectrum of disease, measure the effect of new control measures or clinical interventions, assess the usefulness of microbiologic or other biological markers, or evaluate the utility of new diagnostic tests.

Recognition of newly emergent or reemerging diseases often prompts aggressive investigations because of the potential for extensive, life-threatening illness. Certain diseases are initially recognized only on the occasion of an epidemic, although subsequent investigations and studies enable retrospective diagnosis of earlier occurrences, as well as more complete characterization of the spectrum of clinical manifestations and epidemiology. For example, as referred to earlier, after *L. pneumophilia* was discovered and a serologic test developed, subsequent studies showed that, in addition to the severe illness manifest in the 1976 Philadelphia outbreak, *Legionella* infection commonly results in mild disease or asymptomatic infection. Often, when new diseases are detected, they are recognized in their most severe or distinctive stage, followed later by recognition of a broader spectrum of illness. The initial recognition of certain other problems—such as toxic shock syndrome, influenza A(H1N1)pdm09, AIDS, Hantavirus pulmonary syndrome, West Nile virus disease, and SARS—was followed by aggressive investigations that enabled analogous understanding of the natural history and disease spectrum of these infections. One caveat is that dramatic outbreaks and investigations that identify previously unrecognized pathogens and that yield a wealth of new scientific insights are unusual; more commonly, field investigations of outbreaks identify familiar pathogens and modes of transmission. Yet, even for familiar diseases and modes of exposure or transmission, investigations are warranted to interrupt outbreaks and understand the evolving context in which outbreaks occur. For example, the changing prevalence of underlying conditions (e.g., obesity, diabetes, and cardiovascular disease) among the US population and demographic characteristics (e.g., cultural determinants and age) of the population have the potential to alter host susceptibility and, indeed, the epidemiologic consequences of exposure to pathogens and other hazards.

Certain outbreaks that initially appear to be routine might lead to important epidemiologic discoveries. For example, in 1983, investigators pursued a cluster of diarrhea cases, an extremely common problem, to extraordinary lengths (17). As a result, the investigators were able to trace the chain of transmission of a unique strain of multiply antibiotic-resistant *Salmonella* back from the affected persons to hamburger they ate, to the meat supplier, and, ultimately, to the specific animal source herd. This investigation played a key role in clarifying the link between antibiotic use in the cattle industry and subsequent antibiotic-resistant infection in humans.

Legal Obligations

Field investigations frequently require access to patients' private medical records, queries about private behaviors, analyses of private enterprises putatively responsible for illness-causing exposures, reviews of proprietary information, or assessments of reported putative errors of healthcare providers or health product manufacturers. These tasks may be necessary to complete an objective, defensible field investigation, but each is also fraught with considerable ethical and legal overtones (see Chapter 13).

Findings from some investigations are likely to be used as testimony in civil or criminal trials (18). In these situations, investigations might be carried further than they otherwise would be. For example, investigations in situations where criminal actions might be suspected to have played a role (19) might carry additional legal requirements for establishing a chain of custody of evidence, which is necessary for criminal prosecutions. The anthrax attacks during fall 2001 and related concerns about bioterrorism have stimulated other advanced and carefully designed legal measures to facilitate joint epidemiologic and criminal investigations. An example of such measures is a protocol developed by the New York City Department of Health and Mental Hygiene, New York City Police Department, and Federal Bureau of Investigation to guide in the interviewing of patients during joint investigations by public health and law enforcement professionals representing those agencies (20). Similar collaborations exist at the federal level (21).

Training Needs

By analogy to clerkships in medical school and postgraduate residencies, outbreak investigations provide opportunities for training in basic epidemiologic skills. Just as clinical training often is accomplished at the same time patient care is delivered, training in field epidemiology often simultaneously assists in developing skills in and the delivery of disease control and prevention. For example, since 1951, CDC's EIS Program has provided assistance to state and local health departments while simultaneously training health professionals in the practice of applied epidemiology (22,23). Changes in the epidemiologic capacities of state and local health departments (24) also highlight the need for workforce training and education on an expanded set of skills, such as bioinformatics, health economics, communications, systems thinking, and laboratory techniques. Globally, more than 70 Field Epidemiology Training Programs have been modeled after EIS but are owned by individual countries and ministries of health. These Field Epidemiology Training Programs provide similar on-the-job training but within the context of specific cultures, partners, capacities, and public health systems (25).

UNIQUE CHALLENGES TO EPIDEMIOLOGISTS IN FIELD INVESTIGATIONS

An epidemiologist investigating problems in the field faces unique challenges that sometimes constrain the ideal use of scientific methods. In contrast to prospectively planned studies, which generally are based on carefully developed and refined protocols, field investigations must rely on data sources that are immediately available, less readily controlled, and subject to change with successive hours or days. In addition to possible limitations in data sources, factors that pose challenges for epidemiologists during field investigations include sampling considerations, availability of specimens, effects of publicity, reluctance of persons to participate, and conflicting pressures to intervene. New technologies hold the promise of mitigating some of these challenges.

Data Sources

Field investigations often use information abstracted from different sources, such as hospital, outpatient medical, or school health records. These records vary substantially in completeness and accuracy among patients, healthcare providers, and facilities because entries are made for purposes other than conducting epidemiologic studies. Moreover, rapid and substantive transitions have occurred for several key information sources—as, for example, in the growing use of electronic medical records, hospital and managed-care data systems, and laboratory information management systems. These automated systems can facilitate access to needed records but might not be compatible with meeting the needs of or supporting specific record access by external investigators. Thus, the quality of such records as sources of data for epidemiologic investigations can be substantially less than the quality of information obtained when investigators can exert greater control through the use of standardized, pretested questionnaires; physical or laboratory examinations; or other prospectively designed, rather than retrospective, data collection methods. These transitions necessitate that epidemiologists involved in field investigations increasingly might need to know how to use these data sources and, therefore, possess the requisite skills needed to analyze them.

The increasing use of social media and email can facilitate outreach to and queries of persons who might have common exposures in an outbreak situation, such as participants in an organized event linked to a common-source exposure. Recently, social media networks have been used to assist in identifying contacts of persons with sexually transmitted diseases who might be at high risk and should be considered for targeted prophylaxis. These communication tools have provided added insight into social links and high-risk behaviors and have been used to guide and augment data collected from traditional case investigation methodologies (26).

Small Numbers

In a planned prospective study, the epidemiologist determines appropriate sample sizes that are based on statistical requirements for power to draw conclusions about associations between exposures and health outcomes. In contrast, outbreaks can involve a relatively small number of persons, thereby imposing substantial restrictions on study design, statistical power, and other aspects of analysis. These restrictions, in turn, place limitations on the inferences and conclusions that can be drawn from a field investigation. However, communication technologies between jurisdictions can now be used to help alleviate this problem. For example, the electronic Epidemic Information Exchange (Epi-X) was developed for CDC officials, state and local health departments, poison control centers, and other public health professionals to access and share preliminary health surveillance information (27). Although a primary motivation for this system was to enhance the recognition of multistate events or the multistate dispersion of persons with disease exposures in a single state or outside the United States, the resulting cross-jurisdictional collaboration has the additional benefit of increasing potential sample sizes for field investigations.

Specimen Availability

Because the field investigator usually arrives on the scene after the fact, collection of necessary environmental or biological specimens is not always possible. For example, suspected food items might have been entirely eaten or discarded, a suspected water system might have been flushed, or ill persons might have recovered, thereby precluding collection of specimens during the acute phase of illness when certain tests are most likely to be informative. Under these conditions, the epidemiologist depends on the diligence of healthcare providers who are first to evaluate the affected persons and on the recall of affected persons, their relatives, or other members of the affected community.

This challenge increasingly is counterbalanced by expanding technologies in the laboratory to help in using routinely collected specimens to determine sources of outbreaks. For example, PulseNet is a national laboratory network that enables the use of DNA fingerprinting to detect thousands of local and multistate outbreaks (28), thereby enabling epidemiologists to rapidly implement control measures for food safety problems that would not otherwise be recognized. As another example, in 2015, epidemiologists investigated the largest HIV outbreak in the United States since 1996. Phylogenetic analyses of target genes within the human immunodeficiency and hepatitis C viruses enabled epidemiologists to retrospectively determine and intervene in the link between specific outbreak strains and local needle-sharing networks using contaminated equipment (29).

Effects of Publicity

Acute disease outbreaks often generate considerable local attention and publicity. In this regard, media coverage can assist the investigation by helping to develop information, identify cases, or promote and help implement control measures. Conversely, such publicity can cause affected persons and others in the community to develop preconceptions about the source or cause of an outbreak, which in turn can lead to potential biases in comparative studies or failure to fully explore alternate hypotheses.

As government employees, field epidemiologists are obligated to communicate with the public about what is known, what is unknown, and what actions are being taken to assess public health threats. Many reporters, in turn, endeavor to find and bring this information to the public's attention. That said, reporters in pursuit of the most current information on the investigation can demand a considerable amount of epidemiologists' time to the detriment of the field investigation itself. Ensuring that a member of the response team has the time and skills to communicate effectively with reporters can be essential to the success of a field investigation and to disease control and prevention efforts, particularly in high-profile situations. Frequently during the course of an event, as information unfolds and as field epidemiologists test, reject, or accept and reshape and retest hypotheses, recommendations for interventions might evolve or become more focused. Apprising affected parties and the public of the rationale for these changes is important to ensure the credibility of the field epidemiologists and of public health recommendations (see Chapter 12).

In recent years, CDC and other public health agencies have used social media tools to disseminate health messages. Although unskilled use of this medium during an ongoing investigation can pose challenges, such as spreading misperceptions or fostering information biases, social media also can be an effective means for expanding the reach of pertinent evidence-based health messages (30).

Reluctance to Participate

Although health departments are empowered to conduct investigations and gain access to records, voluntary and willing participation of involved parties (e.g., case-patients, persons potentially exposed to pathogens, owners or operators of settings in which exposure or transmission might have occurred) is more conducive to successful investigations than compelled participation. In addition, persons whose livelihoods or related interests are at risk might be reluctant to cooperate voluntarily. This reluctance often can be the case for common-source outbreaks associated with restaurants and other public establishments, in environmental or occupational hazard investigations, or among healthcare providers suspected as being sources for transmission of infectious diseases, such as hepatitis B. When involved parties do not willingly cooperate, delays can compromise access to and quality of information (e.g., by introducing bias and by decreasing statistical power).

Conflicting Pressures to Intervene

Epidemiologists who conduct field investigations are often working in a fishbowl-type of environment. Epidemiologists conducting field investigations and the public health officials under whose direction they work must weigh the need for further investigation against the need for immediate intervention, often in the face of strong and varying opinions of affected persons and others in the community. In the absence of definitive information about the source, cause, or potential impact of a problem, the various parties affected by a particular situation might view implementation of a plausible control measure differently. The action might be welcomed by those who favor erring on the side of protecting health and challenged by those who question the rationale for interventions absent definitive information about the cause or source of illness, particularly if their economic or other personal interests are threatened. Delaying interventions might allow time to obtain more definitive information, but such delays also might lead to additional illness. Although this dilemma is not unique to field epidemiology within the realm of public health practice, the heightened urgency of acute situations can elevate the emotional impact on all involved parties.

STANDARDS FOR EPIDEMIOLOGIC FIELD INVESTIGATIONS

Field investigations are sometimes perceived to represent what is sometimes called "quick and dirty" epidemiology. This perception might reflect the inherent nature of circumstances for which rapid responses are required. However, these requirements for action do not justify epidemiologic shortcuts. Rather, they underscore for the field epidemiologist the importance of combining good science with prudent judgment. A better description of a good epidemiologic field investigation would be "quick and appropriate."

In judging an epidemiologic field investigation, consideration should be given to the quality of the science, opportunities and constraints that shaped the context of the investigation, *and* judgment applied in using the findings to take public health actions. The goal should be to maximize the scientific quality of the field investigation in the face of the full range of limitations, pressures, and responsibilities imposed on the investigator(s). Thus, the standards for an epidemiologic field investigation are that it (1) is timely; (2) addresses an important public health problem in the community, as defined by standard public health measures (e.g., attack rates, apparent or potential serious illness, or death) or community concern; (3) examines resource needs early and deploys them appropriately; (4) uses appropriate methods of descriptive and/or analytic epidemiology that make optimal use of all appropriate available data; (5) engages expertise, when indicated, from other public health sciences, such as microbiology, toxicology, psychology, anthropology, informatics, economics, laboratory sciences, or statistics; (6) probes causality to enable identification of the source and/or etiology of the problem (31); (7) identifies evidence-based options for immediate control and long-term interventions; and (8) is conducted in active collaboration with colleagues who have policy, legal, programmatic, communication, or administrative roles to ensure that the evidence from the investigation is used optimally.

CONCLUSION

This chapter has provided a definition of and framework for field epidemiology in a modern and evolving context. Key developments in public health practice during recent decades reflect the growing recognition and formalization of field epidemiology, including establishment of field epidemiology training programs in affiliation with ministries of health and other national-level public health agencies around the world (32).

Other examples of this trend include the development of field epidemiology courses and tracks within curriculum offerings of schools of public health (33); undergraduate programs, and even middle school and high school programs in the United States; the emergence of organizations that promote or link national-level field epidemiology programs (34); and the growth of a body of literature related to the field epidemiology worldwide (35,36). CDC's own workforce development program in field epidemiology, EIS, has operated continuously since its creation in 1951 and has helped to train more than 4,500 professionals in this discipline (37,38).

As the discipline of field epidemiology continues to evolve, new developments and trends are shaping its ongoing incorporation within public health practice. Examples of these developments include the following.

- The importance of global epidemiologic capacity building to protect the United States and other populations in an era of expanded travel and population connectivity.
- The potential for parties affected in outbreaks to threaten or actually bring lawsuits and how threatened or actual litigation might affect an ongoing investigation (e.g., complicate or otherwise interfere with data collection or create or increase response bias).
- The importance of ethical public health practice, including the ongoing need to respect privacy and protect confidentiality in the face of the ever-evolving landscape of culture, policy, law, and technology.
- The persistent awareness of and concerns about intentionality as a cause of disease outbreaks, including lower thresholds for considering intentional actions as a primary or contributing determinant for an outbreak and, when criminal or terrorist acts are suspected, the resulting need for public health and law enforcement agencies to coordinate investigations.
- Uses during field investigations of Internet-based and other advanced information technologies for connecting jurisdictions, identifying cases and contacts, conducting surveys or collecting electronically stored health data, and communicating findings and control measures.
- The use of new laboratory methods for multipathogen detection, genetic sequencing, and environmental testing to increase opportunities for detecting and investigating epidemics, emphasizing the need for increased close communication between epidemiologists and laboratory scientists.
- The increasing expectation from the public for government transparency and for timely information about unfolding events, combined with the advent of social

media and the 24-hour news cycle for transmitting instant, if not consistently accurate, information, each of which underscores the heightened importance of evidence-based decision-making and enhanced communication skills.

Field epidemiology draws on general epidemiologic principles and methods, and field epidemiologists face questions that are familiar to all epidemiologists regardless of where they work, including questions about how study methods are shaped by logistical constraints and about the amount of information necessary to recommend or take action. Likewise, field epidemiologists are affected by trends that influence the practice of epidemiology in general, such as public concerns about the privacy of health information, the increasing automation of health information, and the growth in use of the Internet. Field epidemiology is unique, however, in compressing and pressurizing these concerns in the context of acute public health emergencies and other events and in thrusting the epidemiologist irretrievably into the midst of the administrative, legal, and ethical domains of policy-making and public health action.

ACKNOWLEDGMENTS

Portions of this chapter as incorporated within previous editions of this book were adapted from Goodman RA, Buehler JW, Koplan JP. The epidemiologic field investigation: science and judgment in public health practice. *Am J Epidemiol.* 1990;132:91–96.

REFERENCES

1. Fraser DW, Tsai TR, Orenstein W, et al. Legionnaires' disease: description of an epidemic of pneumonia. *N Engl J Med.* 1977:297:1189–97.
2. CDC. Follow-up on respiratory illness—Philadelphia. *MMWR.* 1997;46:49–56.
3. CDC. 2014 Ebola outbreak in West Africa—case counts. https://www.cdc.gov/vhf/ebola/outbreaks/2014-west-africa/case-counts.html
4. World Health Organization. Situation report—Ebola virus disease. June 10, 2016. http://apps.who.int/iris/bitstream/10665/208883/1/ebolasitrep_10Jun2016_eng.pdf?ua=1
5. Fasina O, Shittu A, Lazarus D, et al. Transmission dynamics and control of Ebola virus disease outbreak in Nigeria, July to September 2014. *Euro Surveill.* 2014;19:pii=20920.
6. CDC. *Manual for the Surveillance of Vaccine-Preventable Diseases.* Atlanta: CDC; 2008.
7. Jernigan DB, Raghunathan PL, Bell BP, et al. Investigation of bioterrorism-related anthrax, United States, 2001: epidemiologic findings. *Emerg Infect Dis.* 2002;8:1019–28.
8. Butler JC, Cohen ML, Friedman CR, Scripp RM, Watz CG. Collaboration between public health and law enforcement: new paradigms and partnerships for bioterrorism planning and response. *Emerg Infect Dis.* 2002;8:1152–6.
9. Treadwell TA, Koo D, Kuker K, Khan AS. Epidemiologic clues to bioterrorism. *Public Health Rep.* 2003;118:92–118.

10. Diaz MH, Cross KE, Benitez AJ, et al. Identification of bacterial and viral codetections with *Mycoplasma pneumoniae* using the TaqMan Array Card in patients hospitalized with community-acquired pneumonia. *Open Forum Infect Dis*. 2016;3:1–4.

11. Mandl KD, Overhage MJ, Wagner MM, et al. Implementing syndromic surveillance: a practical guide informed by the early experience. *J Am Med Inform Assoc*. 2004;11:141–50.

12. Institute of Medicine, National Research Council. *BioWatch and Public Health Surveillance: Evaluating Systems for the Early Detection of Biological Threats—Abbreviated Version*. Washington, DC: National Academies Press; 2011.

13. Steere AC, Malawista SE, Snydman DR, et al. Lyme arthritis: an epidemic of oligoarticular arthritis in children and adults in three Connecticut communities. *Arthritis Rheum*. 1977;20:7–17.

14. Schulte PA, Ehrenberg RL, Singal M. Investigation of occupational cancer clusters: theory and practice. *Am J Public Health*. 1987;77:52–6.

15. CDC. Investigating suspected cancer clusters and responding to community concerns: guidelines from CDC and the Council of State and Territorial Epidemiologists. *MMWR*. 2013;62(RR-8):1–24.

16. Rosenberg ML, Koplan JP, Wachsmith IK, et al. Epidemic diarrhea at Crater Lake from enterotoxigenic. *Escherichia coli*: a large waterborne outbreak. *Ann Intern Med*. 1977;86:714–8.

17. Holmberg SD, Osterholm MT, Senger KA, Cohen ML. Drug-resistant *Salmonella* from animals fed antimicrobials. *N Engl J Med*. 1984;311:617–22.

18. Goodman RA, Loue S, Shaw FE. Epidemiology and the law. In: Brownson RC, Petitti DB, editors. *Applied Epidemiology: Theory to Practice*. 2nd ed. New York: Oxford University Press; 2006:289–326.

19. Goodman RA, Munson JW, Dammers K, Lazzarini Z, Barkley JP. Forensic epidemiology: law at the intersection of public health and criminal investigations. *J Law Med Ethics*. 2003;31:684–700.

20. Miller J. City and FBI reach agreement on bioterror investigations. *The New York Times*. November 21, 2004. https://mobile.nytimes.com/2004/11/21/nyregion/city-and-fbi-reach-agreement-on-bioterror-investigations.html?_r=0

21. FBI, CDC. Joint criminal and epidemiological investigations handbook. 2015 Domestic edition. https://stacks.cdc.gov/view/cdc/34556

22. Langmuir AD. The Epidemic Intelligence Service of the Centers for Disease Control. *Public Health Rep*. 1980;104:170–7.

23. Thacker SB, Dannenberg AL, Hamilton DH. Epidemic Intelligence Service of the Centers for Disease Control and Prevention: 50 years of training and service in applied epidemiology. *Am J Epidemiol*. 2001;154:985–92.

24. Boulton ML, Hadler JL, Ferland L, Marder E, Lemmings J. The epidemiology workforce in state and local health departments—United States, 2010. *MMWR*. 2012;61:205–8.

25. CDC Division of Global Health Protection. Field Epidemiology Training Program: disease detectives in action. https://www.cdc.gov/globalhealth/healthprotection/pdf/factsheet_fieldepidemiologytrainingprogram.pdf

26. Isaac BM, Zucker JR, MacGregor J, et al. Notes from the field: use of social media as a communication tool during a mumps outbreak—New York City, 2015. *MMWR*. 2017;66;60–1.

27. CDC. Epi-X. The Epidemic Information Exchange. https://www.cdc.gov/epix/

28. CDC. PulseNet. https://www.cdc.gov/pulsenet/

29. Galang RR, Gentry J, Conrad C, et al. Phylogenetic analysis of HIV and hepatitis C virus co-infection in an HIV outbreak among persons who inject drugs. 65th Annual Epidemic Intelligence Service (EIS) Conference. May 2–5, 2016, Atlanta. [Abstract at page 23]. https://www.cdc.gov/eis/downloads/eis-conference-2016.pdf

30. CDC. The health communicator's social media toolkit. https://www.cdc.gov/socialmedia/Tools/guidelines/pdf/SocialMediaToolkit_BM.pdf

31. Rothman KJ, Greenland S, Lash TL. *Modern Epidemiology*. 3rd ed. Philadelphia: Lippincott; 2008.

32. CDC. Career Paths to Public Health (CPP). https://www.cdc.gov/careerpaths/

33. University of North Carolina Gillings School of Global Public Health. Public Health Leadership Program online certificate in field epidemiology. http://sph.unc.edu/phlp/phlp-degrees-and-certificates/certificate-in-field-epidemiology/

34. European Programme for Intervention Epidemiology Training (EPIET). EPIET fellowships. http://ecdc.europa.eu/en/epiet/Pages/HomeEpiet.aspx

35. Dabis F, Drucker J, Moren A. *Epidémiologie d'intervention*. Paris: Arnette; 1992.

36. Iamsirithaworn S, Chanachai K, Castellan D. Field epidemiology and One Health: Thailand's experience. In: Yamada A, Kahn LH, Kaplan B, Monath TP, Woodall J, Conti L, editors. *Confronting Emerging Zoonoses: The One Health Paradigm*. Tokyo: Springer; 2014:191–212.

37. Langmuir AD, Andrews JM. Biological warfare defense: the Epidemic Intelligence Service of the Communicable Disease Center. *Am J Public Health*. 1952;42:235–8.

38. CDC. Epidemic Intelligence Service. https://www.cdc.gov/eis/diseasedetectives.html

/// 2 /// INITIATING OPERATIONS

DUC J. VUGIA, RICHARD A. GOODMAN, JAMES L. HADLER, AND DANICE K. EATON

INTRODUCTION

In the United States, the responsibility for public health rests primarily with city or county and state public health agencies. All states and many large counties and cities have their own public health departments. Although many public health investigations are conducted with local resources, a city, county, or state health department can request field epidemiologic or laboratory assistance from the next higher level public health agency in response to a large or complex outbreak or problem that requires additional staff, expertise, or other resources. In the United States, the Centers for Disease Control and Prevention (CDC) is the highest level public health agency. Federal prisons, military bases, and tribal reservations have their own independent health systems but also can request assistance from CDC. Globally, countries can request assistance for field investigations from the World Health Organization, which coordinates with its members for needed resources.

An epidemiologic field investigation entails considerably more effort than simply following the recommended, scientifically oriented steps as enumerated and described in Chapter 3. Numerous operational concerns must be addressed in addition to the necessary data collection, tabulation, and analyses. This chapter describes crucial operational and management steps and principles that apply before, during, and after the field work, often to both invitees and inviters.

INITIAL REQUEST, COMMUNICATIONS, AND FORMAL INVITATION

Initial Request and Communications

When requesting epidemiologic assistance, inviters should gather as much information as possible about the outbreak or problem and communicate the details, along with a formal invitation, to the invited agency to prepare for initial teleconference meetings. At the initial teleconference meeting, invitees and inviters should attempt to answer the following questions:

- What is the purpose of the investigation?
  - Is the local or state health department simply requesting additional staff to complete the investigation?
  - Has the local or state health department been unable to determine the source of disease or the mode of spread?
  - Does the local or state health department want to share the responsibility of the investigation with others to more fully address the political or scientific pressure?
- What specifically is the investigation expected to accomplish? The field team might be asked to confirm findings from data already collected or perform an entirely new investigation and develop new recommendations.
- What authority does the inviter have to request assistance? Occasionally, field investigations have been aborted simply because persons requesting assistance had no authority to do so.

Formal Invitation

An essential consideration is the need for a formal request for assistance from an official who is authorized to request help. In the United States, each state has a State Epidemiologist. This official usually has the authority and responsibility for major epidemiologic field investigations of acute public health problems and for deciding whether to investigate independently within the state or to request CDC assistance on behalf of the state or a local health department. However, a State Epidemiologist first needs to inform his or her State Health Officer and, depending on the sociopolitical context, obtain permission to proceed with a formal invitation. At the city or county health department level, a senior city or county public health officer usually has authority to invite assistance from the state health department. For international problems, determining who has authority to extend a request can be more complicated and might involve, for example, senior officials from ministries of health requesting assistance from the World Health Organization.

CLARIFICATION OF OBJECTIVES, ROLES, AND RESPONSIBILITIES

Depending on the extent and complexity of the outbreak or problem and the main purpose(s) of the field investigation initially discussed, subsequent communications between invitees and inviters should focus on clarifying the investigation's main objectives and the roles and responsibilities of key persons.

- What are the main public health questions the field investigation needs to answer? The primary purpose of field investigations in response to outbreaks or other urgent public health events is to identify control and prevention measures.
- What is the status of the Incident Command System (ICS) and local Emergency Operations Center (EOC) (see also under Other Issues)? Have they already been activated or are likely to be activated? If so, what will be the role of the field team?
- What epidemiology, laboratory, and other resources (including personnel) will the jurisdiction requesting assistance provide?
- What resources will the visiting team and responding agency provide?
- Who will supervise the day-to-day investigation?
- Who will provide overall direction and ultimately be responsible for the investigation?
- Who will be the media point person for the investigation?

- Who will be responsible for data analyses, and how will data be shared?
- Who will write a report of the findings, if needed? To whom will it be disseminated?
- Who will be the lead and senior authors, if field investigation results warrant publication in a peer-reviewed journal or presentation at a scientific venue?

Not all of these crucial problems can be resolved before the field team arrives or the investigation concludes. However, they must be addressed, discussed openly, and agreed on as soon as possible.

FIELD TEAM PREPARATION

Many field investigations require laboratory support. Even if local laboratories are available and capable of processing and testing specimens, invited epidemiologists should immediately contact their laboratory counterparts within their agency to share details of the problem and discuss specimen types, collection, processing and testing, and potential basic or applied research questions that can be appropriately addressed and answered during the field investigation. Early enlistment of laboratory collaboration and support, at both the local level and at the invited agency, is crucial to the success of many field investigations.

The same early consideration applies to statistical support and contacting other health professionals, such as behavioral scientists, veterinarians, mammalogists, entomologists and vector-control specialists, environmental health specialists, and infection prevention and control practitioners, whose expertise can be crucial to a successful field investigation. The invited agency should consider including such professionals on the field team so that appropriate data and environmental specimens can be collected at the same time as other relevant epidemiologic information.

After the field team is chosen, the invited agency should take the following key measures to prepare the team:

- Identify the team leader and the senior staff at the agency home base to whom the team leader should report.
- Meet with all proposed field team members and home-based staff to review details of the public health problem, nature of the request for assistance, current knowledge of any suspected pathogen or disease, goals and objectives for the field investigation, and preliminarily agreed-on roles and responsibilities.
- Arrange in advance an initial in-person meeting with the requestor (e.g., the State Epidemiologist) or persons designated by the requestor (e.g., local senior health

officials and epidemiologists). This contact ensures that local authorities are not surprised by an unexpected arrival and underscores for all parties the need for advance planning and orderliness in the investigation, which will set the tone for the conduct of the investigation.

- Write a memorandum for the record or to relevant key officials, which should be done by a senior member of the team before leaving for the field that summarizes the following points:
  - How and when the request was made.
  - What information the requesting health agency has provided.
  - What the agreed-on purpose is of the investigation.
  - What the commitments are of both the visiting team and requesting health officials.
  - Who will be members of the field team.
  - When the team is expected to arrive in the field.

This memorandum should be distributed to key personnel in the offices of the visiting team and the requesting host agency and to others who need to know. The memo serves not only as notification to everyone, but also as a method to prevent redundant responses. It will also identify expertise and resources from other programs that might contribute to the investigation. Even when a problem does not directly involve a state (for example, an investigation on tribal land or at a federal facility), an array of state and local officials typically are notified because of possible ramifications to populations in surrounding communities.

- Review a basic checklist with each team member before departing to ensure they have materials and aids essential for field operations and have covered fundamental travel and logistic considerations. A partial list includes the following items:
  - Cell phones with key contacts
  - Laptop computers with appropriate software (e.g., Epi Info, SAS, or R)
  - Digital cameras
  - Credit cards
  - Travel and lodging reservations
- Review with each team member before leaving the need for any necessary personal protective measures, such as vaccinations; antimalarial prophylaxis; antimicrobials or antivirals for postexposure prophylaxis; and personal protective equipment, including face masks or respirators, gloves, and gowns.

INITIAL IN-PERSON MEETING OF FIELD TEAM WITH LOCAL HEALTH OFFICIALS

The field team needs to keep in mind its role as consultant or collaborator. The guiding principle should be that the field team is there to provide help but not to take charge. Equally important is the need to balance the focus of the investigation with the competing priorities of the requesting jurisdiction. Although the immediate problem is the team's sole concern, local health officials must continue to address a myriad of other local priorities and ongoing problems. The team needs to try to understand and appreciate the local viewpoint early in the investigation.

After arriving on site, the team should meet promptly with the official who requested assistance and his or her key staff. At this meeting, essential steps include the following items:

- Review and update the status of the problem.
- Identify or review the primary points of contact.
- Identify a principal local collaborator who also can serve as what might be termed a "guardian angel" to facilitate and coordinate local contacts and team needs.
- Identify or confirm availability of local resources (e.g., office space, clerical support, assistance for surveys, and laboratory support).
- Create a method and schedule for the team to update local officials and home base.
- Review sensitivities, including potential problems with institutions and individuals (e.g., hospitals, administrators, practitioners, and local public health staff) likely to be encountered during the investigation. Meeting the requesting official at the outset should ensure that key doors will be opened, rather than spending valuable time later in the investigation mending fences.

Because large outbreaks are likely to attract media attention, the presence of an experienced and knowledgeable public information officer (PIO) who can respond to public inquiries and regularly meet the media is invaluable. In the United States, the inviting local or state health department often has its own PIO who can serve as the media point person for the investigation. During the initial meeting, the local PIO should be identified. The field team should avoid direct contact with the news media and defer to local health officials. The field team essentially is working at the request and under the authority of the local health officials. The local officials not only know and appreciate the local situation, but also are the appropriate persons to comment on the investigation.

MANAGEMENT OF FIELD TEAM ACTIVITIES

Because of the potential complexity of field investigations, as well as the distracting circumstances under which they typically are conducted, the field team leader might want to take the following approaches to ensure the systematic and orderly progression of the investigation:

- Maintain lists of necessary tasks, check off completed actions, and update the list at least daily.
- Communicate frequently with other field team members, requesting official, and designated media contact, and hold a team meeting each day at a regularly scheduled time. Communicate with home base senior staff as often as needed.
- Request additional help, without hesitation, as required by the circumstances.
- Avoid setting a departure date in advance or succumbing to the pressure of team family members to return earlier to ensure the investigation will be completed.

Investigations of large and complex problems can be particularly challenging for field teams and require even more rigorous organization of field operations. The following practical pointers can help designated team leaders manage key aspects of the investigation:

- Record the team's decisions as they are made. This will help to ensure consistency and make the investigation reproducible, a consideration particularly important to case definitions and why certain criteria were used.
- Remember the need for quality control measures, such as training and monitoring of data collectors and abstractors, including conducting error checks, validating data independently, and evaluating nonrespondents and missing records.
- Resist collecting more data than are needed (e.g., excessive clinical details); focus on accomplishing the investigation objectives.
- Write continually while the investigation is ongoing and before key details are forgotten.
  - Write the background section of the report.
  - Write the methods as they are being defined and developed by team members; keeping a decision log helps.
  - Maintain and retain an inventory of data files.
- Assess data continually to determine when enough is known to make or update recommendations for control and prevention measures (see Chapter 11).

- Make a special effort to maintain morale and to provide ongoing encouragement, positive reinforcement, and appreciation to participating investigators. Because field investigations are often difficult and associated with long hours and stress, the necessity might arise to give team members breaks or periods of rest to maintain productivity.

Occasionally, after some time in the field, an investigation does not yield definite results or it identifies additional questions that require one or more subsequent investigations to address. At that point, the team leader, in consultation with home base senior staff, should assess the team's morale and capacity to persevere to determine whether the team should continue or a fresh team should prepare to extend the investigation.

DEBRIEFING AND DEPARTURE MEETING

After concluding the on-site field investigation, the team leader and the local senior official should organize a debriefing or departure meeting that includes the requestor, local collaborators, other key officials, and field team members. This meeting enables the team to debrief the requesting official and local partners about preliminary findings of the investigation, review preliminary recommendations, provide acknowledgments, and express appreciation to local hosts and collaborators. The team should obtain any additional names, titles, and street and email addresses for follow-up communications. If possible, the team should leave on site a preliminary report and commit to providing a complete written report within an agreed-on, specified time.

The departure meeting also might be the most appropriate occasion for planning follow-up activities with the requesting official and agency. Such activities include additional data collection, implementation and evaluation of control measures, analysis and maintenance of data collected during the investigation, plans for final reports and manuscripts (including discussion of authorship), and determination of who is responsible for each follow-up activity.

DRAFTING OF REPORTS

Written summaries of the investigation include both preliminary and final reports. The preliminary report fulfills the immediate obligation to the requesting official and agency. It should summarize the methods used to conduct the investigation, preliminary epidemiologic and laboratory findings, recommendations, clearly delineated tasks and activities to be completed, and acknowledgments. In addition to the preliminary report, which optimally should be delivered to the requestor on departure or earlier, the team should prepare follow-up emails or letters to other principals (e.g., local health officials or coinvestigators) to inform them and to reinforce long-term relations.

The final reports with complete and final data should be written as quickly as possible—before team members are called out to another epidemiologic field investigation! In addition to a written final report, field team members should consider other methods for communicating the findings of the investigation. Options include formal presentations in person, teleconference, or videoconference at professional meetings; presentations or media communication to local communities affected by the public health event or to the general public; and written reports for public health bulletins intended for public health practitioners (e.g., CDC's *Morbidity and Mortality Weekly Report*) or comprehensive articles for peer-reviewed journals.

OTHER ISSUES

Human Subjects and Privacy Concerns

Investigators must ensure that data collections comply with all requirements for human subjects protection. Field investigations conducted in response to outbreaks or other urgent public health events usually are determined to be public health response rather than research. However, an appropriate human subjects institutional review board must approve data collections determined to be research. Investigators must adhere to privacy requirements and confidentiality concerns throughout all phases of the field investigation. In addition to federal requirements regarding information privacy (see Chapter 13), each state has its own laws that cover privacy and confidentiality of information obtained during epidemiologic investigations (1). The stringency of these laws varies by state. Reports should be written in a manner that prevents identification of persons—and occasionally places—that were the subject of or implicated during the field investigation. After the investigation is complete, all records containing identifying information should be given to the inviting state or local jurisdiction for management according to the jurisdiction's laws. In addition to protecting the privacy interests of persons who were subjects of the investigation, this approach also minimizes the likelihood that members of the invited field team would have information that might be subject to subpoena or freedom of information requests that normally would be denied by the state or local jurisdiction.

Suspected Bioterrorism

Suspected bioterrorism raises a spectrum of general operational and other practical considerations about the coordination of concurrent and overlapping investigations involving officials from both public health and law enforcement agencies (2) (see Chapter 24). A paramount operational consideration is determination of what sector and persons might be in charge of a given site; this is a function of several factors, including the extent to which information or evidence indicates that the site is a crime scene or has public health intervention implications in terms of preventing further exposures or identifying and managing potentially exposed persons.

In addition to determining who is in charge of the site, other key operational considerations are the approaches to interviewing persons who might be affected, either with active disease or with exposure, or who might be targeted by the criminal investigation as potential suspects, and to collecting biological samples from such persons and environmental samples from the site. For a concurrent investigation of suspected bioterrorism, interviews of affected persons are best conducted jointly by public health and law enforcement officials. Epidemiologists and criminal investigators must adhere to procedures that serve the interests of public health and safety and respect laws that safeguard the rights of persons, including those who are or might become suspects in a criminal investigation. When biological specimens and environmental samples are collected, field team members must recognize that physical information-gathering steps taken by law enforcement officials as part of an ongoing criminal investigation must adhere strictly to the process of establishing a chain of custody of evidence. A key purpose for this process is to ensure that specimens and samples presented as evidence during a criminal prosecution and trial in court can withstand challenge by the defense.

Incident Command Systems

Finally, regardless of whether an acute public health problem resulted from a natural or unintentional occurrence or from suspected bioterrorism, it might be serious enough to involve multiple jurisdictions (i.e., local, state, and federal) and multiple government agencies (e.g., emergency medical services, law enforcement, public health, or environmental health) and might require a standardized, coordinated response encompassing jurisdictions beyond public health. In the United States, ICS is a standardized command structure to manage incidents across jurisdictional boundaries (see Chapter 16). ICS enables personnel from different agencies and disciplines to work together in a common management structure with a clear chain of command or unified commands and provides logistical and administrative support to operational staff. In recent years, as part of bioterrorism preparedness, public health personnel at local, state, and federal levels have been engaged in emergency preparedness, and many are trained in ICS. In addition, ICS increasingly is used at all levels of public health to coordinate responses to large outbreaks or other acute situations with substantial political and public interest.

During the 2001 anthrax attacks in the United States, local, state, and federal public health field investigators worked with investigators from other agencies under an ICS set up at state and federal levels while the EOC was activated at CDC (3). In recent years, ICS and EOCs have been activated at CDC or states in response to pandemic influenza A(H1N1) (4) and outbreaks of Ebola virus disease (5) and Zika virus infection (6). Field investigators should be familiar with ICS and EOC, as well as their roles when a local EOC is activated. Use of ICS should simplify the defining of roles for all involved and optimize use of all resources and expertise across jurisdictions during management of emergency incidents.

CONCLUSION

Epidemiologic field investigations are important public health responses that can be enhanced through consideration of and adherence to certain key operational principles and practices. They will proceed more smoothly and productively if both inviters and invitees adequately address operational aspects before, during, and after the investigation.

ACKNOWLEDGMENTS

The authors gratefully acknowledge the late Michael B. Gregg, Robert A. Gunn, and Jeffrey J. Sacks, whose work on this chapter in previous editions of this book contributed in part to this chapter.

REFERENCES

1. Hodge JG, Hoffman RE, Tress DW, Neslund VS. Identifiable health information and the public's health: practice, research, and policy. In: Goodman RA, Hoffman RE, Lopez W, Matthews GW, Rothstein MA, Foster KL, eds. *Law in public health practice.* 2nd ed. New York: Oxford University Press; 2007:238–61.
2. Goodman RA, Munson JW, Dammers K, Lazzarini Z, Barkley JP. Forensic epidemiology: law at the intersection of public health and criminal investigations. *J Law Med Ethics.* 2003;31:684–700.

3. Perkins BA, Popovic T, Yeskey K. Public health in the time of bioterrorism. *Emerg Infect Dis.* 2002;8:1015–8.
4. Chamberlain AT, Seib K, Wells K, et al. Perspectives of immunization program managers on 2009–10 H1N1 vaccination in the United States: a national survey. *Biosecur Bioterror.* 2012;10:142–50.
5. Frieden TR, Damon IK. Ebola in West Africa—CDC's role in epidemic detection, control, and prevention. *Emerg Infect Dis.* 2015;21:1897–905.
6. CDC. Zika virus. About Zika: what CDC is doing. http://www.cdc.gov/zika/about/whatcdcisdoing.html

/// 3 /// CONDUCTING A FIELD
INVESTIGATION

MICHAEL E. KING, DIANA M. BENSYL,
RICHARD A. GOODMAN,
AND SONJA A. RASMUSSEN

INTRODUCTION

When a threat to the public's health occurs, epidemiologists are ready responders who investigate the problem so they can identify causes and risk factors, implement prevention

and control measures, and communicate with everyone involved. Epidemiologic field investigations are a core function of epidemiology and perhaps the most obvious way information is transformed into action to ensure public health and safety (see Chapter 1). This chapter describes the step-by-step process required in performing an epidemiologic field investigation. The 10 steps covered here build on and further refine the steps that have been taught traditionally in the Centers for Disease Control and Prevention's (CDC) annual Epidemic Intelligence Service courses, in the three previous editions of this manual (the textbook *Field Epidemiology*), and in other CDC instructional programs. The 10 steps discussed here are similar to those found in other epidemiology instructional publications (1–5). Lists, take-home points, and examples are provided to clarify key aspects and improve the practical utility of the discussion. This chapter describes a field investigation in the context of a public health response to a presumed acute infectious disease outbreak, although this approach also applies to other scenarios and problems.

BACKGROUND CONSIDERATIONS

An *outbreak* is defined as "the occurrence of more cases of disease than expected in a given area or among a specific group of people over a particular period of time" (1). When there are clearly many more cases than usual that are distributed across a larger geographic area, the term *epidemic* can be used. An outbreak is a situation that usually needs a rapid public health response. Notification of a suspected outbreak can come from different sources, including astute clinicians, laboratory scientists, public health surveillance data, or the media.

After the decision is made to start an investigation, clearly defining the objective of the investigation is crucial. Field investigations of common outbreak scenarios have standard objectives and time-tested methods that can be implemented rapidly. For example, because transmission modes associated with foodborne and waterborne outbreaks are well-known (i.e., spread by contact with infected persons, animals, or contaminated food or water), epidemiologists have developed the National Hypothesis Generating Questionnaire (6), a standardized questionnaire to help develop hypotheses and collect information from ill persons regarding demographics and specific exposures. In contrast, at the time of initial recognition, many outbreaks have no obvious or known cause, which challenges the epidemiologist to establish a clear objective early—albeit one that is broad and can be revised as the investigation evolves—and to generate hypotheses (Box 3.1).

BOX 3.1

HOW CASE DEFINITION AND OUTBREAK FOCUS CHANGE: ZIKA VIRUS INFECTION

Zika was first identified in nonhumans in 1947 and associated with mosquito transmission. Since then, researchers have continued to learn and adapt to new information about Zika transmission. Before 2007, when the first larger scale outbreak occurred, Zika was not a disease of special concern given the small number of people affected. In 2008, sexual transmission was suspected as a mode of transmission, but with so few cases, confirming it was not possible. Then Zika virus cases increased exponentially in 2015. Preliminary investigations indicated mother-to-child transmission among pregnant women, and a case of sexual transmission was confirmed. Each time researchers learned new information, case definitions had to be adapted and the focus of information gathering had to expand to account for multiple transmission modes.

Source: Adapted from Reference 7.

Finally, a certain urgency to field investigations and pressure to find an answer quickly will always exist. For example, rapid surveys or other study designs used in outbreak investigations might lack the level of statistical power or proof of causality that often are possible in prospectively planned research studies. Likewise, delays caused by waiting for all laboratory samples to be tested can delay determination of pathogens or modes of spread and, consequently, implementation of control measures. However, the goal is to be both timely and accurate. Because of these considerations, coordinating with all partners and establishing priorities early is key to a successful investigation.

THE INVESTIGATION

Epidemiologists use a systematic multistep approach to field investigations (Box 3.2). Although these steps are presented here in a numeric order, they might be conducted out of order or concurrently to meet the demands of the investigation. For example, in certain circumstances, implementing a control measure soon after notification and confirmation of an outbreak might be possible and even advisable. Often, Steps 2 (Confirm the Diagnosis) and 3 (Determine the Existence of an Outbreak) are performed at the same time. These two steps highlight the need for increased collaboration (or teamwork)

BOX 3.2
TEN STEPS OF A FIELD INVESTIGATION

1. Prepare for field work.
2. Confirm the diagnosis.
3. Determine the existence of an outbreak.
4. Identify and count cases (i.e., create a case definition and develop a line listing).
5. Tabulate and orient the data in terms of time, place, and person (i.e., descriptive epidemiology).
6. Consider whether control measures can be implemented now. (Note: control measures should be considered again after more systematic studies are completed.)
7. Develop and test hypotheses.
8. Plan for more systematic studies.
9. Implement, if not already done, and evaluate control and preventive measures.
10. Communicate findings (i.e., summarize investigation for requesting authority and prepare written reports).

Source: Adapted from Reference 8.

---

early in the investigation among public health officials, laboratory personnel, clinicians, and other stakeholders.

Step 1. Prepare for Field Work

An important first step in any field investigation is addressing the operational aspects related to preparing for field work (see Chapter 2). This preparation includes ensuring that all persons involved agree on the purpose of the investigation and that the required official approvals for the field investigation have been received. A formal invitation for assistance must be received from an authorized official; for example, when a state requests assistance from CDC to conduct an investigation, the Governor or an appropriate public health officer like the state epidemiologist would be authorized to extend that invitation. In addition, roles and responsibilities of those involved in the investigation must be delineated. For most investigations, laboratory testing will play a crucial role; thus, discussions with laboratory colleagues about types of testing and specimens need to occur before the field investigation begins. Concerns related to the safety of the field team (e.g., whether personal protective equipment will be needed) also should be considered during this first step. Ensuring that this early preparation for the field investigation is completed will prevent misunderstandings and other problems later.

Step 2. Confirm the Diagnosis

Confirming or verifying the diagnosis ensures, to the extent possible, that you are addressing the problem that was reported initially and rules out misdiagnosis and potential laboratory error. For example, in a communicable disease outbreak, the real clustering of false infections—a consequence of misdiagnosis and laboratory error—can result in a pseudoepidemic. The term *pseudoepidemic* refers to a situation in which there is an observed increase in positive test results or the incidence of disease related to something other than a true increase in disease. Diagnoses can be confirmed by implementing some or all of the following activities:

- Interviewing the affected persons;
- Clinical examination of the affected persons by health-care personnel when indicated and possible;
- Reviewing medical records and other pertinent clinical information (e.g., radiography and other imaging studies); and
- Confirming the results of laboratory testing; if the epidemiologist does not have the expertise to assess the adequacy, accuracy, or meaning of the laboratory findings, laboratory scientists and other personnel should be consulted.

Although laboratory data might be the best and only link between a putative cause and case, not every case requires laboratory confirmation before further action can be taken. A related step to confirming diagnoses is the need to obtain specimens (e.g., microbiologic strains already isolated) before they have been discarded so that they are available for further analysis if new questions arise later in an investigation.

Step 3. Determine the Existence of an Outbreak

Determining the existence of an outbreak is a sometimes difficult step that should be completed before committing program resources to a full-scale investigation. This step also is necessary to rule out spurious problems (e.g., pseudoepidemics or reporting increases caused by surveillance artifacts). As noted previously, pseudoepidemics might result from real clustering of false infections (e.g., inadvertent contaminants of laboratory specimens) or artifactual clustering of real infections (e.g., increases in the number of reported cases because of changes in surveillance procedures introduced by the health department or implemented by a healthcare delivery system) (9). Problems potentially associated with pseudoepidemics include risks related to unnecessary or inappropriate treatment and unnecessary diagnostic procedures.

To confirm the existence of an outbreak, the field investigation team must first compare the number of cases during the suspected outbreak period with the number of cases that would be expected during a nonoutbreak timeframe by

- Establishing a comparison timeframe in the suspected epidemic setting by considering, for example, whether it should be the period (e.g., hours, days, weeks, or months) immediately preceding the current problem or the corresponding period from the previous year;
- Taking into account potential problems or limitations in determining comparison timeframes (e.g., lack of data, varying or lack of case definitions, incomplete reporting, and other reasons for inefficient surveillance); and
- Calculating occurrence rates, when possible, between the period of the current problem and a comparator period.

For certain problems, an outbreak can be rapidly confirmed through use of existing surveillance data. For others, however, substantial time lags might occur before a judgment can be made about the existence of an outbreak (Box 3.3).

BOX 3.3
ESTABLISHING A BASELINE FOR CONFIRMING AN OUTBREAK

After the initial June 1981 *Morbidity and Mortality Weekly Report* of a cluster of cases of *Pneumocystis* pneumonia among men in Los Angeles, the ensuing investigation required approximately 6 months to establish surveillance and a baseline that confirmed the early phase of what eventually came to be known as the national epidemic of human immunodeficiency virus/acquired immunodeficiency syndrome (HIV/AIDS).

Source: Adapted from References 10, 11.

Step 4. Identify and Count Cases

The aim of this step is to identify, or ascertain, as many cases as possible without including noncases. As a practical matter, this entails casting a broad net through use of a classification scheme—the *case definition* (see the following discussion)—that maximizes sensitivity (i.e., correctly identifies persons who have cases of the condition [true-positives]) and optimizes specificity (i.e., does not include persons who do not have cases of the condition [false-positives]) (see Box 3.4).

BOX 3.4
SIMPLE VERSUS COMPLEX CASE DEFINITIONS

EXAMPLE OF A SIMPLE CASE DEFINITION

The 2007 Zika virus (ZIKV) outbreak in Yap used the following case definition:

> *Case definition*: A patient with suspected disease had acute onset of generalized macular or papular rash, arthritis or arthralgia, or nonpurulent conjunctivitis during the period from April 1 through July 31, 2007.
>
> *Case classification*: We considered a patient to have confirmed Zika virus disease if Zika virus RNA was detected in the serum or if all the following findings were present: IgM antibody against Zika virus (detected by ELISA), Zika virus PRNT90 titer of at least 20, and a ratio of Zika virus PRNT90 titer to dengue virus PRNT90 titer of at least 4. A patient was classified as having probable Zika virus disease if IgM antibody against Zika virus was detected by ELISA, Zika virus PRNT90 titer was at least 20, the ratio of Zika virus PRNT90 titer to dengue virus PRNT90 titer was less than 4, and either no Zika virus RNA was detected by RT-PCR or the serum sample was inadequate for the performance of RT-PCR.

EXAMPLE OF A COMPLEX CASE DEFINITION

Note how the case definition changed from 2007 as researchers learned more about ZIKV transmission.

Laboratory Criteria for Diagnosis

Recent ZIKV Infection
- Culture of ZIKV from blood, body fluid, or tissue; *OR*
- Detection of ZIKV antigen or viral ribonucleic acid (RNA) in serum, cerebrospinal fluid (CSF), placenta, umbilical cord, fetal tissue, or other specimen (e.g., amniotic fluid, urine, semen, saliva); *OR*

- Positive ZIKV immunoglobulin M (IgM) antibody test in serum or CSF with positive ZIKV neutralizing antibody titers and negative neutralizing antibody titers against dengue or other flaviviruses endemic to the region where exposure occurred.

Recent Flavivirus Infection, Possible ZIKV
- Positive ZIKV IgM antibody test of serum or CSF with positive neutralizing antibody titers against ZIKV and dengue virus or other flaviviruses endemic to the region where exposure occurred,
- Positive ZIKV IgM antibody test AND negative dengue virus IgM antibody test with no neutralizing antibody testing performed.

Epidemiologic Linkage
- Resides in or recent travel to an area with known ZIKV transmission; *OR*
- Sexual contact with a confirmed or probable case within the infection transmission risk window of ZIKV infection or person with recent travel to an area with known ZIKV transmission; *OR*
- Receipt of blood or blood products within 30 days of symptom onset; *OR*
- Organ or tissue transplant recipient within 30 days of symptom onset; *OR*
- Association in time and place with a confirmed or probable case; *OR*
- Likely vector exposure in an area with suitable seasonal and ecological conditions for potential local vectorborne transmission.

See Also Subtype Case Definitions
- Zika virus disease, congenital
- Zika virus disease, noncongenital
- Zika virus infection, congenital
- Zika virus infection, noncongenital

Source: Adapted from Duffy MR, Chen TH, Thane Hancock W, et al. Zika virus outbreak on Yap Island, Federated States of Micronesia. *N Engl J Med* 2009;360:2536–2543; and Centers for Disease Control and Prevention. National Notifiable Disease Surveillance System (NNDSS). Zika virus disease and Zika virus infection, 2016 case definition. https://wwwn.cdc.gov/nndss/conditions/zika/case-definition/2016/06/.

The case definition is a statement consisting of three elements that together specify a person

1. With a condition consisting of (a) a set of symptoms (e.g., myalgia or headache) or (b) signs (e.g., elevated temperature, maculopapular rash, or rales) or (c) laboratory findings (e.g., leukocytosis or positive blood culture); and

2. With the condition occurring during a particular period, usually referred to as the *epidemic period*; and

3. With the condition occurring after the person was in one or more specific settings (e.g., a hospital, school, place of work, or community or neighborhood, or among persons who participated in a gathering, such as a wedding or meeting).

Although the case definition might be broad at the onset of an epidemiologic field investigation, it is a flexible classification scheme that often is revised and narrowed as the investigation progresses.

To minimize the likelihood of ascertainment bias (i.e., a systematic distortion in measurement due to the way in which data are collected), cases ideally are sought and counted through systematic searches of a multiplicity of potential sources to identify the maximum number, or a representative sample, of cases. Examples of sources include

- Public health agency surveillance data;
- Medical system records from hospitals, laboratories, or ambulatory care settings;
- Institutional setting records (e.g., school and workplace attendance records); and
- Special surveys.

Information about identified cases (e.g., coded patient identifiers, age, sex, race/ethnicity, date of illness onset or diagnosis, symptoms, signs, laboratory findings, or other relevant data) should be systematically recorded in a spreadsheet or through other means (e.g., a *line listing* or similar epidemiologic database) for subsequent analysis and for use in conducting further investigative studies (e.g., hypothesis testing). All staff involved in data collection and maintenance should be trained to use the forms and questionnaires (whether these be on paper or electronic) and to store the forms to protect personal information while facilitating rapid data analysis.

Depending on the nature, scope, and extent of the outbreak, consideration should be given to the need for additional active case finding and surveillance once sufficient information has been collected to support prevention and control efforts. Specifically, ongoing or intensified surveillance can be paramount in subsequent efforts to evaluate the effectiveness of control measures for curbing and terminating the epidemic (see Step 9).

Step 5. Tabulate and Orient the Data in Terms of Time, Place, and Person

This step involves translating and transforming data from the line listing into a basic epidemiologic description of the outbreak. This description characterizes the outbreak in terms of time, place, and person (referred to as descriptive epidemiology). Through systematic review of data in the line listing, key actions typically involve

- Drawing epidemic curves,
- Constructing spot maps or other special spatial projections, and
- Comparing groups of persons.

In addition, these key actions contribute to developing initial hypotheses for explaining the potential cause, source, and mode of spread of the outbreak's causative agent(s).

Time

Establishing the time of the outbreak or epidemic requires the following actions:

- Develop a chronologic framework by collecting information about and ordering key events identified during creation of the line listing or through other inquiry, including
  - Time of onset of illness (symptoms, signs, or laboratory test positivity) among affected persons;
  - Period of likely exposure to the causal agent(s) or risk factor(s);
  - Time when treatments were administered or control measures were implemented; and
  - Time of potentially related events or unusual exposures.

Chapter 6 includes examples of epidemic curves displaying the types of information that can be analyzed to aid in conducting a field investigation.

- Develop an epidemic curve by graphing the number of cases on the y-axis in relation to units of time (e.g., hours, days, months) on the x-axis—note that time intervals conventionally should be less than (i.e., one-fourth to one-third) the known or suspected incubation period.
- Use the epidemic curve configuration to make preliminary inferences about the modes of spread (e.g., person-to-person, common-source, or continuing point source) of a suspected causative agent.
  - If the agent is known, use knowledge of the incubation period to look retrospectively at the period of likely exposure among affected persons.
  - If the agent is unknown, but a common event or exposure period is likely, consider potential causal agents on the basis of the possible incubation period.

- When indicated, construct epidemic curves relative to specific sites (e.g., workplace settings, hospital units, classrooms, or neighborhoods) or groups identified by other potential risk characteristics.

Place

Use information collected for the line listing and through other inquiry to orient cases in relation to locations, including

- Place of residence,
- Place of occupation,
- Venues for recreational activity;
- Activity sites (e.g., rooms or units in which persons were hospitalized; rooms visited during a convention or meeting; or seating or activity locations on transportation conveyances, such as planes or cruise ships).

Using information about place, construct spot maps (Figures 3.1, 3.2, 3.3) or other visual methods to depict locations of cases at time of onset of illness or possible exposure to causal agents or factors, including

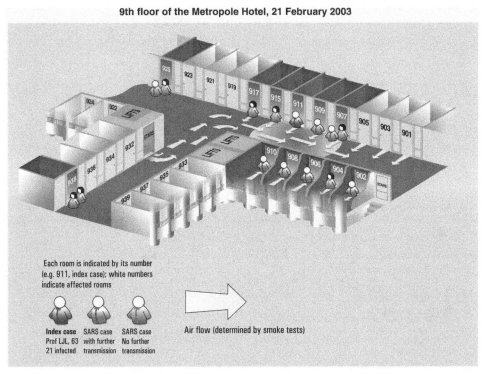

9th floor of the Metropole Hotel, 21 February 2003

FIGURE 3.1 Spot map of residents on the ninth floor of the Metropole Hotel, Hong Kong, February 21, 2003, who had symptoms later identified as severe acute respiratory syndrome.

Source: Reference 12. Reprinted with permission from the World Health Organization, February 5, 2018.

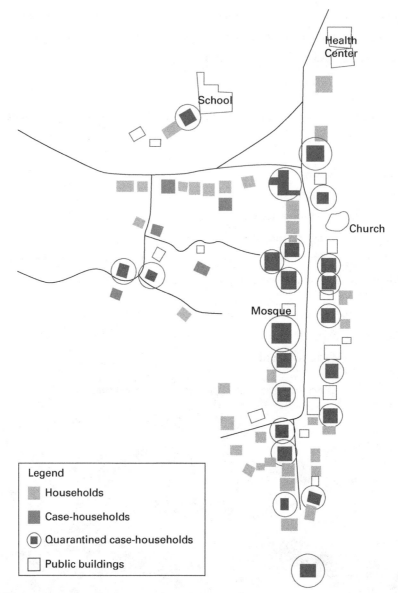

FIGURE 3.2 Schematic map of village X, Sierra Leone, indicating cumulative Ebola virus infection household status and quarantine status, August 1–October 10, 2014.

Source: Reference 13.

- Within buildings
- City blocks or neighborhoods, or
- Geographic or geopolitical areas (e.g., cities, counties, states, or regions).

Person

Use information collected for the line listing to describe cases in relation to such factors as

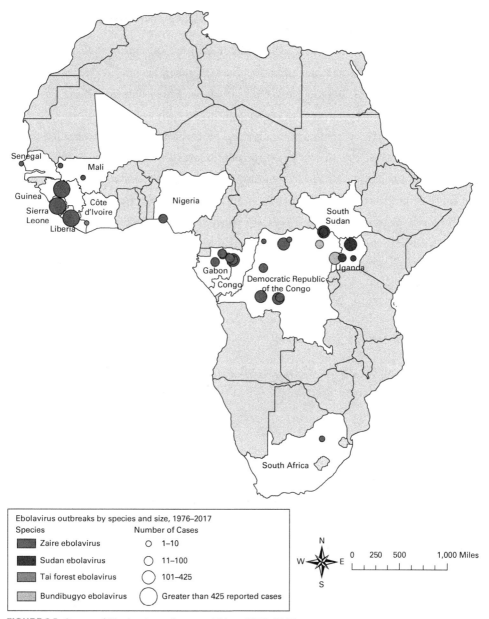

FIGURE 3.3 Cases of Ebola virus disease, Africa, 1976–2017.

Source: Reference 14.

- Demographic characteristics (e.g., age, sex, and race/ethnicity), occupation, and diagnoses; and
- Features shared by affected persons.

When possible and where indicated, obtain denominator data (e.g., total cook-out attendees in a foodborne disease outbreak) to develop preliminary estimates of rates of illness in relation to demographic, exposure, and other characteristics.

Step 6. Consider Whether Control Measures Can Be Implemented Now

Control measures include two categories of interventions: (1) those that can be directed at the source(s) of most infectious and other disease-causing agents (e.g., treating infected persons and animals or isolating infected persons who are contagious) and (2) those that can be directed at persons who are susceptible to such agents (administering post-exposure prophylaxis, vaccinating in advance, or employing barrier techniques) (see Chapter 11 and Box 3.5). In concept, control measures are implemented only after the preceding and subsequent steps—including developing and testing hypotheses about the cause or mode of spread—have been implemented. In practice, however, decisions about control measures might be necessary at any step in the sequence, and preliminary control measures can be instituted on the basis of limited initial information and then modified as needed as the investigation proceeds. Control measures should be considered again after more systematic studies are complete.

Step 7. Develop and Test Hypotheses

Hypotheses about the disease-causing agent, source or reservoir of the agent, transmission mode, and risk factors for disease can be developed based on information from multiple sources including:

BOX 3.5
PUBLIC HEALTH EXAMPLE: CONTROLLING AN OUTBREAK OF HEPATITIS A IN A CHILD DAY CARE SETTING

When the etiology and mode of spread, as well as interventions, are known at the time an outbreak is recognized, control measures can begin immediately. For example, before hepatitis A vaccine was routinely administered to children starting at age 1 year, a single case of hepatitis A in a child day care setting led to administration of immune globulin prophylaxis to an entire cohort of exposed children and staff. This was performed because of the known epidemiologic associations between asymptomatic and symptomatic cases; it directed efforts toward prophylaxis of exposed persons while minimizing the need for an extensive investigation to specifically identify infected persons. The response was predicated on routine policy and guidelines developed by experts on the basis of studies and previous outbreak experience and virtual certainty about the etiology of the problem and its mode of spread.

Source: Adapted from Reference 15.

- Expert subject-matter knowledge by field epidemiologists, laboratory colleagues, and others;
- Descriptive epidemiologic findings resulting from analysis of the line listing of identified affected persons;
- Information obtained from interviews of individuals or groups of affected persons by using structured questionnaires or open-ended questioning;
- Anecdotes, impressions, and ideas from affected persons or others in the affected area; and
- Consideration of outlier cases (i.e., cases with onset occurring at the beginning or end of the outbreak period).

In certain instances, descriptive epidemiologic findings alone, or results of cross-sectional survey data or other studies will be sufficient for developing hypotheses. Often, however, analytic epidemiologic methods—especially cohort or case–control studies—will be needed for identifying possible risk and other causative factors and for testing the strength of the association of the factors with the disease. The process of hypothesis testing, therefore, can entail multiple iterations of hypothesis generating and testing, serial studies, and collection, analysis, and management of considerable additional data. See Chapter 7 for description of how cohort and case–control studies can be used effectively in foodborne or waterborne disease outbreaks and other types of field investigations (Box 3.6).

Typically, statistically significant (e.g., small p value) findings of associations alone do not constitute an adequate body of evidence to support conclusions about the validity of hypotheses and to implement interventions to terminate an outbreak. Instead, all key information and investigative findings should be viewed as a whole in relation to such standards as the Bradford Hill tenets of causation (17) (Box 3.7).

Step 8. Plan One or More Systematic Studies

At this stage of most epidemiologic field investigations, the purposes of systematic or other studies might include improving the quality of information underlying the investigation's conclusions about the problem (e.g., improving the quality of numerators or denominators). Additional examples include refining the accuracy of the estimates of persons at risk and examining other germane concerns (e.g., expanding characterization of the causative agent and its epidemiology).

BOX 3.6
PUBLIC HEALTH EXAMPLE: HYPOTHESIS FORMULATION

In a nationwide foodborne outbreak, the descriptive results of interviews based on the National Hypothesis Generating Questionnaire were used to identify institutional settings (e.g., hospitals and schools), peanut butter, and chicken as potential sources of salmonellosis. The high percentage of respondents with exposure to institutional settings (58%) and exposure to peanut butter (71%) and chicken (86%) enabled them to focus further investigation activities in these three areas. As the investigation continued, cases from institutional settings indicated a common food distributor. A particular brand of peanut butter was distributed to the facilities, and an open tub of this brand of peanut butter was available for *Salmonella* testing. The outbreak strain was isolated from the sample.

Source: Adapted from Reference 16.

Step 9. Implement and Evaluate Control and Prevention Measures

The ultimate purpose of an epidemiologic field investigation is to implement scientifically rational and advisable control measures for preventing additional outbreak-associated morbidity or mortality. Control measures implemented in outbreaks will vary based on the causative agent; modes of spread; size and characteristics of the population at risk; setting; and other considerations, such as available resources, politics, and community concerns. Categories of control measures used for terminating outbreaks are described in this chapter in Step 6 and are further addressed in Chapter 11.

Evaluating the impact of control measures is essential. Therefore, evaluation efforts should be implemented concurrently with control measures to assess their effectiveness

---

BOX 3.7
BRADFORD HILL CRITERIA

- Strength of association.
- Consistency with other studies.
- Temporality (exposure precedes effect [illness]).
- Biologic plausibility.
- Biologic (dose-response) gradient.

Source: Adapted from Reference 17.

in attenuating and ultimately terminating the outbreak. If not yet in place, active surveillance should be initiated to monitor for new cases and for evidence of effect of the control measures and to guide decision-making about additional needs (e.g., further investigation, additional studies, or modifications to the control measures).

Regardless of the intervention, the ethical implications of any action must be considered. Because outbreak investigations typically involve collection of private, personally identifiable information from individual persons, and often from their families, coworkers, or other acquaintances, epidemiologists should be familiar with applicable local, state, and federal laws regarding privacy protections.

Step 10. Communicate Findings

Field epidemiologists must be diligent and effective communicators throughout and after outbreak investigations. The information they provide helps keep the public and stakeholders accurately apprised during an outbreak, informs decisions about actions to halt the outbreak, and documents the investigation.

This step requires the following actions:

1. Establish a communications plan at the onset of the investigation (see also Chapter 2).
   - Identify and designate a spokesperson or a consistent point of contact who will serve as the primary communicator for the investigative team. This will optimize the team's efficiency by concentrating the communications role in one person who is accessible to the news media and others. This also minimizes the potential for confusion or misunderstanding by ensuring consistency in messaging throughout the investigation.
   - Provide oral briefings and written communications, as might be indicated.
     - Written reports can be customized for multiple purposes, including formally conveying recommendations, meeting institutional requirements for documentation, providing a record for future reference, and facilitating rapid dissemination of investigation findings to the requesting authority, stakeholders, scientific colleagues, and others.
     - Before departing the field, the investigative team should provide a preliminary written report and oral briefing to the requesting authority and local stakeholders that documents all activities, communicates the findings, and conveys recommendations. A final, more detailed, report might be provided later, especially if additional analyses and studies are planned.

- Brief reports published rapidly in public health bulletins (e.g., *Morbidity and Mortality Weekly Report*) can help alert colleagues about the problem.

CONCLUSION

This chapter presents a 10-step approach to conducting an epidemiologic field investigation. Although no steps should be skipped, they might be conducted concurrently or out of order depending on the circumstances of the investigation. Although descriptive epidemiologic findings are sufficient for supporting initiation of public health action in certain investigations, more extensive inquiry, including analytic studies, often is required to provide a scientifically rational basis for interventions. Regardless of complexity, the list of steps that organize epidemiologic field investigations helps to ensure focus and thoroughness throughout the investigative response.

ACKNOWLEDGMENTS

The authors thank the late Michael B. Gregg who served as Editor-in-Chief for the first three editions of *Field Epidemiology*; he also authored the initial version of this chapter. For many years, Dr. Gregg taught this subject in the Epidemic Intelligence Service Summer Course.

REFERENCES

1. CDC. Self-study course SS1978. Principles of epidemiology in public health practice, third edition. An introduction to applied epidemiology and biostatistics. Lesson six: investigating an outbreak. https://www.cdc.gov/ophss/csels/dsepd/ss1978/lesson6/section2.html
2. Gertsmann BB. Outbreak investigation. In: Gertsman BB, ed. *Epidemiology kept simple: an introduction to traditional and modern epidemiology.* 2nd ed. Hoboken, NJ: Wiley-Liss, Inc.; 2003:351–64.
3. Brownson RC. Outbreak and cluster investigations. In: Brownson RC, Petitti DB, eds. *Applied epidemiology: theory to practice.* New York: Oxford University Press; 1998:71–104.
4. Reingold AL. Outbreak investigations—a perspective. *Emerg Infect Dis.* 1998;4:21–7.
5. CDC. Multistate and nationwide foodborne outbreak investigations: a step-by-step guide. https://www.cdc.gov/foodsafety/outbreaks/investigating-outbreaks/investigations/index.html
6. CDC. Foodborne disease outbreak investigation and surveillance tools: national hypothesis generating questionnaire. http://www.cdc.gov/foodsafety/outbreaks/surveillance-reporting/investigation-toolkit.html
7. Imperato PJ. The convergence of a virus, mosquitoes, and human travel in globalizing the Zika epidemic. *J Community Health.* 2016;41:674–9.
8. Gregg MB. Conducting a field investigation. In: Gregg MB, ed. *Field epidemiology.* 3rd ed. New York: Oxford University Press; 2008:81–96.
9. Weinstein RA, Stamm WE. Pseudoepidemics in hospital. *Lancet.* 1977;310:862–4.

10. CDC. Pneumocystis pneumonia—Los Angeles. *MMWR*. 1981;30:250–2.

11. CDC. Task Force on Kaposi's Sarcoma and Opportunistic Infections. Epidemiologic aspects of the current outbreak of Kaposi's sarcoma and opportunistic infections. *N Engl J Med*. 1982;306:248–52.

12. World Health Organization. SARS: how a global epidemic was stopped. WHO Regional Officer for the Western Pacific Region. Manila, Philippines: World Health Organization; 2006. http://www.yncdc.cn/newsview.aspx?id=19185

13. Gleason B, Foster S, Wilt G, et al. Geospatial analysis of household spread of Ebola virus in a quarantined village—Sierra Leone, 2014. *Epidemiol Infect*. 2017;145:2921–9.

14. CDC. Ebola virus disease distribution map. https://www.cdc.gov/vhf/ebola/outbreaks/history/distribution-map.html

15. Goodman RA, Buehler JW, Koplan JP. The epidemiologic field investigation: science and judgment in public health practice. *Am J Epidemiol*. 1990;132:9–16.

16. Cavallaro E, Date K, Medus C, et al. *Salmonella* Typhimurium infections associated with peanut products. *N Engl J Med*. 2011;365:601–10.

17. Hill AB. The environment and disease: association or causation? *Proc R Soc Med*. 1965;58:295–300.

/// 4 /// COLLECTING DATA

KATRINA HEDBERG AND JULIE MAHER

INTRODUCTION

Epidemiologic data are paramount to targeting and implementing evidence-based control measures to protect the public's health and safety. Nowhere are data more important than during a field epidemiologic investigation to identify the cause of an urgent public health problem that requires immediate intervention. Many of the steps to conducting a field investigation rely on identifying relevant existing data or collecting new data that address the key investigation objectives.

In today's information age, the challenge is not the lack of data but rather how to identify the most relevant data for meaningful results and how to combine data from various sources that might not be standardized or interoperable to enable analysis. Epidemiologists need to determine quickly whether existing data can be analyzed to inform the investigation or whether additional data need to be collected and how to do so most efficiently and expeditiously.

Epidemiologists working in applied public health have myriad potential data sources available to them. Multiple factors must be considered when identifying relevant data sources for conducting a field investigation. These include investigation objectives and scope, whether requisite data exist and can be accessed, to what extent data from different sources can be practically combined, methods for and feasibility of primary data collection, and resources (e.g., staff, funding) available.

Sources of data and approaches to data collection vary by topic. Although public health departments have access to notifiable disease case data (primarily for communicable diseases) through mandatory reporting by providers and laboratories, data on chronic diseases and injuries might be available only through secondary sources, such as hospital discharge summaries. Existing data on health risk behaviors might be available from population-based surveys, but these surveys generally are conducted only among a small proportion of the total population and are de-identified. Although some existing data sources (e.g., death certificates) cover many disease outcomes, others are more specific (e.g., reportable disease registries).

Accessing or collecting clean, valid, reliable, and timely data challenges most field epidemiologic investigations. New data collected in the context of field investigations should be evaluated for attributes similar to those for surveillance data, such as quality, definitions, timeliness, completeness, simplicity, generalizability, validity, and reliability (1). Epidemiologists would do well to remember GIGO (garbage in, garbage out) when delineating their data collection plans.

DATA COLLECTION ACTIVITIES

Collecting data during a field investigation requires the epidemiologist to conduct several activities. Although it is logical to believe that a field investigation of an urgent public health problem should roll out sequentially—first identification of study objectives, followed by questionnaire development; data collection, analysis, and interpretation; and implementation of control measures—in reality many of these activities must be conducted in parallel, with information gathered from one part of the investigation informing the approach to another part. Moreover, most, if not all, field investigations will be done by a larger team. The importance of developing a protocol, identifying roles and responsibilities of team members, and documenting all activities and processes should not be underestimated.

DETERMINE DECISIONS REGARDING CONTROL MEASURE IMPLEMENTATION

The epidemiologist must keep in mind that the primary purpose of a field investigation into an urgent public health problem is to control the problem and prevent further illness. The range of public health control measures is broad (see Chapter 11). Many of these control measures, such as recalling contaminated food products, closing business establishments, recommending antibiotic prophylaxis or vaccination, and requiring isolation of an infectious person, considerably burden individuals, businesses, or the community. Therefore, it is incumbent on the epidemiologists to determine up front which decisions need to be made and what information is needed to support these decisions.

DEFINE THE INVESTIGATION'S OBJECTIVES AND DETERMINE DATA NEEDED

Determining whether an urgent public health problem exists (i.e., an excess of observed cases of illness above what is expected) depends on knowing the expected background rate of endemic disease. The background rate generally is determined by accessing existing data sources, such as reportable disease registries or vital statistics. For foodborne outbreaks, most states and local jurisdictions publish data at least annually; however, for chronic diseases (e.g., cancer) or birth outcomes (e.g., microcephaly), expected baseline rates might have to be extrapolated by applying previously published rates to the population of concern. Although not specific, data from syndromic surveillance systems (e.g., from emergency departments) can be useful in determining background rates of prediagnostic signs or symptoms, such as fever, respiratory illness, or diarrhea.

After the epidemiologist has confirmed the existence of an urgent public health problem, the next important task in a field investigation is to define the specific objectives and determine what data are necessary and sufficient to justify the control measures. Is the objective to identify a point source (e.g., a contaminated food item) of an outbreak to recall the product? Is the objective to identify specific behaviors that put people at

increased risk (e.g., cross-contamination during food handling)? Is the objective to identify factors in the environment that might be causing disease (e.g., elevated lead levels in
drinking water)?

Although engaging stakeholders, such as other public health agencies, community
partners, industry leaders, affected businesses, healthcare practitioners, customers, and
regulatory agencies, early in an investigation is time-consuming, including them is essential. Discussing up front the purpose of the investigation and the data collection processes
will prove invaluable in the long run when collaborators are needed during case finding,
data collection, implementation of control measures, and communication with affected
populations and the public.

DEVELOP A STUDY PROTOCOL

The ability to conduct an epidemiologic field investigation efficiently and effectively
depends on understanding the interconnectedness of its parts. Many investigation activities must be conducted in parallel and are interdependent and iterative, with results
informing edits or amendments. For example, available resources will influence how
complex data collection efforts can be; the timeline for an investigation of an infectious
disease outbreak needing urgent control measures might require a quick-and-dirty data
collection process, whereas an investigation of a cancer cluster that has unfolded over
several years may permit more in-depth data collection and analysis. Therefore, writing a
protocol before embarking on any data collection is paramount.

The urgency of most field investigations requires that the epidemiologist act quickly
but thoughtfully. An important and potentially time-saving step is to review prior epidemiologic investigations of similar illnesses and, whenever possible, use or adapt existing
protocols, including standard data collection approaches and case definitions. Doing so
facilitates data exchange with other systems if the outbreak extends to other jurisdictions.

A field investigation protocol does not have to be long, but it must include the
following:

- Investigation objectives.
- Study design (e.g., cohort study, case–control study).
- Study population, case definition, sample size, and selection.
- Data collection procedures, variables to be collected, procedures to safeguard
  participants.
- Data security, privacy, confidentiality, information technology controls.
- Analysis plan.

- Logistics, including budget, personnel, and timeline.
- Legal considerations, including statutes, rules, and regulations.

Identifying up front which software package(s) will be used for questionnaire development, data collection, data entry, and analysis also is useful. One such tool, Epi Info, was developed by the Centers for Disease Control and Prevention (CDC) and is a public domain suite of interoperable software tools designed for public health practitioners (available at https://www.cdc.gov/epiinfo/index.html) (see Chapter 5).

Considering all the different elements of an investigation from the beginning will minimize error that potentially can lead to inconclusive results. Major sources of error that need to be considered during data collection include the following:

- Lack of generalizability because of selection bias, variable participation rates.
- Information bias, such as measurement error, self-report bias, and interviewer bias.
- Uncontrolled confounding or bias introduced in the association between exposure and outcome because of third variable.
- Small sample size, resulting in inadequate power to detect differences between groups.

IDENTIFY POSSIBLE DATA SOURCES

Keeping in mind the investigation objectives, the epidemiologist should evaluate whether existing data sources (e.g., vital statistics, notifiable disease registries, population surveys, healthcare records, environmental data) are useful for addressing the investigation objectives, whether these data are accurate and readily accessible for analysis, whether existing data systems are interoperable, and what additional data, if any, need to be collected de novo.

Mortality Statistics

Collecting mortality statistics and classifying the causes of death dates to the 1500s in London, when the Bill of Mortality was periodically published (2). During the 1800s, Dr. William Farr developed a disease classification system that ushered in the era of modern vital statistics (3). During the same period, Dr. John Snow, known as the father of modern epidemiology, mapped deaths from cholera in London and determined the Broad Street Pump as the source of contaminated water (4). The story of removing the pump handle is the quintessential public health intervention based on scientific data.

Vital statistics remain an important source of data for understanding leading and unusual causes of death (e.g., childhood influenza-associated, viral hemorrhagic fever, variant Creutzfeldt-Jakob disease), and their timeliness is improving thanks to the electronic death reporting system, which many states have implemented (5).

Notifiable Diseases Reporting

In the United States, the legal framework for reporting infectious diseases to public health authorities for investigation and control dates to 1878, when Congress authorized the Public Health Service to collect reports of cholera, smallpox, plague, and yellow fever from consuls overseas to implement quarantine measures to prevent introduction into the United States (6).

In 1951, the first conference of state epidemiologists determined which diseases should be nationally notifiable to the Public Health Service and later to CDC. This process continues today; the Council of State and Territorial Epidemiologists determines which diseases and conditions are designated as nationally notifiable to CDC, but each state and territory legally mandates reporting in its jurisdiction. Although the list comprises primarily infectious diseases, in 1995, the first noninfectious condition—elevated blood lead levels—was added (7).

Laboratory Data

Data from laboratories are critical for investigating infectious disease outbreaks. By law, most states require laboratories that identify causative agents of notifiable diseases to send case information electronically to state public health agencies. In addition, most states require laboratories to send cultures to the public health laboratory in their jurisdiction for confirmation, subtyping, and cataloging results in state and national databases. These data are invaluable for determining whether an apparent cluster of cases might be linked and require further investigation or caused by a random clustering of events. Genotyping data on specific infectious agents (e.g., *Salmonella* strains) produced by state public health laboratories are loaded to CDC's PulseNet database to enable identification of cases across jurisdictions that might have a common source (Box 4.1) (9).

Ongoing Population Surveys

Ongoing population surveys are important for understanding the prevalence of health risk behaviors in the general population. The predominant survey conducted in all states

BOX 4.1

MULTISTATE OUTBREAK OF SALMONELLA TYPHIMURIUM INFECTIONS ASSOCIATED WITH PEANUT BUTTER–CONTAINING PRODUCTS, 2008–2009

Public Health Problem: In November 2008, CDC's PulseNet staff noted a multistate cluster of *Salmonella enterididis* serotype Typhimurium isolates with an unusual DNA fingerprint (pulsed-field gel electrophoresis [PFGE] pattern). The outbreak grew to involve 714 case-patients in 46 states; 166 (23%) were hospitalized and 9 (1%) died.

Public Health Response: The broad scope of the outbreak and severity of illness required coordination of data collection across jurisdictions and use of multiple data sources to identify a common source.

- *Case ascertainment: Salmonella* is a reportable infection in all 50 states; laboratory subtyping of isolates (i.e., PFGE) identified outbreak-associated cases across multiple jurisdictions.
- *Data collection*: The initial investigation included detailed, open-ended questions to generate hypotheses; case–control studies used common questionnaires of 300 possible food items; studies identified peanut butter products as common exposure.
- *Product tracing*: Environmental testing of unopened packages and Food and Drug Administration product trace-back identified a single brand of peanut butter products.

Take-Home Point: This outbreak involved many jurisdictions and evolved over a several months. Coordination of epidemiologic studies (e.g., common methods, questionnaires), having a national database of PFGE patterns to identify outbreak-associated isolates, and an FDA product trace-back were key to identifying the cause, which resulted in a widespread product recall (and eventual criminal liability of the peanut butter producer).

———————————

Source: Reference 8.

is the Behavioral Risk Factor Surveillance System, a random-digit–dialed household survey of noninstitutionalized US adults. Other ongoing surveys include the Youth Risk Behavior Survey, Pregnancy Risk Assessment Monitoring System, and National Health and Nutrition Examination Survey. Several states conduct population-based food preference surveys; such surveys are valuable in assessing the background rate of consumption of various food items and can help the field epidemiologist determine whether a foodborne outbreak in which many case-patients report eating a particular food item needs to be investigated further.

Environmental Exposure Data

Distribution of Vectors

Many emerging infectious diseases are zoonotic in origin, so related data are needed. For example, understanding the distribution of vectors for each infection and patterns of the diseases in animals is paramount. During the 2016 epidemic of Zika virus infection, understanding the ecologic niche for the *Aedes* mosquito vector was important when investigating an increase in febrile rash illnesses (Box 4.2) (12).

BOX 4.2
ZIKA VIRUS INFECTION: AN EMERGING VECTORBORNE DISEASE

Public Health Problem: In early 2015, an outbreak of Zika virus, transmitted by *Aedes* spp. mosquitoes was identified in northeastern Brazil. This area also had been affected by an outbreak of dengue fever. By September, an increased number of infants with microcephaly was reported from Zika virus–affected areas.

Public Health Response:

- *Laboratory testing*: To identify the association between Zika virus and illness, samples were tested of amniotic fluid from two women whose fetuses had microcephaly and from several body tissues of an infant with microcephaly who died. Samples tested positive for Zika virus RNA.
- *Case investigation*: Brazil's Ministry of Health developed a protocol for investigating infants with microcephaly and pregnant women infected with Zika virus. Data included pregnancy history (exposure, symptom, laboratory test) and physical examination. A standard case definition for microcephaly was developed.
- Distribution of the mosquito vector throughout the Americas led to recognition of the potential further spread of the virus.

Take-Home Point: Increase in an unusual syndrome (microcephaly) prompted government health agencies to coordinate efforts to collect systematic case data, develop a standard case definition to use across jurisdictions, and conduct uniform laboratory testing for possible etiologic agents. Since this outbreak was recognized, the epidemic has spread through the mosquito vector as well as through sexual and perinatal transmission to multiple countries and continents around the world.

Source: References 10, 11.

Environmental Contaminants

Illness resulting from exposure to environmental contaminants is another area of public health importance requiring surveillance. For example, elevated childhood blood lead levels are a reportable condition, prompting investigation into possible environmental sources of lead. During 2014–2015, a sharp increase in the percentage of children with elevated blood lead levels in Flint, Michigan, resulted from exposure to drinking water after the city introduced a more corrosive water source containing higher levels of lead (Box 4.3) (14).

BOX 4.3

ENVIRONMENTAL: CHILDHOOD LEAD POISONING AND DRINKING WATER

Public Health Problem: During April 2014–October 2015, residents of Flint, Michigan, were exposed to elevated lead levels in drinking water after the water source was switched from the Detroit Water Authority from Lake Huron to the Flint Water System (FWS) from the Flint River. Because corrosion control was not used at the FWS water treatment plant, the levels of lead in Flint tap water increased over time. Exposure to lead has significant adverse health effects (e.g., developmental delays) particularly for young children with developing brains.

Public Health Response:

- To assess the impact of drinking contaminated water on blood lead levels (BLLs), the distribution of BLLs 5 µg/dL or higher among children less than 6 years of age before, during, and after the switch in water source was assessed.
- Among 9,422 blood lead tests conducted during April 2013–March 2016, 284 (3.0%) BLLs were 5 µg/dL or higher; the probability of having BLLs of 5 µg/dL or greater was 46% higher during the period after the switch from Detroit Water Authority to FWS than before the switch to FWS. The probability of having an elevated BLL when the FWS was the source of water remained after controlling for covariates (e.g., age, race, season).

Take-Home Point: Collecting data over time and understanding changes in environmental exposures (e.g., various drinking water sources) was key to identifying a source of communitywide elevated BLL in children and supporting recommended control measures (e.g., filters on tap water).

Source: Reference 13.

Additional Existing Sources of Data

Additional existing data sources can help identify cases, determine background rates of human illness, or assess exposures to disease-causing agents (e.g., pathogenic bacteria, vectors, environmental toxins) in a field investigation. Examples of clinical data sources include medical record abstraction, hospital discharge data (e.g., for cases of hemolytic uremic syndrome) (15), syndromic surveillance systems (16) (e.g., for bloody diarrhea during an Shiga toxin–producing *Escherichia coli* outbreak) (17), poison control center calls (e.g., exposure to white powder during anthrax-related events) (18), and school and work absenteeism records (e.g., New York City school absenteeism in students traveling to Mexico at the beginning of the influenza A[H1N1] pandemic) (19). Examples of data sources for assessing possible exposures include sales receipts (e.g., meals ordered online or food items purchased from a particular store) (20) and law enforcement data (e.g., drug seizures involving illicit fentanyl in conjunction with opioid overdose deaths due to fentanyl) (21).

Newer Sources of Data

Electronic health records (EHRs) appear to be a promising newer source of data for public health surveillance and for assessing the prevalence of disease or behavioral risk factors in the population seeking healthcare (22). Furthermore, EHRs contain potentially useful data on healthcare use, treatment, and outcomes of a disease—elements not typically assessed by more traditional public health data sources.

With the advent of personal computers in most households and smartphones in many pockets (23), epidemiologists are evaluating the utility of the Internet and social media as data sources for identifying outbreaks or case finding during outbreak investigations. Many of these data sources are promising in theory, and epidemiologists are busy evaluating their utility in outbreak detection and case identification. Examples of these data sources include Google hits for antidiarrheal or antipyretic medications to detect outbreaks of gastrointestinal illness or influenza (24) and social media (e.g., Facebook, Twitter, blogs) to identify contacts of patients with sexually transmitted infections, restaurants where case-patients ate or products they ate before becoming sick, or levels of disease activity during influenza season (25). Online order forms or electronic grocery receipts may be useful in identifying names of customers to contact to determine illness status.

DETERMINE DATA COLLECTION METHOD

After evaluating whether existing data can address the study objectives, the field epidemiologist must determine whether additional data need to be collected and, if so, what and how (Box 4.4). This chapter focuses on the collection of quantitative data (see Chapter 10 for qualitative data collection). Information was drawn in part from the "Surveys and Sampling" chapter in the earlier edition of this book (27) and from *Designing Clinical Research* (28).

BOX 4.4
COMPARISON OF SURVEY METHODS IN NOROVIRUS
OUTBREAK INVESTIGATION

Public Health Problem: To support a rapid response, field epidemiologists need to determine the most efficient, timely, and cost-effective method for data collection during an outbreak. In September 2009, the Oregon Public Health Division investigated an outbreak of gastroenteritis that occurred among more than 2,000 participants of a week-long, 475-mile bicycle ride. Participants came from throughout Oregon and other states, and were of higher socioeconomic status and technology-savvy. Norovirus (GII) infection was confirmed as the causative agent.

Public Health Response:

- To determine the most efficient means of collecting data, epidemiologists administered a questionnaire using Internet- and telephone-based interview methods to directly compare data regarding response rates, attack rates, and risk factors for illness.
- Survey initiation, timeliness of response, and attack rates were comparable.
- Participants were less likely to complete the Internet surveys.
- The Internet survey took more up-front time and resources to prepare but less staff time for data collection and data entry.

Take-Home Points: Internet-based surveys permit efficient data collection but should be designed to maximize complete responses. The field epidemiologist must understand the characteristics of the study population and their ability and willingness to respond to various survey methods (e.g., access computers and Internet-based surveys).

Source: Reference 26.

An important initial step in collecting data as part of a field investigation is determining the mode of data collection (e.g., self-administered, mailed, phone or in-person interview, online survey) (29). The mode in part dictates the format, length, and style of the survey or questionnaire.

Factors to consider when deciding on data collection methods include the following:

- The feasibility of reaching participants through different modes. What type of contact information is available? Do participants have access to phones, mailing addresses, or computers?
- Response rate. Mailed and Internet surveys traditionally yield lower response rates than phone surveys; however, response rate for phone surveys also has declined during the past decade (30).
- Sensitivity of questions. Certain sensitive topics (e.g., sexual behaviors) might be better for a self-administered survey than a phone survey.
- Length and complexity of the survey. For example, for a long survey or one with complex skip patterns, an interviewer-administered survey might be better than a self-administered one.
- Control over completeness and order of questions. Interviewer-administered surveys provide more control by the interviewer than self-administered ones.
- Cost (e.g., interviewer time). A mixed mode of survey administration (e.g., mailed survey with phone follow-up) might be less expensive to conduct than a phone-only survey, but it also increases study complexity.

DEVELOP THE QUESTIONNAIRE OR SURVEY INSTRUMENT

Before developing a survey instrument, review the investigation objectives (i.e., study questions) to identify the specific variables that need to be collected to answer the questions. Similar to developing a protocol, the most efficient and effective means for developing a survey instrument might be to identify an existing survey questionnaire or template that can be adapted for current use. Pay special attention to ensuring that survey instruments can be used across multiple sites in the event that the outbreak involves multiple jurisdictions.

Information and variables to include in a survey instrument are

- Unique identifier for each record.
- Date questionnaire is completed.

- A description of the purpose of the investigation for participants.
- Participant demographics.
- Outcome measures.
- Measures of exposure.
- Possible confounders and effect modifiers.
- Information about who participants should contact with questions.

If the survey is interviewer-administered, it should include fields for interviewer name and interview date. A cover sheet with attempts to contact, code status of interview (e.g., completed), and notes can be helpful.

In writing survey questions, borrow from other instruments that have worked well (e.g., that are demonstrated to be reliable and accurate) whenever possible. Write questions that are clear and use vocabulary understandable to the study population and that contain only one concept.

Three basic types of questions are

- *Close-ended questions.* These questions ask participants to choose from predetermined response categories. An "other (specify) _____" field can capture any other responses. They are quick for participants to respond to and easy to analyze.
- *Open-ended questions.* These questions enable participants to answer in their own words and can provide rich information about new topics or context to close-ended questions; however, responses to these questions can be time-consuming to code and analyze.
- *Precoded, open-ended questions.* These questions can be used on interviewer-administered surveys. They enable participants to answer unprompted, but the interviewer selects from precoded response categories.

Close-ended questions usually are used for outbreak investigations. They can have various response categories (e.g., nominal, numeric, Likert scales). Consider including "don't know" and "refused" response categories. Ideally, code response categories in advance and on the instrument to facilitate data entry and analysis (e.g., yes = 1, no = 0). Close-ended questions could include cascading questions, which can be an efficient way to get more detailed information as one filters down through a hierarchy of questions (e.g., first you ask the participant's state of residence, then a menu of that state's counties drops down).

In compiling questions, consider the flow, needed skip patterns, and order (e.g., placing more sensitive questions toward the end). For self-administered surveys, the format needs to be friendly, well-spaced, and easy to follow, with clear instructions and definitions.

Content experts should review the draft questionnaire. The epidemiologist should pilot the questionnaire with a few colleagues and members of the study population and edit as necessary. This will save time in the long run; many epidemiologists have learned the hard way that a survey question was not clear or was asking about more than one concept, or that the menu of answers was missing a key response category.

CALCULATE THE SAMPLE SIZE AND SELECT THE SAMPLE

Good sample selection can help improve generalizability of results and ensure sufficient numbers of study participants. Information about determining whom to select is covered in study design discussions in Chapter 7, but sample size is worth briefly mentioning here. If the study comprises the entire study population, it is a *census*; a subset of the study population is a *sample*. A sample can be selected through probability sampling or nonprobability sampling (e.g., purposive sampling or a convenience sample). Probability sampling is a better choice for statistical tests and statistical inferences. For probability sampling procedures other than a simple random sample (e.g., stratified or cluster sampling), consult with a survey sampling expert.

How large a sample to select depends on resources, study timeline (generally the larger the sample, the more expensive and time-consuming), the analyses to be conducted, and the effect size you want to detect. For example, to detect a difference in proportions between two groups using a chi-square test, consider how much of a difference needs to be detected to be meaningful.

REVIEW LEGAL AUTHORITY, RULES, AND POLICIES GOVERNING DATA COLLECTION

Generally, government public health agencies have the authority to access healthcare system data (with justification). The Health Insurance Portability and Accountability Act (HIPAA) of 1996 (31) has specific language allowing for the use of personal health information by government agencies to perform public health activities.

Nonetheless, accessing data sources that are not specifically collected and maintained by public health authorities can be challenging. Many outside parties are not familiar with the legal authority that public health agencies have to investigate and control diseases and exposures that affect the public's health and safety. The field epidemiologist may find it useful to consult his or her agency's attorney for legal counsel regarding data collection during a specific public health event.

Other scenarios that challenge epidemiologists trying to access external data include concern by healthcare systems that requests for data on hospitalizations, clinic visits, or emergency department visits breach privacy of protected health information; concern by school officials that access to information about children during an outbreak associated with a school activity violates provisions of the Family Educational Rights and Privacy Act (32); and concerns by businesses that case-patients in an outbreak associated with a particular food item or establishment might pursue legal action or lawsuits. Legal counsel can help address these concerns.

COLLECT THE DATA

Having a written data collection section as part of the overall study protocol is essential. As with survey development, borrowing from previous data collection protocols can be helpful. This protocol can include the following:

- Introductory letter to participants.
- Introductory script for interviewers.
- Instructions for recruiting and enrolling participants in the survey, including obtaining consent for participation. Although field epidemiologic investigations of an urgent public health problem are legally considered to be public health practice and not research (33), including elements of informed consent might be useful to ensure that participants are aware of their rights, participation is voluntary, and the confidentiality of their health information will be protected (see the US Department of Health and Human Services informed consent checklist [34]).
- Instructions on conducting the interviews, especially if there are multiple interviewers: Include the importance of reading the questions verbatim, term definitions, the pace of the interview, answers to frequently asked questions, and ways to handle urgent situations.
- Instructions related to protection of participants (e.g., maintaining confidentiality, data security).

Train staff collecting data on the protocol, reviewing instructions carefully and modifying as needed. Involve interviewers in pilot testing the survey instrument and provide feedback. Have a plan for quality checks during questionnaire administration (if the survey is not computer-based). Review the first several completed surveys to check completeness of fields, inconsistencies in responses, and how well skip patterns work. In addition, debrief interviewers about issues they might have encountered (e.g., if participants cannot understand certain questions, those questions might need rewording).

Similarly, data entry must have quality checks. When starting data entry, check several records against the completed survey instrument for accuracy and consider double data entry of a sample of surveys to check for errors.

Subsequent chapters discuss the details of data analysis. However, it is important to consider conducting some preliminary data analysis even before data collection is complete. Understanding how participants are interpreting and answering questions can enable corrections to the wording before it is too late. Many an epidemiologist has bemoaned a misinterpreted question, confusing survey formatting, or a missing confounding variable resulting in study questions without meaningful results.

ISSUES AND CHALLENGES WITH DATA COLLECTION

The important attributes of a public health surveillance system can and should be applied to data collected in response to an urgent event (see Introduction). In field investigations, tradeoffs exist between these attributes; for example, a more timely collection of data might lead to lower quality data, fewer resources might mean less complete data, and retrospective analysis of preexisting data might be more cost-effective, although prospective data collection from case-patients might enable more targeted questions about specific exposures.

The media can play important and sometimes conflicting roles during an outbreak. The media can be useful in alerting the public to an outbreak and assisting with additional case finding. In contrast, if the public believes an outbreak resulted from eating a specific food item or eating at a specific restaurant, that belief can preclude the field epidemiologist's ability to obtain accurate data after a press release has been issued because it might cause self-report bias among study participants. In addition, with the current calls for government transparency and accountability, field epidemiologists might be reluctant to release information too early, thereby risking additional exposures to the suspected source.

Changes in technology also challenge data collection. Such changes range from laboratories moving to nonculture diagnostic methods for isolating infectious pathogens, which decreases the epidemiologist's ability to link cases spread out in space and time, to increasing use of social media to communicate, which limits response rates from time-honored methods of data collection, such as landline telephones. Conversely, many new sources of data are opportunities made possible by the expanded use of computer technology by individuals, businesses, and health systems. It is incumbent upon field epidemiologists to adapt to these changes to be able to investigate and control urgent public health threats.

CONCLUSION

Responding to urgent public health issues expeditiously requires balancing the speed of response with the need for accurate data and information to support the implementation of control measures. Adapting preexisting protocols and questionnaires will facilitate a timely response and consistency across jurisdictions. In most epidemiologic studies the activities are not done linearly and sequentially; rather, the steps frequently are conducted in parallel and are iterative, with results informing edits or amendments. The analyses and results are only as good as the quality of the data collected (remember GIGO!).

REFERENCES

1. CDC. Updated guidelines for evaluating public health surveillance systems. *MMWR*. 2001;50 (RR13):1–35.
2. Declich S, Carter AO. Public health surveillance: historical origins, methods, and evaluation. *Bull World Health Organ*. 1994;72: 285–304.
3. Lilienfeld DE. Celebration: William Farr (1807–1883)—an appreciation on the 200th anniversary of his birth. *Int J Epidemiol*. 2007;36:985–7.
4. Cameron D, Jones IG. John Snow, the Broad Street pump and modern epidemiology. *Int J Epidemiol*. 1983;12:393–6.
5. Westat. Electronic Death Reporting System online reference manual. 2016. https://www.cdc.gov/nchs/data/dvs/edrs-online-reference-manual.pdf
6. CDC. National Notifiable Diseases Surveillance System (NNDSS). History. https://wwwn.cdc.gov/nndss/history.html
7. CDC. National Notifiable Diseases Surveillance System (NNDSS). 2017 National notifiable conditions (historical). https://wwwn.cdc.gov/nndss/conditions/notifiable/2017/
8. Cavallaro E, Date K, Medus C, et al. *Salmonella* Typhimurium infections associated with peanut products. *N Engl J Med*. 2011;365:601–10.
9. Swaminathan B, Barrett TJ, Hunter SB, et al. PulseNet: the molecular subtyping network for foodborne bacterial disease surveillance, United States. *Emerg Infect Dis*. 2001;7:382–9.
10. Schuler-Faccini L, Ribeiro EM, Feitosa IML, et al. Possible association between Zika virus infection and microcephaly—Brazil, 2015. *MMWR*. 2016;65:59–62.
11. França GVA, Schuler-Faccini L, Oliveira WK, et al. Congenital Zika virus syndrome in Brazil: a case series of the first 1501 livebirths with complete investigation. *Lancet*. 2016;388:891–7.
12. Gardner L, Chen N, Sarkar S. Vector status of *Aedes* species determines geographical risk of autochthonous Zika virus establishment. *PLoS Negl Trop Dis*. 2017;11:e0005487.
13. Kennedy C, Yard E, Dignam T, et al. Blood lead levels among children aged <6 years—Flint, Michigan, 2013–2016. *MMWR*. 2016;65:650–4.
14. Hanna-Attisha M, LaChance J, Salder RC, Schnepp AC. Elevated blood lead levels in children associated with the Flint drinking water crisis: a spatial analysis of risk and public health response. *Am J Public Health*. 2016;106:283–90.

15. Chang H-G, Tserenpuntsag B, Kacica M, Smith PF, Morse DL. Hemolytic uremic syndrome incidence in New York. *Emerg Infect Dis.* 2004;10:928–31.

16. Yoon PW, Ising AI, Gunn JE. Using syndromic surveillance for all-hazards public health surveillance: successes, challenges, and the future. *Public Health Rep.* 2017;132 (suppl I):3S–6S.

17. Hines JA, Bancroft J, Powell M, Hedberg K. Case finding using syndromic surveillance data during an outbreak of Shiga toxin–producing *Escherichia coli* O26 infections, Oregon, 2015. *Public Health Rep.* 2017;132:448–50.

18. Watson WA, Litovitz T, Rubin C, et al. Toxic exposure surveillance system. *MMWR.* 2004;53 (Suppl):262.

19. CDC. Swine-origin influenza A (H1N1) virus infections in a school—New York City, April 2009. *MMWR.* 2009;58;1–3.

20. Wagner MM, Robinson JM, Tsui F-C, Espino JU, Hogan WR. Design of a national retail data monitor for public health surveillance. *J Am Med Inform Assoc.* 2003;10:409–18.

21. Rudd RA, Aleshire N, Zibbell JE, Gladden RM. Increases in drug and opioid overdose deaths—United States, 2000–2014. *MMWR.* 2016;64:1378–82.

22. Birkhead GS, Klompas M, Shah NR. Uses of electronic health records for public health surveillance to advance public health. *Ann Rev Public Health.* 2015;36:345–9.

23. File T, Ryan C. Computer and internet use in the United States: 2013. American Community Survey Reports. https://www.census.gov/content/dam/Census/library/publications/2014/acs/acs-28.pdf

24. Thompson LH, Malik MT, Gumel A, Strome T, Mahmud SM. Emergency department and "Google flu trends" data as syndromic surveillance indicators for seasonal influenza. *Epidemiol Infect.* 2014;42:2397–405.

25. Signorini A, Segre AM, Polgreen PM. The use of Twitter to track levels of disease activity and public concern in the US during the influenza A H1N1 pandemic. *PLoS ONE.* 2011;6:e19467.

26. Oh JY, Bancroft JE, Cunningham MC, et al. Comparison of survey methods in norovirus outbreak investigation, Oregon, USA, 2009. *Emerg Infect Dis.* 2010;16:1773–6.

27. Herold JM. Surveys and sampling. In: Greg M, ed. *Field epidemiology.* 3rd ed. New York: Oxford University Press; 2008:97–117.

28. Hulley SB, Cummings SR, Browner WS, Grady DG, Newman TB. *Designing clinical research.* 4th ed. Philadelphia: Lippincott Williams & Wilkins; 2013:277–91.

29. Dillman DA, Smyth JD, Christian LM. *Internet, phone, mail and mixed-mode surveys: the tailored design method.* 4th ed. Hoboken, NJ: John Wiley; 2014.

30. Czajka JL, Beyler A. Declining response rates in federal surveys: trends and implications. *Mathematic Policy Research Report.* 2016. https://aspe.hhs.gov/system/files/pdf/255531/Decliningresponserates.pdf

31. Health Insurance Portability and Accountability Act of 1996. Pub. L. 104–191, 110 Stat. 1936 (August 21, 1996).

32. Family Educational Rights and Privacy Act, 20 USC § 1232g; 34 CFR Part 99 (1974).

33. CDC. HIPAA privacy rule and public health: guidance from CDC and the US Department of Health and Human Services. *MMWR.* 2003;52:1–12.

34. US Department of Health and Human Services, Office for Human Research Protections. Informed consent checklist (1998). http://www.hhs.gov/ohrp/regulations-and-policy/guidance/checklists/

/// 5 /// USING TECHNOLOGIES FOR DATA COLLECTION AND MANAGEMENT

JANET J. HAMILTON
AND RICHARD S. HOPKINS

INTRODUCTION

Technologies and surveillance systems play an integral, increasing, and evolving role in supporting public health responses to outbreaks or other urgent public health events. The functions supported might include event detection, event characterization, enhanced surveillance, situational awareness, formal epidemiologic investigations, identification and management of exposed persons, and monitoring of the response itself and its effectiveness. In any field investigation, decisions need to be made early and strategically regarding methods, data sources, systems, and technologies. Skillful initial selection of optimal tools and approaches improves the investigation.

To the extent possible, anticipate whether an investigation will be a low-profile and localized or might result in a large, possibly multicentric investigation of considerable public health importance and public interest. This early forecast guides system and technology selections. Anticipate that methods or technologies can change or evolve during the investigation as the scope or direction of the investigation changes. Plan regular reviews of the adequacy of the methods in use, and, if needed, make a transition from one data collection platform or process to another.

Previously, all components of a field investigation were likely to be performed actually in the field. Developments in information systems, data integration, and system interoperability have now made possible and sometimes desirable for some components (e.g., data collection, data cleaning, data analysis) of "field" investigations to be performed off-site (e.g., by central office staff). Access by both office and field staff to systematically collected data often simultaneously or in near–real time, improves support of the field investigation. Broader investments in health information technology (IT) and widespread adoption of electronic health records (EHRs), spurred by the Health Information Technology for Economic and Clinical Health Act in the United States enacted as part of the American Recovery and Reinvestment Act of 2009, have expanded the role technology can play in supporting a public health response (1).

DEFINITIONS AND ASSUMPTIONS

For the purposes of this chapter, the terms *outbreak* and *field investigation* represent any acute public health problem requiring urgent epidemiologic investigation, including

- Infectious disease outbreaks;
- Clusters of cancers, birth defects, or poisonings;

- Environmental exposures;
- Diseases or conditions of unknown etiology;
- Natural disasters; or
- Threats arising from events elsewhere in the world.

During larger and higher profile investigations, the field response most likely will occur in the context of the country's organized approach to emergency management—for example, in the US the National Incident Management System (https://www.fema.gov/pdf/emergency/nims/nimsfaqs.pdf) or the country's equivalent approach to emergency management.

In this chapter, the term *technology* refers broadly to

- Computers,
- Software applications,
- Mobile devices,
- Personal health status monitoring devices,
- Laboratory equipment,
- Environmental monitors and sensors, and
- EHRs.

Technology is also used in regard to

- Public health surveillance systems;
- Ongoing public health databases;
- Purpose-built databases for specific investigations; and
- Technologies that enable storing, managing, and querying data and sharing data among these devices and databases.

GUIDING PRINCIPLES FOR SELECTING AND USING TECHNOLOGIES

Emergency situations typically create increased demands for epidemiologic and laboratory resources. Important factors that affect data collection and management during an event response—compared with business as usual—include time constraints; immediate pressure to both collect and instantaneously summarize substantial amounts of data, typically in fewer than 24 hours; limited human resources; often insufficient data preparedness infrastructure; and unfamiliar field deployment locations and logistics (see also Chapter 2).

Two guiding principles for selecting and using technologies during a field response are:

- Technologies for data collection and management should streamline and directly support the workflow of field investigations rather than disrupt or divert resources and staff time away from epidemiologic investigations and related laboratory testing activities (2).
- Technologies should facilitate more time for epidemiologists to be epidemiologists—to find better data, acquire them, clean them, and use data to better characterize the event, monitor its progress, or monitor the implementation or effectiveness of control measures—and more time for laboratorians to perform testing.

The choice of technology platforms should be driven by the

- Goals of the investigation;
- Training and skills of available staff;
- Existing infrastructure for gathering and managing case reports and other surveillance data;
- Number of geographically distinct data collection sites or teams expected and the number of jurisdictions involved;
- Speed and frequency with which interim summaries or situation reports are needed;
- Types of formal or analytic epidemiologic investigations expected (e.g., surveys, longitudinal studies, or additional human or environmental laboratory testing); and
- Other factors that will be evident in the situation.

The chosen technologies and systems should be subjected to periodic review as the investigation continues.

EVOLVING APPROACH AND CONCEPTUAL SHIFT IN FIELD DEPLOYMENTS

Technologic devices (e.g., mobile and smart devices, personal monitoring devices), EHRs, social media and other apps, automated information systems, and improved public health informatics practices have opened exciting opportunities for more effective and efficient public health surveillance. They are transforming how field teams approach the collection, management, and sharing of data during a field response.

Traditionally in field investigations, a public health agency deploys personnel to the geographic area where the investigation is centered, and the investigation is largely led and managed in the field, with periodic reports sent to headquarters. Although site visits are necessary to identify crucial information and establish relationships necessary for the investigation, a shift is occurring to a new normal in which field response data collection is integrated with existing infrastructure, uses jurisdictional surveillance and informatics staff, and uses or builds on existing surveillance systems, tools, and technologies.

Field data collection can be supported by management and analysis performed off-site or by others not part of the on-site team. Data collection, management, and analysis procedures often can be performed by highly skilled staff without spending the additional resources for them to be on-site. For example, active case finding by using queries in an established syndromic surveillance system (e.g., ESSENCE, which is part of the National Syndromic Surveillance Program [https://www.cdc.gov/nssp/news.html#ISDS]) or reviewing and entering case and laboratory data in a state electronic reportable disease surveillance system can be performed from any location where a computer or smart device and Internet connectivity are available. Data collected in the field electronically can be uploaded to central information systems. When data are collected by using paper forms, these forms can be scanned and sent to a separate data entry location where they can be digitized and rapidly integrated into a surveillance information system.

This approach enables the field team to focus on establishing relationships necessary for supporting epidemiologic investigation and data collection activities or on laboratory specimen collection that can only be accomplished on-site. Specialized staff can be assigned to the team; these staff remain at their desks to collect, manage, or analyze data in support of the field investigation. Staff might include data entry operators, medical record abstractors, data analysts, or statistical programmers. Implementing coordinated field and technology teams also enables more and highly skilled staff across multiple levels (local, state, or federal) to contribute effectively to an investigation. How to coordinate data activities in multiple locations needs to be planned for early in the response.

Field investigations often are led by personnel with extensive epidemiologic, disease, and scientific subject-matter expertise who are not necessarily expert in informatics and surveillance strategies. From a data perspective, such leadership can result in the establishment of ineffective data collection and management strategies. To support effective data collection and management, for all outbreaks, field investigators should

- Identify a role (e.g., chief data scientist or chief surveillance and informatics officer) that reports to a position at a senior level in the incident command structure (e.g., incident commander or planning section chief); and
- Identify and establish the role at the start of the response.

Whatever title is assigned to the role, the person filling the role should have clearly delineated duties and responsibilities, including

- Coordinating the full spectrum of data collection and management processes and systems used during the response;
- Being familiar with existing surveillance systems, processes, procedures, and infrastructure and how they are used currently;
- Identifying when and where existing systems can be modified to support the response or if temporary systems or processes need to be established;
- Anticipating that data collection methods or technologies might need to evolve or change during the investigation as the scope or direction of the investigation changes;
- Preventing creation of divergent, one-off, or disconnected data collection, management, and storage;
- Meeting regularly with response staff to identify additional system needs or modifications and ensuring that data collection and management activities support the progressing response;
- Regularly reviewing the adequacy of the surveillance systems, methods, and technology in use during the response and, if needed, plan for and implement a transition from one data collection strategy or platform to another; and
- Communicating surveillance system needs to the incident commander so that decisions and adequate resources for supporting surveillance efforts can be secured.

PACKING EQUIPMENT AND PREPARING FOR DEPLOYMENT

When preparing and packing for field deployments, two technology items are essential for each investigator: a portable laptop-style computer and a smartphone (essentially a pocket computer providing access to a camera, video, geolocating and mapping services, and data collection capacities). Depending on power availability and Wi-Fi or network connectivity, extra batteries or battery packs/mobile charging stations capable of charging multiple devices, such as laptops and phones, can be crucial. A mobile hotspot device to create an ad hoc wireless access point, separate from the smartphone, can be useful in certain situations. For example, after Hurricane Irma made landfall in Florida during September 2017, widespread power losses lasted for days. Deployed epidemiology staff were housed in locations without consistent power and had to travel to established command centers to charge phones, laptops, and rechargeable batteries once a day. Portable printers or scanners are other optional items to consider. Car-chargers for laptops and phones are also useful, although gas shortages can be a constraint and make car-chargers less optimal during certain types of responses.

As far as possible, responders should be deployed with items similar to ones they have been using on a regular basis. This will ensure that the investigator is familiar with the equipment and how it functions in different settings (e.g., how it accesses the Internet and device battery life), that it has all the expected and necessary software installed, and, perhaps most importantly, that it can be connected to the network (e.g., how it accesses the deploying agency's intranet). Equipment caches of laptops, tablets, or other devices purchased only for use during events can lead to considerable deployment problems (e.g., lack of training in how to use the specialized equipment, network compatibility, or obsolescence of either hardware or software).

Field investigators responding to out-of-jurisdiction locations most likely will need to be issued temporary laptops from within the response jurisdiction to ensure network and software compatibility, connectivity, and adherence to jurisdictional security requirements. Temporary access (log-ins and passwords) to key surveillance system applications or updates to an investigator's existing role-based access to these applications will also need to be considered.

ESTABLISHING WORKING RELATIONSHIPS AND INITIAL ARRIVAL

Data often move at the speed of trust. A field team should establish strong working relationships at the start of the response with those who invited the epidemiologic assistance. On-site visit time should be used to ensure that the relationship will, among other tasks, facilitate gathering data and meet the needs of local authorities. Plans need to be made at the outset for sharing regular, timely data summaries and reports with local partners.

Upon initial arrival, the field team should assess existing surveillance systems and the processes for data submission to these systems. The assessment should address

- Data types already collected and available,
- Data timeliness,
- Data completeness,
- How easily and rapidly systems or processes can be modified or changed,
- Equipment available (e.g., laptops and phones),
- Available surveillance system staffing, and
- Known or anticipated problems and concerns with data quality, availability, and timeliness.

If the team is deploying out of its own jurisdiction, the team leader should seek assistance and consultation from someone at the jurisdictional level who fills a role like that of the chief surveillance and informatics officer (see previous section).

USING TECHNOLOGIES ACROSS OUTBREAK INVESTIGATION PHASES

An outbreak investigation and response has defined steps and phases (see Chapter 3), and each has specific technology and information needs. In recent years, public health agencies have benefitted from technologic advances that support outbreak detection—whether the outbreak is caused by a known or unknown agent. For example, to detect reportable disease clusters effectively, the New York City Department of Health and Mental Hygiene each day prospectively applies automated spatiotemporal algorithms to reportable disease data by using SaTScan (Harvard Medical School and Harvard Pilgrim Health Care Institute, Boston, MA). This system enabled detection of the second largest US outbreak of community-acquired legionellosis by identifying a cluster of eight cases centered in the South Bronx days before any human public health monitor noticed it and before healthcare providers recognized the increase in cases (3). The identification led to an extensive epidemiologic, environmental, and laboratory investigation to identify the source—a water cooling tower—and then implement measures to remediate it. Although technology is revolutionizing approaches to cluster detection, this chapter assumes the field team will be responding after a known event or outbreak has been detected; thus, the following discussion focuses on using technologies for conducting initial characterization, active case finding, enhanced surveillance, supporting and evaluating control measures, and situational awareness, and for monitoring the response and its effectiveness.

Conducting Initial Characterization, Active Case Finding, and Monitoring

In an outbreak setting, routine data management often changes because of new stressors or novel circumstances, particularly the need to almost immediately gather data, produce reports, and inform decision makers and the public (see also Chapters 2 and 3). To assess population groups at highest risk, geographic extent, and upward or downward trends of disease incidence throughout a confirmed outbreak, investigators can use existing surveillance mechanisms. However, such mechanisms might need to be enhanced; for example, investigators might need to

- Create a new syndrome or add new queries to an existing syndromic surveillance system;
- Ask physicians and laboratorians to report suspected and probable, as well as confirmed, cases;
- Conduct active case finding; and
- Provide laboratories with diagnostic direction or reagents or ask them to send specimens meeting certain criteria to the state public health laboratory.

Regardless of whether case detection is enhanced, the technology used should support production of a line-listing for tracking cases that are part of the investigation. The system should also document what changes are made to individual cases and when those changes are made, including changes that result from new information gathered or learned or from epidemiologic findings. The system should ensure that laboratory data are easily made relational (Box 5.1). Even if investigation data are collected entirely or partially on paper, those data usually are keypunched into electronic data systems for further analysis, and the paper forms are scanned and stored electronically. As stated in a review of the 2003 severe acute respiratory syndrome (SARS) outbreak in Toronto, an important step in achieving seamless outbreak management is "uniform adoption of highly flexible and interoperable data platforms that enable sharing of public health information, capture of clinical information from hospitals, and integration into an outbreak management database platform" (5, p. 112).

BOX 5.1

USING EPI INFO 7 AND BIOMOSAIC TO SUPPORT THE FIELD INVESTIGATION OF THE SECOND CONFIRMED US CASE OF MIDDLE EAST RESPIRATORY SYNDROME: FLORIDA, 2014

On May 9, 2014, the Florida Department of Health in Orange County received notification from a hospital infection preventionist about a man with suspected Middle East respiratory syndrome (MERS). Specimens tested at CDC confirmed this was the second reported, confirmed US MERS case. (4)

The investigation determined that the patient possibly exposed others in four general settings: airplanes during travel from Saudi Arabia to Orlando, Florida; at home (household contacts and visiting friends); a hospital outpatient waiting room while accompanying a relative for an unrelated medical reason; and later, an emergency department waiting room where he sought care for his illness. Multiple levels of contacts were tracked by the four exposure settings and risk for exposure (e.g., healthcare workers at high or low risk depending on procedures performed). The Epi Info 7 (CDC, Atlanta, Georgia) database that was created supported easy generation of line listings for tracking contacts and linking contact and laboratory information, including associated exposure settings, tracking isolation periods, contact method, attempts, signs and symptoms, final outcome, persons who should provide a clinical specimen, number and types of specimens collected (multiple and over time), whether specimens were received for testing, and laboratory results. The novel nature of the investigation required that additional data fields be captured as the scope of the investigation shifted. Because field investigators can control Epi Info 7 database management, these needed shifts were able to be met rapidly with no technical support. As a result, the progress of the contact investigation was able to be monitored in real time to identify priorities, optimally use personnel resources, and ensure leadership had current information on which to base decisions. Because of the ongoing reported MERS cases in the Middle East, CDC used BioMosaic, a big-data analytics application, to analyze International Air Transport Association travel volume data to assess potential high-exposure areas in the United States on the basis of US-bound travel. Effective database management and linking of epidemiologic and laboratory information in a single location supported the investigation.

ITs can be used to improve the quality, completeness, and speed of information obtained in a field investigation and the speed and sophistication of reports that can be generated from that information at the individual or aggregate level. To ensure that the full benefits of these technologies are realized, investigators need to perform the following actions:

- Begin with the type of output desired, create mock reports, and work backward to define the necessary input elements, ideally at the outset before any data collection begins; however, in reality this process often is iterative.

- Test the data export features and ensure the analytic software can easily access the necessary data.

- Carefully consider the questions leadership will need to have answered and ensure that the collected data elements answer the overarching questions. Completing this step may directly affect the underlying table structure of the database.

- Develop a flowchart detailing the steps associated with data gathering, information sharing, data management, and data technology. This flow chart will also help to identify processes that must be or should be manual and to identify and remove duplications of data transfer and entry (Figure 5.1).

- Recognize that field setups typically need rapid creation and modification of the database and to allow for creation of case records from laboratory results and for addition of multiple laboratory results to case records.

- Ensure the database can track both cumulative data (total cases) and temporal data changes (what occurred during the previous 24 hours or previous week). Collect status changes (i.e., change-history status and date-time stamps when the data changed) for priority data elements to ensure accurate reporting of information that changed and when (e.g., the number of new cases, the number of cases that changed from probable to confirmed, or the number of suspected cases that have been ruled out).

- Ensure the database supports user-defined data extraction and query capabilities. Do not underestimate the need for easy access to the data by the field investigators for data entry and rapid data summary and for planning the next day's field operations (e.g., completed interviews, number of houses to revisit, number of non-English interviewers, number of persons with specimens collected, and number of specimen collection containers or other laboratory supplies on hand and needed). Field investigators should not have to be experts in formulating relational database queries.

- Plan to test field data collection equipment and applications (see also Chapter 2). For example, if interviews and data collection are to be performed in a door-to-door sampling effort, are the laptop computers too heavy to hold while completing an interview? Can the screens be viewed in direct sunlight? Does the system screen navigation match the flow of the interview? Will Internet connectivity be available?

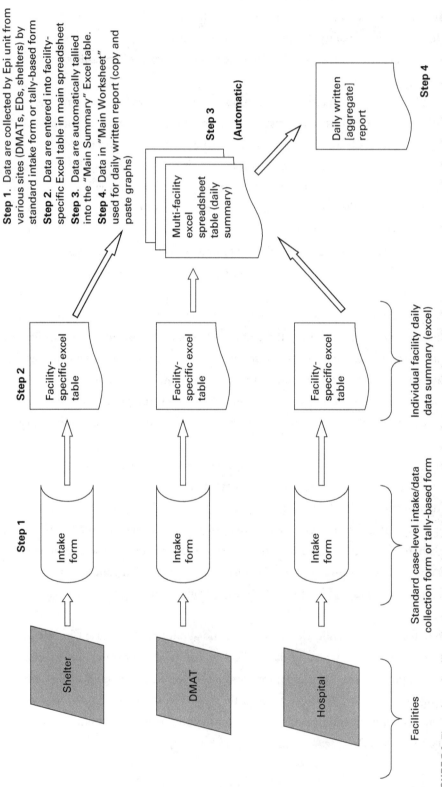

Step 1. Data are collected by Epi unit from various sites (DMATs, EDs, shelters) by standard intake form or tally-based form
Step 2. Data are entered into facility-specific Excel table in main spreadsheet
Step 3. Data are automatically tallied into the "Main Summary" Excel table.
Step 4. Data in "Main Worksheet" used for daily written report (copy and paste graphs)

FIGURE 5.1 Flow chart detailing the steps associated with data-gathering for manual data collection post-storm when conducting drop-in syndromic surveillance from reporting facilities, Florida Department of Health.

Note: DMAT: Disaster Medical Assistance Team; ED: Emergency Department

Source: Reference 6.

- Use programmed data quality and validity checks to identify and resolve discrepancies at the time of data collection. For example, date fields should only accept valid dates within a given range, or pregnancy should be available as a valid value for women only.

- Be aware that, typically, the more complex the data entry checks or programmed skip patterns in place, the more time that is needed to set up the form itself; during field responses, setup time can be an important tradeoff against other uses of investigators' time and against data quality concerns.

- Recognize that structured data collection techniques and standardization processes can minimize data quality problems, although even highly structured data collection techniques do not eliminate data errors. The standardization process that facilitates computer-readable data forms risks losing the richness of information identified within unstructured documents (i.e., clinicians' notes or field observations). How data elements are collected (e.g., structured drop-down lists, free text, check boxes when multiple selections are possible, or radio buttons for single-choice selections) dictates data storage format and table structures and can dictate how the data can be analyzed (e.g., symptoms being reported by interviewees can be stored in a comma-delimited string, or each symptom can be stored as yes/no choices in separate columns).

Using Routine Surveillance Data and Systems

The value and use of routine surveillance data systems should not be underestimated during outbreak investigations and ideally will be managed within a data preparedness framework. Many state reportable disease surveillance systems (both commercially available or state- or in-house–designed) now have outbreak management components (7). To avoid duplicating efforts or processes, field investigators should understand and assess existing surveillance systems that support outbreak management before determining which technologies to use (Box 5.2).

In addition to public health electronic disease surveillance systems supporting outbreak management components, reportable disease electronic laboratory reporting (ELR) is now a mainstay of reportable disease surveillance. Every state health department has operational ELR systems (9). Although ELR was designed for supporting individual identification and reporting of disease events, it can also be used to support outbreak response activities. Using existing surveillance systems, including ELR processes, supports outbreak detection, characterization, outbreak identification, and control measure evaluation (Box 5.3).

USING AN EXISTING STATE HEALTH DEPARTMENT– DEVELOPED REPORTABLE DISEASE SURVEILLANCE SYSTEM'S OUTBREAK MANAGEMENT FUNCTION DURING THE ZIKA VIRUS RESPONSE: FLORIDA, 2016

Following the identification of the initial case of Zika virus infection attributed to likely local mosquito-borne transmission in Florida, the Florida Department of Health conducted active surveillance in selected areas of the state to identify locally acquired Zika virus infections and to assess whether ongoing transmission was occurring (8). Data collected during these field surveys were managed in the outbreak module (OM) of the state health department–developed reportable disease surveillance application, Merlin. Three types of OM events were used: *index*, cases and their contacts; *urosurvey* (i.e., survey administration paired with urine sample collection), participants of residential, business, or clinic urosurveys; and *other*, nonindex cases. Data regarding residential urosurveys (persons within a 150-meter radius of a locally acquired index case), business urosurveys (employees at a business or worksite), and clinic urosurveys (persons who lived or worked in the area of interest) were collected and analyzed. For each urosurvey OM event, an event-specific survey was generated in real time and used to capture the collected data. In 2016, door-to-door survey data were collected on a simple paper form. Surveys were faxed nightly to the central office staff in Tallahassee, where existing reportable disease data entry staff entered all the survey data collected; the digitized information was made available to local- and state-level investigators within 24 hours.

In 2016, 87 OM events (49 index, 32 urosurvey, and 6 other) were initiated. These events comprised approximately 2,400 persons, of whom approximately 2,200 (92%) had participated in any urosurvey event. Managing the data within the Merlin system OM was also useful for immediately linking the laboratory data received electronically from the state public health laboratory information system via the state's existing electronic laboratory reporting (ELR) infrastructure. Modifications were made to the ELR feed (e.g., new Zika virus test codes were added) with these changes able to be completed before the first urosurvey was launched, thus ensuring rapid data receipt. For positive laboratory results, case records were created immediately, and those records were linked between the case record and separate survey data collection areas. Merlin continued to support routine case reporting, and the OM facilitated flexible group-specific, event-level investigations. Event surveys comprised core questions and site- or setting-specific questions. Use of core questions enabled comparability within and between urosurvey event data, improving the ability to conduct ad hoc analysis. Managing data electronically within Merlin and OM facilitated easy access to data for export, event-specific analysis, and linking for mapping. The seamless management of case and survey data eliminated duplicate data entry. During the response, modifications were made to automate sending reportable disease case data from Merlin to CDC for national reporting in the ArboNet database (replacing a previously manual data entry process).

> **BOX 5.3**
>
> **USING ROUTINE ELECTRONIC LABORATORY REPORTING TO SUPPORT OUTBREAK IDENTIFICATION AND EVALUATION OF PUBLIC HEALTH RECOMMENDATIONS**
>
> Identification of influenza outbreaks can be challenging, often relying on a healthcare provider to recognize and report that information to the jurisdiction's health department. Influenza infections among certain populations at high risk (e.g., older persons, particularly those in nursing homes or other long-term care facilities) can have more severe outcomes especially if there are delays implementing appropriate antiviral treatment or chemoprophylaxis. To more effectively identify outbreaks in this setting, the Florida Department of Health (FDOH) implemented regulations to require reporting of influenza results through electronic laboratory reporting (ELR).
>
> Following an approach first described by the New York Department of Health and Mental Hygiene (10), FDOH obtained a list of all licensed nursing homes and other long-term care facilities from the state licensing agency. Addresses of these facilities were then matched to the patient address received on the ELR form to determine whether a person in these facilities had an influenza-positive specimen. A single positive result within these high-risk settings triggers an outbreak investigation. Previously unreported outbreaks have been identified through this approach.
>
> As another example, during the FDOH's 2016 response to locally acquired Zika virus infections (8), ELR was vital for evaluating public health recommendations. In Miami-Dade County, FDOH recommended that all pregnant women be tested for Zika virus infection after active local transmission was identified. Laboratories obtaining testing capacity for Zika virus were asked to send *all* Zika laboratory test results to FDOH. The FDOH birth defects program determined the estimated number of live births and pregnant women living in Miami-Dade, and the ELR data (negative and positive results) were used to assess what proportion of pregnant women had actually been tested and where the public or healthcare providers needed additional outreach or education. With the high volume of testing performed (approximately 65,000 results in 2016), using technology (established ELR processes and advanced analytic software) made such an approach feasible.

Syndromic surveillance uses data about symptoms or health behaviors (e.g., substantial increases in over-the-counter medication sales) and statistical tools to detect, monitor, and characterize unusual activity for further public health investigation or response and situational awareness. The most recognized and largest syndromic surveillance data source is patient encounter data from emergency departments and urgent care centers. These data can be monitored in near–real time as potential indicators of an event, a disease, or an outbreak of public health significance or to provide event characterization and monitoring after initial detection. ESSENCE, an established syndromic surveillance

> **BOX 5.4**
>
> **USING AN EXISTING SYNDROMIC SURVEILLANCE SYSTEM, ESSENCE-FL, TO CONDUCT ENHANCED SURVEILLANCE AND ACTIVE CASE FINDING OF ZIKA VIRUS DISEASE: FLORIDA, 2016–2107**
>
> Zika virus disease (Zika) became a widespread public health problem in Brazil in 2015 and quickly spread to other South and Central American countries and eventually to the United States. Zika is associated with increased probability of severe birth defects in babies when their mothers are infected with the virus during pregnancy. Zika also has been associated with Guillain-Barré syndrome.
>
> The primary vector for Zika is the *Aedes aegypti* mosquito, which is present in Florida. With large numbers of tourists visiting Florida annually, including from many of the countries with Zika outbreaks, Florida instituted measures to minimize introduction of this disease into the state (*8*). Identification of persons infected with Zika early in the course of their illness allows for a twofold public health intervention: (1) patient education about how to avoid mosquito bites while viremic to help prevent spread to others and (2) mosquito control efforts that are targeted to the areas where the patient has been (e.g., home or work).
>
> Florida's syndromic surveillance system (ESSENCE-FL) has nearly complete coverage in hospitals that have emergency departments (245/250 hospitals). Queries were created to search the chief complaint, discharge diagnosis, and triage notes field for Zika terms (including misspellings of the words Zika and *microcephaly*) and clusters of symptoms (e.g., rash, fever, conjunctivitis, or joint pain) in individuals who had travel to countries of concern. Dashboards were created by state-level staff and shared with county epidemiologists to facilitate daily review of emergency department visits for which Zika was suspected.
>
> A total of 19 Zika cases (10 in 2016, 7 in 2017, and 2 in 2018) were identified by using ESSENCE-FL. These visits were not reported to public health by using traditional reporting mechanisms and would not have been identified without active case finding using ESSENCE-FL by the public health agency. These identifications were completed by using an existing surveillance system and helped to reduce the probability of introducing locally spread Zika in Florida.

system, was used to quickly facilitate active case finding when Zika virus was introduced in the US in 2016 and 2017 (*8*) (Box 5.4).

Building New Surveillance Systems Versus Modifying Existing Systems

There is a danger that data management in the context of a field investigation can create more, rather than better, data systems. Condition-specific, event-specific, or stand-alone systems that are not integrated or interoperable require burdensome, post hoc coordination that is difficult and time-consuming, if not impossible.

Rather than setting up new stand-alone systems,

- Work to modify existing systems. Making an urgent system modification is typical, and modifying systems often is more sustainable than designing and developing separate, nonintegrated data management approaches.
- Consider stand-alone systems only when no other options are available. If used, immediately implement a plan to retrieve and share the data with other systems.
- Look for opportunities in which the event response can help catalyze surveillance system modifications that will strengthen future surveillance activities.

Using EHRs

With broad implementation of EHRs, opportunities exist for improving links between healthcare providers and public health departments, making data collection during field investigations more effective and timely (*11*). Increasingly, public health agencies have been able to establish agreements with healthcare facilities, often at the local level, to support remote access to EHRs for day-to-day surveillance activities. With such access to EHRs, staff can review medical records remotely to gather additional clinical, exposure, or demographic data about a case whose case report has been received through other channels.

Routine use of such access by local or state health department staff before an event can reduce public health learning curves when EHRs need to be accessed during a response event. Even without routine access, field investigators have been able to get time-limited system-specific EHR access *during* such response events, as happened during the response to the multistate outbreak of fungal meningitis in 2012 (Box 5.5). This benefitted the outbreak team as they conducted active case finding, completed case abstraction after case identification, and characterized the cases. Medical records abstraction can be done remotely by technical experts who are not on the deployed field team. Familiarity with EHR systems and direct contact with vendors can be helpful. Healthcare provider office staff might be knowledgeable about conducting record-level retrieval in the EHR product, but they might be less skilled at producing system extracts or querying *across* records (e.g., all persons receiving a specific procedure during a specific time frame) in ways that clinical users of the EHR have little occasion to do.

BOX 5.5

USING ELECTRONIC HEALTH RECORDS TO SUPPORT DATA COLLECTION DURING A MULTISTATE OUTBREAK OF FUNGAL MENINGITIS: TENNESSEE, 2012

On September 18, 2012, a clinician alerted the Tennessee Department of Health about a patient with culture-confirmed *Aspergillus fumigatus* meningitis diagnosed after epidural steroid injection. This case was the first in a multistate outbreak of fungal infections linked to methylprednisolone acetate injections produced by the New England Compounding Center (Framingham, MA) (*12*). Three lots of methylprednisolone acetate distributed to 75 medical facilities in 23 states were implicated. Medical record abstraction is a common practice during outbreak investigations, but it typically requires on-site abstraction. The Tennessee Department of Health used remote desktop access to electronic health records (EHRs) to review data regarding known affected patients and identify the background rate of adverse events from the procedures of concern. Remote EHR access enabled abstraction of past, current, and follow-up visits and review of medical histories, clinical course of the disease, laboratory test results, imaging results, and treatment data. This was critically important to inform the real-time development and dissemination of CDC guidelines for patient care that evolved with the constantly changing clinical manifestations. Remote EHR access saved health department and facility staff time, enabled staff to return to their offices to complete case ascertainment, and supported multiple highly skilled staff working simultaneously. Assistance from facility information technology staff was needed in certain instances to obtain remote desktop access and provide guidance on using the EHR.

During the investigation, public health authorities needed a substantial amount of information quickly on an ongoing basis and from multiple, disparate institutions, and traveling to obtain the information was impractical. To remedy the challenges of accessing EHRs remotely, areas for improvement include better understanding of privacy policies, increased capability for data sharing, and links between jurisdictions to alleviate data entry duplication.

When data to support an event response might be in an EHR, field teams should

- Use on-site time to establish necessary relationships and agreements to support remote or desk EHR access;
- Have a low threshold for requesting remote EHR access;
- Elevate resolution of any barriers to EHR access that are encountered to jurisdictional leadership and request assistance from privacy and legal teams (see also Chapter 13);

- Expand the response team to include experts in medical data abstraction who can support the response remotely;
- Contact EHR vendors or use health department surveillance and informatics staff to facilitate coordination with vendors and to help with gaining remote access or to performing data extractions or queries across records; and
- Ensure quality EHR data integration into existing surveillance systems.

Using EHRs is new to some public health workers and can present challenges. For example, public health users require time to learn how to access, connect, and navigate systems. Where in the EHR the needed data are stored depends in part on how healthcare facilities use their EHRs; for example, data ideally stored as coded elements or in available system-designated fields might instead be located in free-text boxes. The more system users exist, the more likely the same data element is recorded in different ways or in different places. Data important to the response might even be stored on paper outside the EHR system. Ideally, public health personnel have access to an institution's entire EHR system, but some facilities still require that those personnel request specific records, to whom the facility assigns specific record access; the latter approach slows the process. The benefits of timely data and data access have proved to be worth the effort to overcome these challenges.

Improving Analysis, Visualization, and Reporting

During outbreaks and response events in recent years, demand has increased for rapid turnaround of easily consumable information. This demand is in part driven by cultural changes and expectations, where people now have powerful computers in their pockets (smartphones) and easy access to social media, the Internet, and 24-hour news cycles. The field team must meaningfully summarize the data and produce reports rapidly, turning collected data into information useful for driving public health action.

Regardless of collection method, after data are digitized, analytic and statistical software can be used to manipulate the data set in multiple ways to answer diverse questions. Additionally, advanced analytic software enables use of other types of data (e.g., electronic real-time data about air or water quality or data acquisition or remote sensing systems, such as continual or automated collection and transmission). Combining these data with geographic information system data can facilitate overlay of environmental and person-centric information by time and place (*11*).

The following principles apply to facilitating effective analysis and visualization:

- Data must be easily exportable to other systems for analysis; often this process can be automated. Even when data collection occurs in one primary database, completing data analyses may require use of other, more sophisticated tools or merger of outbreak data with data from other sources.
- Establish a report schedule (e.g., every day at 9 AM) early during the investigation. In larger outbreaks for which data input is managed in multiple or disparate locations, communicating explicitly when data should be entered or updated in the system and what time the daily report will be run is imperative for ensuring that the most up-to-date information is available for analysis. Reports summarizing the cumulative information known, as well as daily or even twice-daily data summaries (i.e., situation reports) (Handout 5.1), might be necessary.
- Use software to automate report production to run at specific times. This function is useful during larger events where situation reports might be needed multiple times each day.

Transitioning from Field Investigations to Ongoing Surveillance

New systems or processes at the local, state, and federal levels often have been developed for supporting outbreak responses. Because of time and resource constraints in outbreak settings, surveillance systems or processes initiated during outbreaks can partially duplicate other processes. They may be time-consuming or staff-intensive in ways that are acceptable during the response but not as part of a routine system and may present integration problems when the outbreak is over. To minimize this potential, field investigators should ensure that processes for reviewing data collection are strictly followed throughout the outbreak. Field investigators should begin transition planning for sustainability with the goal of transitioning as soon as possible to existing mechanisms, keeping in mind related data collection activities that may be needed in future, long-term records management and storage, and continued analyses.

Determining Security, Standards, and Database Backups

Data security is paramount in any uses of technology in a field response. Computers, tablets, and other mobile devices taken into the field must be protected against data loss and unauthorized access. Determinations must be made regarding what types of equipment can interact with the public health agency's internal network. Confidential data

HANDOUT 5.1

EXAMPLE OF A SITUATION REPORT FROM THE FIELD RESPONSE TO ZIKA VIRUS, FLORIDA DEPARTMENT OF HEALTH, 2016

A situation report summarizing epidemiologic activities was produced daily by the Florida Department of Health and provided to the incident commander for decision-making and resource prioritization purposes. Data were extracted from the state reportable disease surveillance system into analytic software, where the report production was automated.

Zika Fever Summary Points
- 112 Zika fever cases have been reported in Florida as of 2:30 pm on 05/12/16
- No cases are new since 2:30 pm on 05/11/16
- 7 cases have been in pregnant women
- 0 cases were acquired in Florida
- 13 cases have been hospitalized during their illness
- 4 cases are currently ill
- 0 cases have been associated with microcephaly, fetal intracranial calcifications, or poor fetal outcomes (after 1st trimester)
- 1 case has been associated with Guillain-Barré syndrome
- 1117 people have been tested by the Bureau of Public Health Laboratories for Zika virus (634 were pregnant women)

Figure 1: Zika Fever Cases Reported in Florida by Characteristics as of 05/12/16 at 2:30 pm (n = 112)

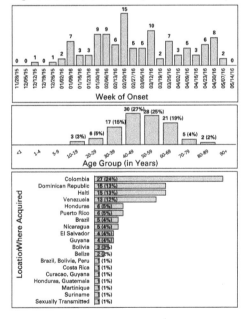
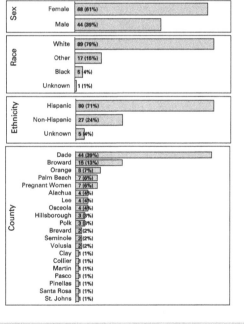

TABLE 1 Zika Fever Cases Reported in Florida by County and Status as of 05/12/16 at 2:30 pm (n=112)

County	Currently Ill	Illness Resolved	Total Cases
Alachua	0	4	4
Brevard	1	1	2
Broward	0	15	15
Clay	0	1	1
Collier	0	1	1
Dade	0	44	44
Hillsborough	0	3	3
Lee	0	4	4
Martin	0	1	1
Orange	2	6	8
Osceola	0	4	4
Palm Beach	0	7	7
Pasco	0	1	1
Pinellas	0	1	1
Polk	0	3	3
Santa Rosa	0	1	1
Seminole	1	1	2
St. Johns	0	1	1
Volusia	0	2	2
Pregnant Women (No County Released)	0	7	7
Total	**4**	**108**	**112**

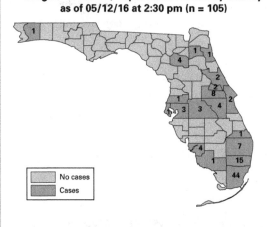

Map 1: Zika Fever Cases (Excluding 7 Cases in Pregnant Women) Reported in Florida by County as of 05/12/16 at 2:30 pm (n = 105)

No cases
Cases

TABLE 2 Zika Fever Cases Reported in Florida by Mosquito Reduction Activities for New Cases

Case ID	County	Date Case Reported	Mosquito Reduction Activities Complete
841144	Volusia	5/9/2016	Yes
841176	Volusia	5/9/2016	Yes

Source: Reference 13.

storage on a local machine should be discouraged, and, if unavoidable, address the need early and through the public health agency's privacy and security standards (see also Chapter 13).

Before data collection or device selection,

- Understand at a high level the public health agency's privacy and security standards;
- Assess whether data security in the field meets the jurisdiction's standards, which might require meeting with the health department's IT director;
- Determine how data collection (and mobile or off-site data collection) will interact with potential firewall and network problems;
- For field deployments where Internet connections or department of health network availability might not be consistently accessible (as was the situation during deployments after Hurricane Irma struck Florida in 2017 and during the Zika response in Miami–Dade County where door-to-door surveying was done inside large apartment buildings), ensure strict security standards are followed; and
- Implement effective database management and rigor by establishing regular and automated backup procedures.

TRACKING AND MANAGING OTHER TYPES OF INFORMATION

Focus first on the *case* information associated with the event. Most often, the field team will also track or manage much other data as well (Box 5.6). For example, in Illinois during a measles outbreak in 2015, in addition to tracking cases, the field team needed to track the number of persons placed in quarantine (*14*) (Box 5.7).

EVALUATING THE ROLE WORKFORCE PLAYS IN TECHNOLOGY USE

Technology will not solve insufficient levels of physical and human resources. Technology decisions to support field deployments often are based, not on the best technology to support the response, but rather on the knowledge and comfort level among staff. The location of the data collection (e.g., from a desk telephone, at a clinic or hospital, or through door-to-door interviews) is a key factor in determining the acceptable technology, as is the acceptance of technology by those under investigation who might be asked to use the instruments or tools directly. If large amounts of data need to be collected manually, not having adequate data entry staff can be a limitation. Necessary data entry staffing is often underestimated, and the data entry process can become a bottleneck. Field team staffing concerns to consider include the following:

BOX 5.6
EXAMPLES OF OTHER, NONCASE DATA THAT FIELD TEAMS MIGHT NEED TO MANAGE DURING INVESTIGATIONS

Field investigators might need to manage noncase data stored in different systems, requiring field teams to have access or collect and aggregate the information; in other situations, the field team might need to create a means of tracking data from multiple sources. For example,

- Current and projected need for laboratory materials, including the number of reagents or laboratory specimen-collection materials (e.g., swabs); specific types of transport media (e.g., stool cans for ova and parasite analysis and bacteriology); or sterile containers.
- Turnaround time from receipt of specimen at the laboratory to availability of results (and by laboratory test type, e.g., culture, polymerase chain reaction [PCR]).
- Availability of crucial supplies (e.g., antiviral drugs, oxygen, or sterile gloves) and equipment (e.g., respirators) and services (e.g., dialysis) in relation to current and projected needs.
- Number of completed surveys conducted each day, number of homes visited, specific residences, and persons needing to be revisited.
- Availability of vaccine, locations offering the vaccine, and doses of vaccine administered (and demographic characteristics of those vaccinated).
- Availability of and access to prophylactic treatments.
- School and workplace attendance and closures.
- Hospital bed availability by bed type, as well as staffing of available beds or staffing issues.
- Documentation of control measures implemented (e.g., number and status of persons isolated or quarantined, number of persons prophylaxed, notification of mosquito control authorities, and if and when spraying occurred).
- Number of persons exposed and exposure location.
- Adequacy of staff for monitoring exposed and isolated persons, status of exclusions, and follow-up testing dates.
- Number of households visited and number of attempts, number of exposed persons contacted, and number of persons responding to contact.
- Distribution of letters and other education materials.
- Status of recalls of food or medical products, continued availability of product at retail or treatment locations, status of contact with facilities receiving implicated products, and assurance products are no longer in use.
- Travel restrictions.

BOX 5.7

USING REDCAP TO SUPPORT MONITORING OF EXPOSED PERSONS DURING A MEASLES OUTBREAK: ILLINOIS, 2015

In January 2015, the Illinois Department of Public Health (IDPH) began investigating a large US measles outbreak comprising 15 confirmed cases and many exposed contacts. The customizable function in REDCap enabled IDPH to rapidly modify the existing Ebola virus disease module to create a measles-specific questionnaire for supporting the measles contact investigation. Within 72 hours, the IDPH measles module in REDCap was ready for use by multiple local health departments. The REDCap survey instrument was offered to 33 (52%) of 63 contacts as a monitoring option alternative to daily telephone calls for reporting body temperature and symptoms, with 17 (52%) of the 33 contacts completing one or more surveys. Postevaluation found REDCap simplified follow-up by reducing staff time and effort for monitoring contacts identified as being at low risk for developing infection. Moreover, the system supported rapid prioritization of persons who needed further follow-up among those contacts failing to report their symptoms daily. To enhance the tool for future use, Spanish and Polish language translation options, a vaccination history data collection tool, and the ability to manage multiple contacts within one household were requested (*14*).

- The number of persons collecting, entering or digitizing data, deployment lengths (from rotating staff leads to the need for multiple trainings), deployment locations, and familiarity with and knowledge of technical tools.
- Available training time. Some level of in-event training is often needed. Training staff for data collection and management *during* the field response can make introducing new technology incredibly difficult and can lead to a lack of acceptance or perceived acceptability of the new tools.
- Interviewing skill sets, languages spoken, and interview locations.
- Team member personal safety and equipment safety.

In addition to epidemiologic, scientific, and disease knowledge, a highly skilled data manager with a firm understanding of public health informatics might be needed on-site as a member of the field team. To be most effective, this person should be familiar with existing surveillance systems, practices, and procedures. Field investigators should have a low threshold for requesting such support if not part of the initial team.

USING PUBLIC HEALTH INFORMATICS

As an emerging field, *informatics* is only vaguely familiar to some professionals in public health. Public health informatics specialists design and implement public health–related systems that efficiently handle data crucial to public health practice. Informatics tools and approaches if applied well can find an appropriate balance between the *ideal* of public health informatics practice and the *reality* of field data collection (*15*).

Public health informaticians are trained to understand public health programs and their data needs as well as information system design—it is this dual training that distinguishes them from most public health agency IT workers. Health IT service professionals are often confused with public health informatics specialists. Health IT service professionals should be able to resolve infrastructure problems such as network connections, whereas trained public health informaticians should be able to support public health decisions by facilitating the availability of timely, relevant, and high-quality information by calling on a broad array of disciplines, including IT architecture and security, statistics, data management science, and systems theory (*11*).

USING TRADITIONAL OR WIDELY USED APPLICATIONS

Because field investigations evolve rapidly, description of specific technologies or programs to support outbreaks, surveillance, and data collections can become outdated quickly (Table 5.1). Ideally, public health agencies should use modern technologies to facilitate public health practice. In reality, public health agencies may struggle to incorporate new technology, in part because of the lack of resources and availability of savvy informatics staff in the field (*15*). Many health departments have restrictive lists of approved software, although exceptions or new approvals can often be expedited during outbreak responses if the need or role the desired software will serve can be demonstrated.

Widely used data collection applications include the Centers for Disease Control and Prevention's (CDC) Epi Info (CDC, Atlanta, Georgia) and, increasingly, REDCap (Research Electronic Data Capture; Vanderbilt University, Nashville, Tennessee). Many state-based reportable disease surveillance systems have integrated outbreak management modules (*7*). Some other free software packages (e.g., SurveyMonkey [San Mateo, CA]) are inadequate for storing and collecting confidential data, and their use must be avoided (see also Chapter 13). Numerous survey tools are designed for handling one-time data collection (e.g., launching a single-use questionnaire), but do not support saving and reusing the same survey.

TABLE 5.1 Examples of commonly used applications that can support epidemiologic field investigations

Application	Comments
Support of survey and questionnaire data collection	
Epi Info (CDC, Atlanta, GA)	• Free public-domain suite of software tools designed and maintained by CDC for public health practitioners and researchers • Easy to set up; can be used to support mobile data collection also Web-based and cloud-optimized components for data collection • Contains customizable data entry forms and database construction • Enables data analyses with epidemiologic statistics, maps, and graphs for public health professionals who lack an IT background • Used in outbreak investigations and for developing small-to-mid–sized disease surveillance systems • Useful for public health field investigators to know and use because of its capabilities • Available for free download at http://www.cdc.gov/epiinfo
Microsoft Access (Microsoft Corp., Redmond, WA)	• Database management system and part of the Microsoft Office suite • Makes data easy to store and manipulate • Limitation: single-user data entry • Additional information available at https://www.microsoft.com/en-us/
REDCap (Vanderbilt University, Nashville, TN)	• Secure Internet application for building and managing online surveys and databases • Used to collect virtually any type of data, including in environments compliant with electronic records legislation (21 Code of Federal Regulations Part 11), the Federal Information Security Management Act of 2002 (44 US Code §3541), and the Health Insurance Portability and Accountability Act of 1996 (Public Law 104–191, 110 Stat 1936) • Specifically designed to support online or offline data capture for research studies and operations • Accessible through computers, tablets, and smartphones • Available at no charge to not-for-profit institutions that join the REDCap Consortium at http://www.project-redcap.org
Outbreak management components of reportable disease surveillance systems	• Might be available as an integrated outbreak management component through the public health agency's reportable disease surveillance system (7). • Might be commercial off-the-shelf products (e.g., Maven [The Apache Software Foundation, Wakefield, MA; https://maven.apache.org/]) or health department–designed and developed (e.g., Florida Department of Health's Merlin system)

(continued)

TABLE 5.1 Continued

Application	Comments
Applications for Analysis, Visualization, and Reporting (AVR)	
SAS (Statistical Analysis System; SAS Institute, Inc., Cary, NC)	• Statistical analysis software suite for advanced analytics, multivariate analyses, business intelligence, data management, and predictive analytics • Highly powerful software application • Additional information available at https://www.sas.com/en_us/home.html
SPSS (IBM Corporation, Armonk, NY)	• Analytic software widely used in social science studies • In addition to statistical analysis, features data management (e.g., selecting cases, reshaping files, or creating derived data) and data documentation (e.g., metadata dictionary stored in the data file) • Additional information available at http://www.ibm.com/spss
R (R Foundation, Vienna, Austria)	• Free, open-source statistical analysis software • Contains graphics capability and can run programs stored in script files • Associated with RStudio, an integrated development environment for R • Additional information is available at http://www.r-project.org and http://www.rstudio.com
ArcGIS (Esri, Redlands, CA)	• Designed to store, manipulate, analyze, manage, and present spatial or geographic data • Includes an excellent mapping tool (see also Chapter 17) • Additional information available at http://www.esri.com
ESSENCE (Electronic Surveillance System for the Early Notification of Community-based Epidemics)	• Syndromic surveillance system operational in many jurisdictions and nationally as part of CDC's National Syndromic Surveillance Program • Jurisdictional versions have different features or data sets • Developed by the Johns Hopkins University Applied Physics Laboratory • Enhancements developed through a collaboration among CDC, state and local health departments, and the Applied Physics Laboratory • Additional information about the National Syndromic Surveillance Program and ESSENCE available at https://www.cdc.gov/nssp/news.html#ISDS
SaTScan (Harvard Medical School and Harvard Pilgrim Health Care Institute, Boston, MA)	• Analyzes spatial, temporal, and space-time data by using scan statistics • Available for free download at http://www.statscan.org

TABLE 5.1 Continued

Application	Comments
BioMosaic (CDC, Atlanta, GA)	• Analytic tool that integrates demography, migration, and health data • Available to designated CDC staff only • Combines information about travel, disease patterns, and location of US settlement of persons from other countries • Combines complex data from multiple sources into a visual format, including maps and other types of graphics • Developed through a collaboration in 2011 among CDC's Division of Global Migration and Quarantine, Harvard University, and the University of Toronto
HealthMap (Boston Children's Hospital, Boston, MA)	• Free mapping utility • Uses informal Internet sources (e.g., online news aggregators, eyewitness reports, expert-curated discussions, and validated official reports) for disease outbreak monitoring and real-time surveillance of emerging public health threats to achieve a unified and comprehensive view of the current global state of infectious diseases • Available for use at http://www.healthmap.org
Emerging or Crowdsourcing Applications	
EpiCollect (Imperial College London, UK)	• Internet and mobile app for generating forms (e.g., questionnaires) and freely hosted project online sites for data collection • Data collected, including global positioning systems and media, by using multiple telephones • All data centrally viewable by using Google Maps, tables, or charts • Additional information available at http://www.epicollect.net/
Apps	• Multiple application tools available or under development to assist field investigators with public health surveillance **Note:** Field investigators should check with the investigating agency's authorities and use extreme caution regarding privacy and confidentiality requirements before using a new application (see also Chapter 13).
Mobile devices	• Data obtained from the device itself, or • Device used to collect data
Single-use online forms	• For example, SurveyMonkey (San Mateo, CA)
Social media	• For example, Yelp (Yelp, Inc., San Francisco, CA), Twitter (Twitter, Inc., San Francisco, CA), and Facebook (Facebook, Inc., Menlo Park, CA)

CDC, Centers for Disease Control and Prevention; REDCap, Research Electronic Data Capture.

Equally important are data management and analysis of collected data. Such software as SPSS (IBM Corporation, Armonk, NY), SAS (Statistical Analysis System; SAS Institute, Inc., Cary, NC), and R (R Foundation, Vienna, Austria) are invaluable analysis and data management applications. Google Maps (Google Inc., Mountain View, CA), and geographic information system data (see Chapter 17) are valuable mapping tools. Be aware, however, that confidentiality can be a serious problem when creating point maps of people with disease, exposure, or injury.

Worldwide adoption of the Internet has enabled a new class of participatory systems that enable people to contribute and share information and collaborate in real time (16). Social media applications (e.g., Facebook [Facebook, Inc., Menlo Park, CA], Yelp [Yelp, Inc., San Francisco, CA], and Twitter [Twitter, Inc., San Francisco, CA]) are increasingly used to conduct surveillance and crowdsourcing, serving both to push out and pull in health-related information. Using social media for both pushing and pulling information can be helpful during outbreaks to support distribution of public health messaging and to support active case finding. These types of data have been used to derive signals of important health trends faster and more broadly than more traditional case reporting systems (11). For example, New York City has used social media for active case finding, contact identification, and evaluation of education and prevention messaging during a community-based outbreak of *Neisseria meningitidis* (17,18) (Box 5.8). Rigorous evaluation of the reproducibility, reliability, and utility of data derived from these new data sources is an area of active research (19).

UNDERSTANDING THE FUTURE OF TECHNOLOGY IN FIELD INVESTIGATIONS

The pervasive use of technology in healthcare and in everyday life will continue to propel and transform public health surveillance and data collection and management during field investigations. Mobile devices hold particular promise for data collection because they can be used as point-of-care devices, perform exposure monitoring, conduct health status monitoring, function in remote locations, and are readily carried and used at any time (20,21). In the future, maturation of data interoperability standards will facilitate more immediate information sharing. The evolution of public health informatics and use of technologies in field responses will continue to require ingenuity and adaptation and provide exciting opportunities during response events.

ACKNOWLEDGMENTS

The authors thank Aaron Kite-Powell, Surveillance and Data Branch, Division of Health Informatics and Surveillance Center for Surveillance, Epidemiology, and Laboratory

> ### BOX 5.8
> ### USING SAS, CELL PHONES, AND SOCIAL MEDIA FOR ACTIVE CASE FINDING, IDENTIFICATION OF CONTACTS, AND EVALUATION OF CONTROL MEASURES DURING A COMMUNITY-BASED OUTBREAK OF *NEISSERIA MENINGITIDIS*: NEW YORK CITY, 2010–2013
>
> In September 2012, the New York City Department of Health and Mental Hygiene (NYC DOHMH) identified an outbreak of *Neisseria meningitidis* serogroup C invasive meningococcal disease among men who have sex with men (MSM). The final tally of cases that occurred during August 2010–February 2013 was 22 cases (7 deaths), of which only 7 cases were in people who were not MSM. Although the attack rate of *N. meningitidis* among MSM in New York City had increased, identifying links among patients and among potentially exposed persons was difficult (*17*).
>
> One approach during the investigation was to use patients' cell phones to identify contacts and links among cases. NYC DOHMH obtained cell phone logs to identify who the case-patients had called, who had called them, and incoming and outgoing text messages. The list of phone numbers was analyzed by a matching program written in SAS code to identify numbers in common (SAS Institute, Inc., Cary, NC). One phone number was common among three persons, and investigators discovered these three men had attended events together (*18*).
>
> Review of cell phones themselves proved effective in identifying common apps among patients and exploring links among them (i.e., mini-networks). NYC DOHMH used social media apps to disperse information to the public regarding getting tested or vaccinated. Information was distributed through Twitter (Twitter, Inc., San Francisco, CA) and approximately 100 Internet sites and blogs that had high MSM viewership, and through NYC DOHMH–sponsored banner and pop-up online advertisements and meet-up apps targeting MSM.
>
> During this outbreak, use of technology and social media was evaluated to assess the effectiveness of education and control measures. "In November 2012, a total of 40,116 (8.2%) of 488,000 pop-ups ads and 2,782 (0.6%) of 463,645 banner ads were clicked on, compared with 87 (14.4%) of 605 e-mail blasts to users of a popular hook-up online site. Of 266 users surveyed, 118 (44%) recalled having received an e-mail about the outbreak; only 77 (29%) users recalled having seen one of the banner ads on the site" (*17*). During this outbreak, use of social media supported the outbreak response through active case finding, contact tracing, and communication of education and prevention messages.

Services, Office of Public Health Scientific Services, Centers for Disease Control and Prevention, for his honest feedback and helpful conversations. For their writing and contributions to field examples presented, the authors thank David Atrubin, Leah Eisenstein, Nicole Kikuchi, Bureau of Epidemiology, Florida Department of Health; Benjamin G. Klekamp, Florida Department of Health—Orange County; Marion

A. Kainer, Healthcare Associated Infections and Antimicrobial Resistance Program, Tennessee Department of Health; and Don Weiss, Bureau of Communicable Disease, New York City Department of Health and Mental Hygiene. For her collaboration and expertise, the authors thank Marcella Layton, Bureau of Communicable Disease, New York City Department of Health and Mental Hygiene. Janet Hamilton is grateful for the understanding, encouragement, and love of her husband, Eric I. Hamilton and her children Jackson and Elaine who allowed mom more weekend and night computer time.

REFERENCES

1. American Recovery and Reinvestment Act of 2009, Pub. L. No. 111-5, 123 Stat. 226. February 17, 2009.
2. Martin SM, Bean NH. Data management issues for emerging diseases and new tools for managing surveillance and laboratory data. *Emerg Infect Dis.* 1995;1:124–8.
3. Greene SK, Peterson ER, Kapell D, Fine AD, Kulldorff M. Daily reportable disease spatiotemporal cluster detection, New York City, New York, USA, 2014–2015. *Emerg Infect Dis.* 2016;22:1808–12.
4. Bialek MD, Allen D, Alvarado-Ramy F, et al. First confirmed cases of Middle East respiratory syndrome coronavirus (MERS-CoV) infection in the United States, updated information on the epidemiology of MERS-CoV infection, and guidance for the public, clinicians, and public health authorities—May 2014. *MMWR.* 2014;63;431–6. Erratum in: *MMWR.* 2014;63:554.
5. Public Health Agency of Canada. Learning from SARS: Renewal of public health in Canada. http://www.phac-aspc.gc.ca/publicat/sars-sras/naylor/index-eng.php
6. Florida Department of Health, Bureau of Epidemiology. County health department epidemiology hurricane response toolkit. Updated April 20, 2015, p. 19.
7. Public Health Informatics Institute. Electronic Disease Surveillance System (EDSS) vendor analysis. http://www.phii.org/resources/view/4409/electronic-disease-surveillance-system-edss-vendor-analysis
8. Likos A, Griffin I, Bingham AM, et al. Local mosquito-borne transmission of Zika virus—Miami–Dade and Broward counties, Florida, June–August 2016. *MMWR.* 2016;65:1032–8.
9. Centers for Disease Control and Prevention. Progress in increasing electronic reporting of laboratory results to public health agencies—United States, 2013. *MMWR.* 2013;61;797–9.
10. Levin-Rector A, Nivin B, Yeung A, Fine A, Greene S. Building-level analyses to prospectively detect influenza outbreaks in long-term care facilities: New York City, 2013–2014. *Am J Infect Control.* 2015;43:839–43.
11. Centers for Disease Control and Prevention. CDC's vision for public health surveillance in the 21st century. *MMWR Suppl.* 2012;61(Suppl):1–44.
12. Centers for Disease Control and Prevention. Multistate outbreak of fungal infection associated with injection of methylprednisolone acetate solution from a single compounding pharmacy—United States, 2012. *MMWR.* 2012;61;839–42.
13. Florida Department of Health, Bureau of Epidemiology. Daily situation report from the field response to Zika virus, 2016. Production Date May 12, 2016, 2:30 PM.
14. Vahora, J, Hoferka, S. How Illinois used REDCap to support contact monitoring for the 2015 measles outbreak. June 11, 2015. http://www.cste.org/blogpost/1084057/219374/How-Illinois-Used-REDCap-to-Support-Contact-Monitoring-for-the-2015.Measles-Outbreak.
15. Fond M, Volmert A, Kendall-Taylor N. *Making public health informatics visible: communicating an emerging field. A FrameWorks Strategic Map the Gaps Report.* Washington, DC: FrameWorks Institute; 2015. https://frameworksinstitute.org/toolkits/informatics/elements/pdfs/informatics_phiistrategic mtgfinalseptember2015.pdf

16. Eysenbach G. Medicine 2.0: social networking, collaboration, participation, apomediation, and openness. *J Med Internet Res.* 2008;10:e22.

17. Kratz MM, Weiss D, Ridpath A, et al. Community-based outbreak of *Neisseria meningitidis* serogroup C infection in men who have sex with men, New York City, New York, USA, 2010–2013. *Emerg Infect Dis.* 2015;21:1379–86.

18. Grounder P, Del Rosso P, Adelson S, Rivera C, Middleton K, Weiss D. Using the Internet to trace contacts of a fatal meningococcemia case—New York City. 2010. *J Public Health Manag Pract.* 2012;18:379–81.

19. Hopkins RS, Tong CC, Burkom HS, et al. A practitioner-driven research agenda for syndromic surveillance. *Public Health Rep.* 2017;132 Suppl:116S–26S.

20. Waegemann CP. mHealth: the next generation of telemedicine? *Telemed J E Health.* 2010;16:23–5.

21. Gerber T, Olazabal V, Brown K, Pablos-Mendez A. An agenda for action on global e-health. *Health Aff (Millwood).* 2010;29:233–6.

/// 6 /// DESCRIBING EPIDEMIOLOGIC DATA

ROBERT E. FONTAINE

INTRODUCTION

As a field epidemiologist, you will collect and assess data from field investigations, surveillance systems, vital statistics, or other sources. This task, called *descriptive epidemiology,* answers the following questions about disease, injury, or environmental hazard occurrence:

- What?
- How much?
- When?
- Where?
- Among whom?

The first question is answered with a description of the disease or health condition. "How much?" is expressed as counts or rates. The last three questions are assessed as patterns of these data in terms of time, place, and person. After the data are organized and displayed, descriptive epidemiology then involves interpreting these patterns, often through comparison with expected (e.g., historical counts, increased surveillance, or output from prevention and control programs) patterns or norms. Through this process of organization, inspection, and interpretation of data, descriptive epidemiology serves multiple purposes (Box 6.1).

ORGANIZING EPIDEMIOLOGIC DATA

Organizing descriptive data into tables, graphs, diagrams, maps, or charts provides a rapid, objective, and coherent grasp of the data. Whether the tables or graphs help the investigator understand the data or explain the data in a report or to an audience, their organization should quickly reveal the principal patterns and the exceptions to those patterns. Tables, graphs, maps, and charts all have four elements in common: a title, data, footnotes, and text (Box 6.2). In this chapter, additional guidelines for preparing these data displays will appear where the specific data display type is first applied.

BOX 6.1
PURPOSES OF DESCRIPTIVE EPIDEMIOLOGY

Descriptive epidemiology

- Provides a systematic approach for dissecting a health problem into its component parts.
- Ensures that you are fully versed in the basic dimensions of a health problem.
- Identifies populations at increased risk for the health problem under investigation.
- Provides timely information for decision-makers, the media, the public, and others about ongoing investigations.
- Supports decisions for initiating or modifying control and prevention measures.
- Measures the progress of control and prevention programs.
- Enables generation of testable hypotheses regarding the etiology, exposure mode, control measure effectiveness, and other aspects of the health problem.
- Helps validate the eventual incrimination of causes or risk factors.

Your analytic findings must explain the observed patterns by time, place, and person.

CHARACTERIZING THE CASES (WHAT?)

Tables are commonly used for characterizing disease cases or other health events and are ideal for displaying numeric values. In addition to the previously mentioned elements in common to all data displays (Box 6.2), tables have column and row headings that identify

---

BOX 6.2
COMPONENTS OF STATISTICAL DATA DISPLAYS

A statistical data display should include, at a minimum,

- A title that includes the what, where, and when that identifies the data it introduces.
- A data space where the data are organized and displayed to indicate patterns.
- Footnotes that explain any abbreviations used, the data sources, units of measurement, and other necessary details or data.
- Text that highlights the main patterns of the data (this text might appear within the table or graphic or in the body of the report).

the data type and any units of measurement that apply to all data in that column or row. A well-structured analytical table that is organized to focus on comparisons will help you understand the data and explain the data to others. In arranging analytical tables, you should begin with the arrangement of the data space by following a simple set of guidelines (Box 6.3) (1).

Cases are customarily organized in a table called a *line-listing* (Table 6.1) (2). This arrangement facilitates sorting to reorganize cases by relevant characteristics. The line-listing in Table 6.1 has been sorted by days between vaccination and onset to reveal the

---

BOX 6.3

GUIDELINES FOR ARRANGING DATA IN TABLES

- Round data to two statistically significant or effective numbers.
  - Using three or more significant figures interferes with comparison and comprehension.
  - More precision is usually not needed for epidemiologic purposes.
  - *Effective figures* refers to numbers that contain additional, leading non-zero digits that do not vary (e.g., 123, 145, 168, or 177) or vary slightly (see BMI columns in Table 6.3) within a column or row.
- Provide marginal averages, rates, totals, or other summary statistics for rows and columns whenever possible.
- Use columns for most crucial data comparisons.
  - Numbers are more easily compared down a column than across a row.
- Organize data by magnitude (sort) across rows and down columns.
  - Use the most important epidemiologic features on which to sort the data.
  - Organizing data columns and rows by the magnitude of the marginal summary statistics is often helpful.
  - When the row or column headings are numeric (e.g., age groups), they should govern the order of the data.
- Use the table layout to guide the eye. For example,
  - Align columns of numbers on the decimal point (or ones column).
  - Place numbers close together, which might require using abbreviations in column headings.
  - Avoid using dividing lines, grids, and other embellishments within the data space.
  - Use alternating light shading of rows to assist readers in following data across a table.

Source: Adapted from Reference 1.

TABLE 6.1 Reported cases of intussusception among recipients of tetravalent rhesus-based rotavirus vaccine,[a] by state—United States, 1998–1999

State	Age (mos.)	Sex	Days[b]	Dose
New York	2	M	3	1
California	3	M	3	1
Pennsylvania	6	M	3	1
Pennsylvania	2	M	4	1
Colorado	4	F	4	1
California	7	M	4	2
Kansas	2	F	5	1
Colorado	3	M	5	1
New York	3	F	5	1
North Carolina	4	F	5	1
Missouri	11	M	5	1
Pennsylvania	3	F	7	1
California	4	F	14	2
Pennsylvania	2	M	29	1
California	5	M	59	1

F, female; M, male.

[a]RotaShield®, Wyeth-Lederle, Collegeville, Pennsylvania

[b]Days from vaccine dose to illness onset

Source: Adapted from Reference 2

pattern of this important time–event association. Commonly in descriptive epidemiology, you organize cases by frequency of clinical findings (Table 6.2) (3). If the disease cause is unknown, this arrangement can assist the epidemiologist in developing hypotheses regarding possible exposures. For example, initial respiratory symptoms might indicate exposure through the upper airways, as in Table 6.2.

COUNTS AND RATES (HOW MUCH?)

Counts

A first and simple step in determining how much is to count the cases in the population of interest. Always check whether data sources are providing *incident* (new events among the population) or *prevalent* (an existing event at a specific point in time) cases. For incident cases, specify the period during which the cases occurred. This count of incident

TABLE 6.2 Prevalence of symptoms and work-related[a] symptoms among hospital environmental services staff reporting use of a new disinfection product—Pennsylvania, August–September 2015 (n = 68)

Symptom	Number with		Percentage with	
	Any	Work-related[a]	Any	Work-related[a]
Watery eyes[b]	31	20	46	29
Nasal problems[b]	28	15	41	22
Asthma-like symptoms[c]	19	10	28	15
Shortness of breath	11	5	16	7
Skin irritation[b]	10	7	15	10
Wheeze[b]	10	5	15	7
Chest tightness[b]	9	2	13	3
Cough	3	1	4	1
Asthma attack[b]	2	1	3	1

[a]Defined as a symptom that improved while away from the facility, either on days off or on vacation.
[b]During the previous 12 months.
[c]Defined as current use of asthma medicine or one or more of the following symptoms during the previous 12 months: wheezing or whistling in the chest, awakening with a feeling of chest tightness, or attack of asthma.
Source: Adapted from Reference 3

cases over time in a population is called *incidence*. Never mix incident with prevalent cases in epidemiologic analyses.

The counts of incident or prevalent cases can be compared with their historical norm or another expected or target value. These case counts are valid for epidemiologic comparisons only when they come from a population of the same or approximately the same size.

Rates, Ratios, and Alternative Denominators

Rates correct counts for differences among population sizes or study periods. Thus, incidence divided by an appropriate estimation of the population yields several versions of incidence rates. Similarly, prevalent case counts divided by the population from which they arose produce a proportion (termed *prevalence*). Strictly speaking, in computing rates, the disease or health event you have counted should have been derived from the specific population used as the denominator. However, sometimes the population is unknown, costly to determine, or even inappropriate. For example, a maternal mortality ratio and infant mortality rate use births in a calendar year as a denominator for deaths in the same calendar year, yet the deaths might be related to births in the previous calendar year. To assess adverse effects from a vaccine or pharmaceutical, consider using total doses distributed as the denominator. Another example is injuries from snowmobile use, which have been calculated both as ratios per registered vehicle and as per crash incident (4). Returning now to counts, you can calculate expected case counts for a population by multiplying an expected (e.g., historical counts, increased surveillance, or output from prevention and control programs) or a target rate by the population total. This expected or target case count is now corrected for the population and can be compared with the actual observed case counts.

Measurements on a Continuous Scale

Disease or unhealthy conditions also can be measured on a continuous scale rather than counted directly (e.g., body mass index [BMI], blood lead level, blood hemoglobin, blood sugar, or blood pressure). You can use empirical cutoff points (e.g., BMI ≥26 for overweight). These can then be counted and the rates calculated. However, a person's measurements can fluctuate above or below these cutoff values. To calculate incidence, special care therefore is needed to avoid counting the same person every time a fluctuation occurs above or below the cutoff point. For prevalence, this fluctuation amplifies the statistical error. A more precise approach involves computing the average and dispersion of the individual measurements. These can then be compared among groups, against expected values, or against target values. The averages and dispersions can be displayed in a table or visualized in a box-and-whisker plot that indicates the median, mean, interquartile range, and outliers (Figure 6.1) (5).

TIME (WHEN?)

Time has special importance in interpreting epidemiologic data in that the initial exposure to a causative agent must precede disease. Often, this will follow a biologically determined interval. The disease or health condition onset time is the preferred statistic for studying time patterns. Onset might not always be available. In surveillance systems, you might have only the report date or another onset surrogate. Moreover, with slowly developing health conditions, a discernable onset might not exist. On the opposite end of the scale, injuries and acute poisonings have instantaneous and obvious onsets.

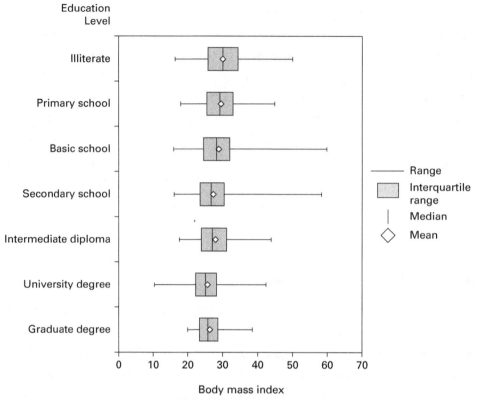

FIGURE 6.1 Mean, median, range, and interquartile range of body mass index measurements of 1,800 residents, by education level: Ajloun and Jerash Governorates, Jordan, 2012.

Source: Adapted from: Ajloun Non-Communicable Disease Project, Jordan, unpublished data, 2017.

Similarly, times of suspected exposures vary in their precision. With acute infections, poisonings, and injuries, you will often have precise exposure times to different suspected agents. Contrast this with chronic diseases that can have exposures lasting for decades before development of overt disease. Other relevant events supplementing a chronologic framework of a health problem include underlying environmental conditions, changes in health policy, and application of control and prevention measures.

Relating disease with these events in time can support calculation of key characteristics of the disease or health event. If you know both time of onset and time of the presumed exposure, you can estimate the incubation or latency period. When the agent is unknown, the time interval between presumed exposures and onset of symptoms helps in hypothesizing the etiology. For example, the consistent time interval between rotavirus vaccination and onset of intussusception (Table 6.1) helped build the hypothesis that the vaccine precipitated the disease (1). Similarly, when the incubation period is known, you can estimate a time window of exposure and identify exposures to potential causative agents during that window.

Depicting Data by Time: Graphs

Graphs are most frequently used for displaying time associations and patterns in epidemiologic data. These graphs can include line graphs, histograms (epidemic curves), and scatter diagrams (see Box 6.4 for general guidelines in construction of epidemiologic graphs).

Contact Diagrams

Contact diagrams are versatile tools for revealing relationships between individual cases in time. In contact diagrams (Figure 6.2, panel A) (5), which are commonly used for visualizing person-to-person transmission, different markers are used to indicate the different groups exposed or at risk.

Epidemic Curves

Epidemic curves (Box 6.5) are histograms of frequency distributions of incident cases of disease or other health events displayed by time intervals. Epidemic curves often have patterns that reveal likely transmission modes. The following sections describe certain kinds of epidemic situations that can be diagnosed by plotting cases on epidemic curves.

Point Source

An epidemic curve with a tight clustering of cases in time (≤ 1.5 times the range of the incubation period, if the agent is known) and with a sharp upslope and a trailing downslope is consistent with a point source (Figure 6.3) (6). Variations in slopes (e.g., bimodal or a broader than expected peak) might indicate different ideas about the appearance, persistence, and disappearance of exposure to the source. Of note, administration of antimicrobials, immunoglobulins, antitoxins, or other quickly acting drugs can lead to a shorter than expected outbreak with a curtailed downslope.

To approximate the time of exposure, count backward to the average incubation period before the peak, the minimum incubation period from the initial cases, and the maximum incubation period from the last cases. These three points should bracket the exposure period. If a rapidly acting intervention was taken early enough to prevent cases, discount the contribution of the last cases to this estimation.

BOX 6.4
GUIDELINES FOR GRAPHICAL DATA PRESENTATION

- Take care in selecting a graph type in computer graphics programs. In Microsoft Excel (Microsoft Corporation, Redmond, WA), for example, you should use "scatter," not "line" to produce numerically scaled line graphs.
- Adhere to mathematical principles in plotting data and scaling axes.
- On an arithmetic scale, represent equal numerical units with equal distances on an axis.
- When using transformed data (e.g., logarithmic, normalized, or ranked), represent equal units of the transformed data with equal distances on the axis.
- Represent dependent variables on the vertical scale and independent variables on the horizontal scale.
- Use alternatives to joining data points with a line. Consider instead
  - No line at all (use data markers only).
  - A trend line of best fit underlying the data markers.
  - A moving average line underlying the data markers.
- Aspect ratios (data space width to height) of approximately 2:1 work well. Extreme aspect ratios distort data.
- Scale the graph to fill the data space and to improve resolution. If this means that you must exclude the zero level, exclude it, but note for the reader that this has been done.
- Do not insist on a zero level unless it is an integral feature of the data (e.g., an endpoint).
- Use graphic designs that reveal the data from the broad overview to the fine detail.
- To compare two lines, plot their difference directly.
- Use visually prominent symbols to plot and emphasize the data.
- Make sure overlapping plotting symbols are distinguishable.
- When two or more data sets are plotted in the same data space
  - Design point markers and lines for visual discrimination; and
  - Differentiate them with labels, legends, or keys.
- To avoid clutter and maintain undistorted comparisons, consider using two or more separate panels for different strata on the same graph.
- When comparing two graphs of the same dependent variable, use scaling that improves comparison and resolution.
- Clearly indicate scale divisions and scaling units.
- Minimize frames, gridlines, and tick marks (6–10/axis is sufficient) to avoid interference with the data.
- Use six or fewer tick mark labels on the axes. More than that becomes confusing clutter.
- Keep keys, legends, markers, and other annotations out of the data space. Instead, put them just outside the data region.
- Proofread your graphs.

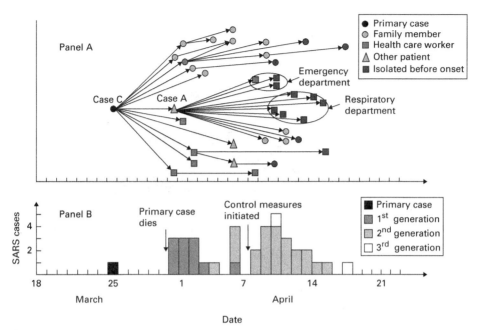

FIGURE 6.2 Contact between severe acute respiratory syndrome (SARS) cases among a group of relatives and health care workers: Beijing, China, 2003.
Source: Adapted from Reference 5.

Point source outbreaks result in infected persons who might have transmitted the agent directly or through a vehicle to others. These secondary cases might appear as a prominent wave after a point source by one incubation period, as observed after a point source hepatitis E outbreak that resulted from repairs on a broken water main

---

BOX 6.5

GUIDELINES FOR EPIDEMIC CURVE HISTOGRAMS

- Time intervals are indicated on the *x*-axis and case counts on the *y*-axis.
- Upright bars in each interval represent the case counts during that interval.
- No gaps should exist between the bars.
- Use time intervals of half an incubation or latency period or less.
- Decrease the time interval size as case numbers increase.
- Indicate an interval of 1–2 incubation periods before the outbreak increases from the background and after it returns to background levels.
- Use separate, equally scaled epidemic curves to indicate different groups.
- Do not stack columns for different groups atop one another in the same graph.
- Use an overlaid line graph, labels, markers, and reference lines to indicate suspected exposures, interventions, special cases, or other key features.
- Compare the association of cases during these pre- and post-epidemic periods with the main outbreak.

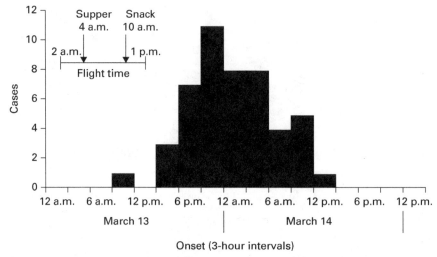

FIGURE 6.3 Cases of salmonellosis among passengers on a flight from London to the United States, by time of onset, March 13–14, 1984.

Source: Adapted from Reference 6.

(Figure 6.4) (7). With diseases of shorter incubation and lower rates of secondary spread, the secondary wave might appear only as a more prolonged downslope.

Continuing Common Source

Outbreaks can arise from common sources that continue over time. The continuing common source epidemic curve will increase sharply, similar to a point source. Rather than increase to a peak, however, this type of epidemic curve has a plateau. The downslope can be precipitous if the common source is removed or gradual if it exhausts itself. The rapid increase, plateau, and precipitous downslope all appeared with a salmonellosis outbreak from cheese distributed to multiple restaurants and then recalled (Figure 6.5).

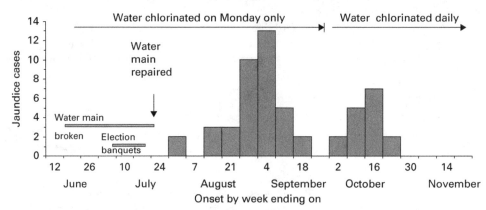

FIGURE 6.4 Cases of jaundice, by week of onset: Jafr, Ma'an Governorate, Jordan, June–October 1999.

Source: Adapted from Reference 7.

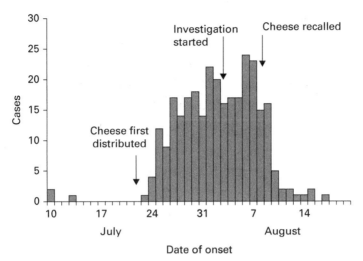

FIGURE 6.5 Cases of *Salmonella enterica* serovar Heidelberg infection, by illness onset date: Colorado, July 10–August 17, 1976.

Propagated

A propagated pattern arises with agents that are communicable between persons, usually directly but sometimes through an intermediate vehicle. This propagated pattern has four principal characteristics (Box 6.6).

The epidemic curve accompanying the severe acute respiratory syndrome (SARS) contact diagram (Figure 6.2, panel B) illustrates these features, including waves with an approximate 1-week periodicity. Certain behaviors (e.g., drug addiction or mass sociogenic illness) might propagate from person to person, but the epidemic curve will not necessarily reflect generation times. Epidemic curves for large geographic areas might not reveal the early periodicity or the characteristic increase and decrease of a propagated outbreak. For these larger areas, stratifying the epidemic curves by smaller subunits can reveal the underlying periodicity.

BOX 6.6
CHARACTERISTICS OF PROPAGATED EPIDEMIC CURVES

- They encompass multiple generation periods for the agent.
- They begin with a single or limited number of cases and increase with a gradually increasing upslope.
- Often, a periodicity equivalent to the generation period for the agent might be obvious during the initial stages of the outbreak.
- After the outbreak peaks, the exhaustion of susceptible hosts usually results in a rapid downslope.

Human–Vector–Human

Vectorborne diseases propagate between an arthropod vector and a vertebrate host. Six biologic differences in human–vector–human propagation affect the size and the shape of the epidemic curve (Box 6.7). The last two factors listed in the box will lead to irregular peaks during the progression of the outbreak and precipitous decreases.

An outbreak of dengue arising from a single imported case in a South China town reveals several of these features (Figure 6.6) (8). After the initial case, 15 days elapsed until the peak of the first generation of new cases. Control measures targeting the larva and adults of the mosquito vectors *Aedes aegypti* and *A. albopictus* began late in the first generation. The line indicates the rapid decrease in *Aedes*-infested houses (house index). A rapid decrease in dengue cases follows this decrease in vector density.

Zoonotic

The epidemic curve for a zoonotic disease among humans typically mirrors the variations in prevalence among the reservoir animal population. This will be modified by the variability of contact between humans and the reservoir animal and, for vectorborne zoonoses, contact with the arthropod vector.

BOX 6.7
FACTORS AFFECTING PATTERNS OF HUMAN–VECTOR–HUMAN TRANSMISSION ACROSS TIME

- Arthropod vectors feed indiscriminately. Contrast this with human social interactions that govern person-to-person transmission. Sequential waves of human–vector–human transmission tend to be larger than person-to-person transmission.
- Generation periods between waves of an outbreak are usually longer than with simple person-to-person transmission because two sequential incubation periods, extrinsic in the vector and intrinsic in the human, are involved.
- Arthropod vectors, after becoming infected, remain so until they perish. This tends to prolong waves of vectorborne outbreaks.
- Increasing environmental temperatures accelerate the multiplication of infectious agents in an arthropod. Consequently, they also accelerate and amplify epidemic development.
- Mean daily temperatures of less than 68°F (<20°C) typically arrest multiplication of infectious agents in the arthropod.
- Arthropod populations can grow explosively and can decline even more rapidly. This will be reflected by an instability of the epidemic curve.

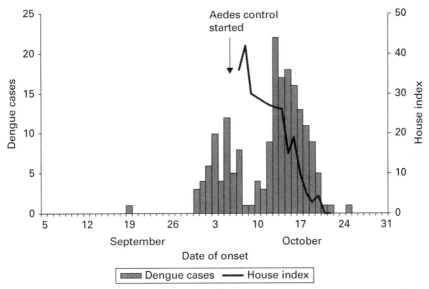

FIGURE 6.6 Date of onset of 185 cases of dengue in a fishing port: Guangdong Province, China, 2007.

Source: Adapted from Reference 8.

Environmental

Epidemic curves from environmentally spread diseases reflect complex interactions between the agent and the environment and the factors that lead to exposure of humans to the environmental source. Outbreaks that arise from environmental sources usually encompass multiple generations or incubation periods for the agent. You should include on the epidemic curve a representation of the suspected environmental factor (e.g., rainfall connected with leptospirosis in Figure 6.7 [9]). In this example, nearly every peak of rainfall precedes a peak in leptospirosis, supporting the hypothesis regarding the importance of water and mud in transmission.

Relative Time

As an alternative to plotting onset by calendar time, plotting the time between suspected exposures and onset can help you understand the epidemiologic situation. For example, a plot of the days between contact with a SARS patient and onset of SARS in the person having contact indicates an approximation of the incubation period (Figure 6.8) (5).

Multiple Strata Display

To reveal distinctive internal patterns (e.g., by exposure, method of case detection, place, or personal characteristics) in time distributions, epidemic curves should be stratified (Figure 6.9). This puts each stratum on a flat baseline, enabling undistorted comparisons.

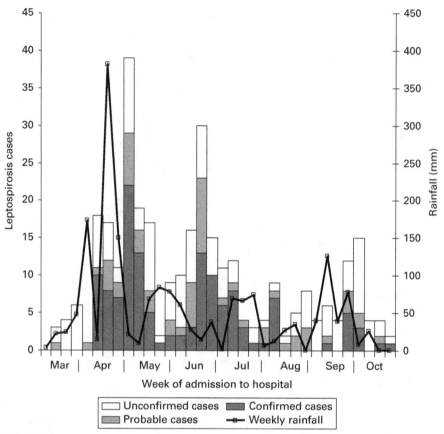

FIGURE 6.7 Cases of leptospirosis by week of hospitalization and rainfall in Salvador, Brazil, March 10–November 2, 1996.

Source: Adapted from Reference 9.

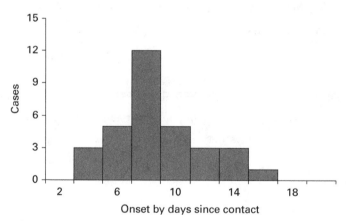

FIGURE 6.8 Days (2-day intervals) between onset of a case of severe acute respiratory syndrome and onset of the corresponding source case: Beijing, China, March–April 2003.

Source: Adapted from Reference 5.

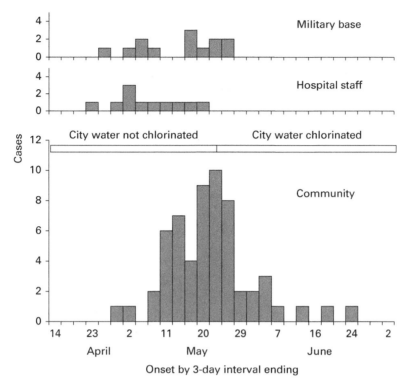

FIGURE 6.9 Cases of typhoid fever by date of onset: Tabuk, Saudi Arabia, April–June 1992.

Stacking different strata atop one another (as in Figure 6.7, which is not recommended) defeats attempts to compare the time patterns by group.

Examining Rates by Time

Temporal disease rates are usually illustrated by using a line graph (Box 6.4). The x-axis represents a period of interest. The y-axis represents the rate of the health event. For most conditions, when the rates vary over one or two orders of magnitude, an arithmetic scale is recommended. For rates that vary more widely, a logarithmic scale for the y-axis is recommended for epidemiologic purposes (Figure 6.10) (10). You should also use a log-arithmic scale for comparing two or more population groups. Equal rates of change in time (e.g., a 10% decrease/year) will yield misleading, divergent lines on an arithmetic plot; a logarithmic scale will yield parallel lines.

Secular Trend

For most conditions, a time characteristic of interest is the secular trend—the rate of disease over multiple years or decades. Secular trends of invasive cervical cancer (Figure 6.11) reveal steady decreases over 37 years (11). New health policies in 1970 and 1995 that broadened coverage of Papanicolaou smear screenings for women were

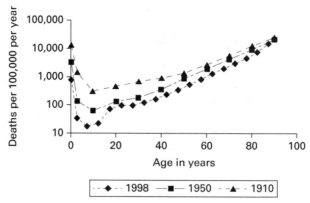

FIGURE 6.10 Age-specific mortality rates per 100,000 population/year: United States, 1910, 1950, and 1998.

Source: Adapted from Reference 10.

initially followed by steeper decreases and subsequent leveling off of the downward trend. This demonstrates how review of secular trends can bring attention to key events, improvements in control, changes in policy, sociologic phenomena, or other factors that have modified the epidemiology of a disease.

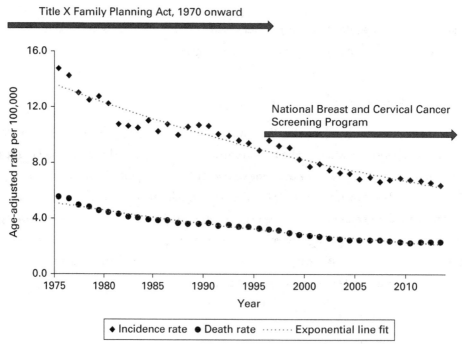

FIGURE 6.11 Cervical cancer (invasive) Surveillance Epidemiology, and End Results Program incidence and death rate: United States, 1999–2013.

Source: Adapted from Reference 11.

Seasonal and Cyclical Patterns

For certain conditions, a description by season, month, day of the week, or even time of day can be revealing. Seasonal patterns might be summarized in a seasonal curve (Box 6.8). Stratifying seasonal curves can further expose key differences by place, person, or other features (Figure 6.12) (12).

EXAMINING DATA BY PLACE (WHERE?)

When creating graphics and interpreting distributions of disease by place, keep in mind Waldo Tobler's first law of geography: "Everything is related to everything else, but near things are more related than distant things" (13). These distance associations of cases or rates are best understood on maps. In addition, maps display a wealth of underlying detail to compare against disease distributions. In creating epidemiologic maps, you should follow certain basic guidelines (Box 6.9).

Information about place of affected persons might include residence, workplace, school, recreation site, other relevant locales, or movement between fixed geographic points. Distinguish between place of onset, place of known or suspected exposure, and place of case identification. They are often different and have distinct epidemiologic implications. Information about place can range in precision from the geographic coordinates of a residence or bed in a hospital to simply the state of residence. Because population estimates or censuses follow standard geographic areas (e.g., city, census tract, county, state, or country), determination of rates is also restricted to these same areas.

BOX 6.8
SEASONAL CURVES

- Use multiple years (≥5) of data.
- Summarize with average rates, average counts, or totals for all the Januarys, Februarys, and so on for each of the 12 months.
- Use other intervals (e.g., weeks or days) accordingly.
- Plot the rate, average, or total for each interval on a histogram or line graph.
- Plot the percentage of the total for the year represented by each interval; however, take care when interpreting the total percentage.
- Use redundant beginning and end points (see Figures 6.9 through 6.14) to visualize the trend between the last and first months of the cycle.
- This type of curve can be made for any time cycle (e.g., time of day, day of week, or week of influenza season).

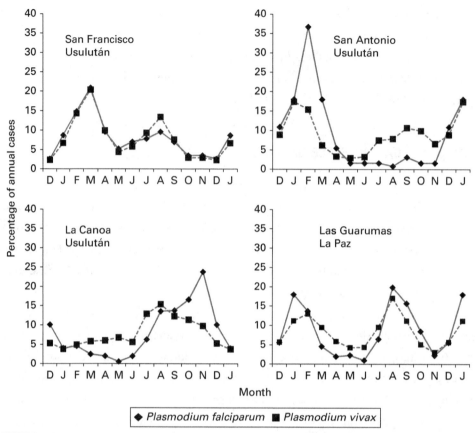

FIGURE 6.12 Seasonal distribution of malaria cases, by month of detection by voluntary collaborators in four villages: El Salvador, 1970–1977.

Source: Adapted from Reference 12.

BOX 6.9

GUIDELINES REGARDING DATA DISPLAY AREA OF EPIDEMIOLOGIC MAPS

- Indicate scaling as a ratio (e.g., 1:100,000), a scale bar (e.g., a 1-cm bar = 50 m), or tick marks on the *x*- and *y*-axes (indicating linear distance or longitude and latitude).
- On maps representing land areas, indicate longitude and latitude and orientation (i.e., by using a northward-pointing arrow).
- Ensure that scaling applies accurately to all features in the map area, especially indicators of location of disease and potential exposures.
- Reduce embellishments that obstruct a clear vision of disease and potential exposures. These might include detailed administrative boundaries or a longitude-latitude grid.

Spot Maps

Use spot maps to reveal spatial associations between cases and between cases and geographic features. Cases can be plotted on a base map (Figure 6.13 [14]), a satellite view of the area, a floor plan, or other accurately scaled diagram to create a spot map. Dots, onset times, case identification numbers for indexing with a line listing, or other symbols might represent disease cases (Box 6.10). The example spot map of a dengue outbreak uses larger dots to represent cases clustered in time and space and numbers these clusters to reference to a table (not shown). It reveals the location of the first case in the business district and the large initial cluster surrounding it (Figure 6.13) (14). Cases not included in clusters are marked with smaller dots. These are widely dispersed, indicating that they did not acquire their infection from their local environs.

You might also use spot maps to represent affected villages, towns, or other smaller population units. If the denominator of the population unit is known, spots of different size or shading (Box 6.10) can represent rates or ratios.

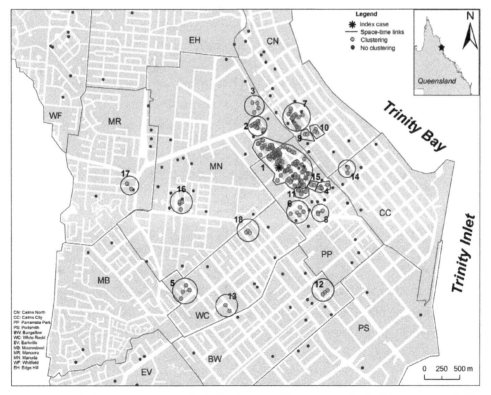

FIGURE 6.13 Significant space–time clustering (assessed by the Knox test) of dengue cases in the city of Cairns, Australia, during January–August 2003.

Source: Adapted from Reference 14.

BOX 6.10

DATA PORTRAYAL ON EPIDEMIOLOGIC MAPS

SPOT MAPS

- Place all spots accurately.
- Ensure that overlapping spots are distinguishable.
- Ensure that potential exposures are easily discerned and labeled.
- Indicate underpopulated or depopulated areas.
- Highlight high-interest cases.

AREA (PATCH OR CHOROPLETH) MAPS

- To indicate numeric intensity, use increasing intensity of gray from white to black. If using color, use increasing intensities of the same hue.
- To indicate divergence from an average range, use white for the center range and deepening intensities of two different hues for divergent strata on opposite extremes.
- To indicate nominative (non-numeric) qualities, use different hues or fill patterns.
- To indicate no data, use a different hue or fill pattern.
- Let the difference in shading of map areas define and replace detailed internal boundary lines.
- Include a legend or key to clarify map features (e.g., disease cases, rates, and exposures).
- Consider indicating the zero-level separately.
- Indicate the data range in the legend; do not leave it open-ended.
- Create multiple maps to indicate associations of cases to different background features to fully communicate the geographic association between disease and exposure.
- Use the smallest possible administrative area that the numerator and denominator will allow.

Spot maps that plot cases have a general weakness. The observed pattern might represent variability in the distribution of the underlying population. When interpreting spot maps, keep in mind the population distribution with particular attention to unpopulated (e.g., parks, vacant lots, or abandoned warehouses) or densely populated areas.

Area Maps and Rates

Rates are normally displayed on area maps (e.g., patch or choropleth). The map is divided into population enumeration areas for which rates or ratios can be computed. The areas are then ranked into strata by the rates, and the strata are shaded (Box 6.10) according to the magnitude of the rate.

Compute and plot rates for the smallest area possible. For example, the map of spotted fever rickettsioses in the United States effectively displays multiple levels of risk for human infection (Figure 6.14) (15). Avoid using area maps to display case counts. Plotting only numerators loses the advantage of both the spot map (indicating exact location and detailed background features) and the area map (indicating rates).

Scatter Plots

Scatter plots are versatile instruments for exploring and communicating data. They indicate the association between two numerically scaled variables (Figure 6.15) (16). Each spot in the plotting area represents the joint magnitude of the two variables. As a convention in plotting epidemiologic or geographic association, the explanatory variable (exposure, environmental, or geographic) is plotted on the x-axis, and the outcome (rate or individual health measurement [e.g., BMI]) is plotted on the y-axis.

When the pattern of the spots forms a compact, linear pattern, suspect a strong association between the two variables. In Figure 6.15, a distinctive pattern of rapidly increasing

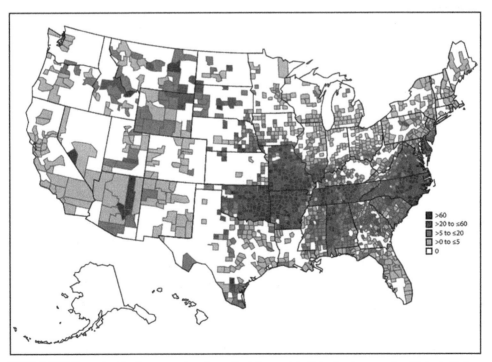

FIGURE 6.14 Reported incidence rate of spotted fever rickettsiosis† by county: United States, 2000–2013.

Source: Adapted from Reference 14.

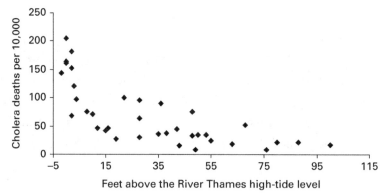

FIGURE 6.15 Cholera deaths per 10,000 inhabitants and altitude above the average high-tide level, by district in London, England, 1849.

Source: Adapted from Reference 15.

cholera death rates is apparent as the altitude approaches the level of the River Thames. This reveals that factor and that an environmental exposure also related to low altitude (e.g., poor drainage of sewage) might have contributed to cholera incidence.

PERSON (AMONG WHOM?)

Recognizing disease patterns by personal attributes (e.g., age, sex, education, income, or immunization status) constitutes the fifth element in descriptive epidemiology. Two important qualifications apply to person data assessments. First, determining rates is more often necessary than for time and place. Second, age is a strong independent determinant for many causes of morbidity and mortality.

Social Groupings and Personal Contact

Social groupings might be as compact as a household or as diffuse as a social network linked by a common interest. The underlying epidemiologic process might produce disease distributions within and among social groupings that range from strong aggregation to randomness or uniformity. Clustered distributions might result from common exposures of group members, an agent that is transmissible through personal contact, an environmental exposure in the living or meeting areas, or localization of houses near or within an environmental area of high risk. Random or uniform distributions indicate that the exposure lies outside the group.

For diseases or behaviors spread through personal contact or association, contact diagrams reveal the pattern of spread plus such key details as index cases and outliers.

In the example diagram, closeness and quality of relationships, timing between onsets, and places of contact are all displayed through different symbols and shading (Figure 6.2) (5). To support person-to-person transmission, you should also see that the timing between onsets of cases approximates the known incubation periods for the disease (Figure 6.8) (5).

Age

In most descriptive analyses, the epidemiologist will determine disease rates by age. This can be as simple as finding that a health event is affecting only a limited age group or as complicated as comparing age-specific rates among multiple groups. Age represents three different categories of determinants of disease risk (Box 6.11). Because age is a pervasive determinant of disease and because population groups often differ in their age structures, age adjustment (standardization) is a useful tool for comparing rates between population groups (17). Age-adjusted rates can be used for comparing populations from different areas, from the same area at different times, and among other characteristics (e.g., ethnicity or socioeconomic status).

An analysis of BMI by age from Ajloun and Jerash Governorates, Jordan, draws attention to increasing BMI and accumulating overweight prevalence for persons aged 18–75 years (Table 6.3) (Ajloun Non-Communicable Disease Project, Jordan, unpublished data, 2017). As an alternative to using tables, charts (Box 6.12) (e.g., dot charts) (Figure 6.16, panel A) or horizontal cluster bar charts (Figure 6.16, panel B) improve perception of the patterns in the data, compared with a table. Cluster bar charts with more than two bars per cluster (e.g., Figure 6.16, panel B) are not recommended.

BOX 6.11

THREE GENERAL INTERPRETATIONS OF AGE DISTRIBUTIONS

- *The condition of the host and its susceptibility to disease.* Persons of different ages often differ in susceptibility or predisposition to disease. Age is one of the most important determinants of chronic diseases, many infectious diseases, and mortality.
- *Differing intensities of exposure to causative agents.*
- *The passage of time.* Older persons have had greater overall time of exposure or might have been exposed at different periods when background exposures to certain agents were greater. A disease with a long latency period (e.g., tuberculosis) might reflect exposures decades in the past.

TABLE 6.3 Body mass index (BMI) and percentage of overweight for 1,800 adults, by age group and sex, Ajloun, Jordan, survey, 2012

Age group (yrs)	Persons			BMI (SD)			BMI ≥ 26 (%)		
	M	F	All	M	F	All	M	F	All
18–29	189	251	440	24.7 (4.9)	24.6 (5.2)	24.6 (5.1)	30	32	31
30–39	242	249	491	27.2 (4.7)	29.1 (6.2)	28.2 (5.6)	54	70	62
40–49	198	182	380	28.4 (4.9)	30.8 (7.6)	29.6 (6.5)	66	77	72
50–59	84	119	203	28.5 (6.4)	30.7 (5.7)	29.8 (6.1)	67	82	76
60–74	90	110	200	29.0 (6.1)	30.9 (7.2)	30.1 (6.8)	71	78	75
75–99	43	43	86	26.9 (3.6)	29.6 (5.7)	28.3 (4.9)	58	70	64
All ages	846	954	1,800	27.2 (5.3)	28.7 (6.8)	28.0 (6.2)	55	64	60

BMI, Body mass index; F, female; M, male; SD, standard deviation.
Source: Ajloun Non-Communicable Disease Project, Jordan, Unpublished data, 2017.

BOX 6.12
GUIDANCE REGARDING PREPARING CHARTS

- Charts present statistical information comparing numeric values for sets of multiple nominative characteristics or grouped numeric characteristics.
- Data presentation is interchangeable with tables. The choice between tables and charts depends on the purpose, the audience, and the complexity of the data.
- The best charts for quick and accurate understanding are dot plots, box-and-whisker plots, and simple bar charts.
- Avoid pie charts, cluster bar charts, stacked bar charts, and other types not presented in this chapter.
- Dot plots, box plots, and bar charts are easier to understand and read if aligned horizontally (with the numeric axis horizontal).
- Sorting nominative categories by the magnitude of the numeric value helps the reader's understanding. If the classification variable is numeric (e.g., age group), sort by the numeric category.
- The dot chart is the most versatile and the easier to understand, particularly as categories increase in number.
- Dot and box-and-whisker charts are plotted against a numeric scale and thus do not need a zero level.
- Bar charts usually need a zero level because viewers judge magnitude by the length of the bar.

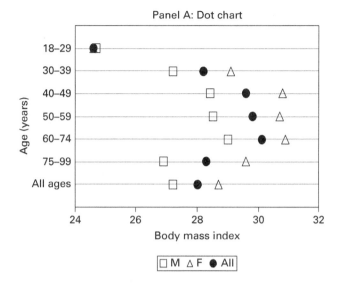

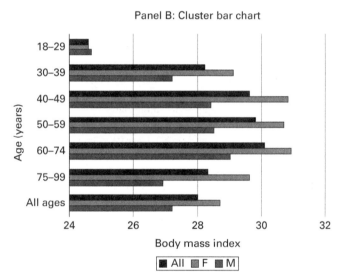

FIGURE 6.16 Dot chart (A) and bar chart (B) comparison of mean body mass index among adults, by age group and sex: Ajloun and Jerash Governorates, Jordan, 2012.

Source: Adapted from Ajloun Non-Communicable Disease Project, Jordan, unpublished data, 2017.

Other Personal Attributes

Analysis by other personal attributes in descriptive epidemiology involves comparing rates or other numeric data by different classes of the attribute. For example, overweight prevalence in the Ajloun data can be compared by using different education levels. A more precise approach to estimating how much for measurements on a continuous scale, discussed earlier in this chapter, might be to compute the average and dispersion of the individual BMI measurements, as shown on a box-and-whisker plot (Figure 6.1).

BEST PRACTICES

The tables, graphs, and charts presented in this chapter have been determined experimentally to perform best in conveying information and data patterns to you and others. Accordingly, less efficient and inaccurate displays, although common, were avoided or noted as not recommended.

REFERENCES

1. Ehrenberg AC. The problem of numeracy. *Am Stat.* 1981;35:67–71.
2. Centers for Disease Control and Prevention. Intussusception among recipients of rotavirus vaccine—United States, 1998–1999. *MMWR.* 1999;48:577–81.
3. Hawley B, Casey ML, Cox-Ganser JM, Edwards N, Fedan KB, Cummings KJ. Notes from the field: respiratory symptoms and skin irritation among hospital workers using a new disinfection product—Pennsylvania, 2015. *MMWR.* 2016;65:400–1.
4. Centers for Disease Control and Prevention. Injuries and deaths associated with use of snowmobiles—Maine, 1991–1996. *MMWR.* 1997;46:1–4.
5. Xie S, Zeng G, Lei J, et al. A highly efficient transmission of SARS among extended family and hospital staff in Beijing, China, April 2003. Presented at the 2nd Southeast Asian and Western Pacific Bi-Regional TEPHINET Scientific Conference, November 24–28, 2003, Borocay, Philippines.
6. Tauxe RV, Tormey MP, Mascola L, Hargrett-Bean NT, Blake PA. Salmonellosis outbreak on transatlantic flights; foodborne illness on aircraft: 1947–1984. *Am J Epidemiol.* 1987;125:150–7.
7. Abu-Sbeih A, Fontaine RE. Secondary water-borne hepatitis E outbreak from water storage in a Jordanian town [abstract LB01]. Presented at the TEPHINET 2000 First International Conference, April 17–21, 2000, Ottawa, Canada.
8. Dou F, Sun H, Wang ZJ. Dengue outbreak at a fishing port: Guangdong Province, China, 2007. Presented at the International Conference on Emerging Infectious Diseases, March 16–19, 2008, Atlanta, Georgia.
9. Ko AI, Galvao Reis M, Ribeiro Dourado CM, Johnson WD, Jr., Riley LW. Urban epidemic of severe leptospirosis in Brazil. Salvador Leptospirosis Study Group. *Lancet.* 1999;354:820–5.
10. Centers for Disease Control and Prevention, National Center for Health Statistics. National Vital Statistics System. Death rates for selected causes by 10-year age groups, race, and sex: death registration states, 1900–32, and United States, 1933–98. https://www.cdc.gov/nchs/nvss/mortality/hist290.htm
11. National Institutes of Health, National Cancer Institute, Surveillance Epidemiology, and End Results Program. SEER*Explorer. http://seer.cancer.gov/explorer/
12. Fontaine RE, van Severin M, Houng A. The stratification of malaria in El Salvador using available malaria surveillance data [Abstract 184]. Presented at the XI International Congress for Tropical Medicine and Malaria, September 16–22, 1984, Calgary, Alberta, Canada.
13. Tobler W. A computer movie simulating urban growth in the Detroit region. *Econ Geogr.* 1970;46(Suppl):234–40.
14. Vazquez-Prokopec GM, Kitron U, Montgomery B, Horne P, Ritchie SA. Quantifying the spatial dimension of dengue virus epidemic spread within a tropical urban environment. *PLoS Negl Trop Dis.* 2010;4:e920.

15. Biggs HM, Behravesh CB, Bradley KK, et al. Diagnosis and management of tickborne rickettsial diseases: Rocky Mountain spotted fever and other spotted fever group rickettsioses, ehrlichioses, and anaplasmosis—United States. *MMWR Recomm Rep.* 2016;65(No. RR-2):1–44.
16. Registrar-General. *Report on the mortality of cholera in England 1848–49*. London, UK: Her Majesty's Stationery Office; 1852.
17. Fleiss JC. *Statistical methods for rates and proportions*. New York: John Wiley & Sons; 1981.

/// 7 /// DESIGNING AND CONDUCTING ANALYTIC STUDIES IN THE FIELD

BRENDAN R. JACKSON
AND PATRICIA M. GRIFFIN

INTRODUCTION

Analytic studies can be a key component of field investigations, but beware of an impulse to begin one too quickly. Studies can be time- and resource-intensive, and a hastily constructed study might not answer the correct questions. For example, in a foodborne disease outbreak investigation, if the culprit food is not on your study's questionnaire, you probably will not be able to implicate it. Analytic studies typically should be used to test hypotheses, not generate them. However, in certain situations, collecting data quickly about patients and a comparison group can be a way to explore multiple hypotheses. In almost all situations, generating hypotheses before designing a study will help you clarify your study objectives and ask better questions.

GENERATING HYPOTHESES

The initial steps of an investigation, described in previous chapters, are some of your best sources of hypotheses. Key activities include the following:

- Describe time, place, and person. Descriptive epidemiology (see Chapter 6) can help develop hypotheses. For example,
  - By examining the sex distribution among persons in outbreaks, US enteric disease investigators have learned to suspect a vegetable as the source when most patients are women. (Of course, generalizations do not always hold true!)
  - In an outbreak of bloodstream infections caused by *Serratia marcescens* among patients receiving parenteral nutrition (food administered through an intravenous catheter), investigators had a difficult time finding the source until they noted that none of the 19 cases were among children. Further investigation of the parenteral nutrition administered to adults but not children in that hospital identified contaminated amino acid solution as the source (1).
- Focus on outliers. Give extra attention to the earliest and latest cases on an epidemic curve and to persons who recently visited the neighborhood where the outbreak is occurring. Interviews with these patients can yield important clues (e.g., by identifying the index case, secondary case, or a narrowed list of common exposures).
- Determine sources of similar outbreaks. Consult health department records, review the literature, and consult experts to learn about previous sources. Be mindful that new sources frequently occur, given ever-changing social, behavioral, and commercial trends.
- Conduct a small number of in-depth, open-ended interviews. When a likely source is not quickly evident, conducting in-depth (often >1 hour), open-ended

interviews with a subset of patients (usually 5 to 10) or their caregivers can be the best way to identify possible sources. It helps to begin with a semistructured list of questions designed to help the patient recall the events and exposures of every day during the incubation period. The interview can end with a "shotgun" questionnaire (see activity 6) (Box 7.1). A key component of this technique is that one investigator ideally conducts, or at least participates in, as many interviews as possible (five or more) because reading notes from others' interviews is no substitute for soliciting and hearing the information first-hand. For example, in a 2009 *Escherichia coli* O157 outbreak, investigators were initially unable to find the source through general and targeted questionnaires. During open-ended interviews with five patients, the interviewer noted that most reported having eaten strawberries, a particular type of candy, and uncooked prepackaged cookie dough. An analytic study was then conducted that included questions about these exposures; it confirmed cookie dough as the source (3).

- Ask patients what they think. Patients can have helpful thoughts about the source of their illness. However, be aware that patients often associate their most recent food exposure (e.g., a meal) with illness, whereas the inciting exposure might have been long before.

- Consider administering a shotgun questionnaire. Such questionnaires, which typically ask about hundreds of possible exposures, are best used on a limited number of patients as part of hypothesis-generating interviews. After generating hypotheses, investigators can create a questionnaire targeted to that investigation. Although not an ideal method, shotgun questionnaires can be used by multiple interviewers to obtain data about large numbers of patients (Box 7.1).

STUDY DESIGNS FOR TESTING HYPOTHESES

As evident in public health and clinical guidelines, randomized controlled trials (e.g., trials of drugs, vaccines, and community-level interventions) are the reference standard for epidemiology, providing the highest level of evidence. However, such studies are not possible in certain situations, including outbreak investigations. Instead, investigators must rely on observational studies, which can provide sufficient evidence for public health action. In observational studies, the epidemiologist documents rather than determines the exposures, quantifying the statistical association between exposure and disease. Here again, the key when designing such studies is to obtain a relevant comparison group for the patients (Box 7.2).

BOX 7.1

GENERATING A HYPOTHESIS IN A LISTERIOSIS OUTBREAK
LINKED TO CARAMEL APPLES

In November 2014, a US surveillance system for foodborne diseases (PulseNet) detected a cluster (i.e., a possible outbreak) of listeriosis cases based on similar-appearing *Listeria monocytogenes* isolates by pulsed-field gel electrophoresis of the isolates. No suspected foods were identified through routine patient interviews by using a *Listeria*-specific questionnaire with approximately 40 common food sources of listeriosis (e.g., soft cheese and deli meat). The outbreak's descriptive epidemiology offered no clear leads: the sex distribution was nearly even, the age spectrum was wide, and the case-fatality rate of approximately 20% was typical. Notably, however, 3 of the 35 cases occurred among previously healthy school-aged children, which is highly unusual for listeriosis. Most cases occurred during late October and early November.

Investigators began reinterviewing patients by using a hypothesis-generating shotgun questionnaire with more than 500 foods, but it did not include caramel apples. By comparing the first nine patient responses with data from a published survey of food consumption, strawberries and ice cream emerged as hypotheses. However, several interviewed patients denied having eaten these foods during the month before illness. An investigator then conducted lengthy, open-ended interviews with patients and their family members. During one interview, he asked about special foods eaten during recent holidays, and the patient's wife replied that her husband had eaten prepackaged caramel apples around Halloween. Although produce items had been implicated in past listeriosis outbreaks, caramel apples seemed an unlikely source. However, the interviewer took note of this connection because he had previously interviewed another patient who reported having eaten caramel apples. This event underscores the importance of one person conducting multiple interviews because that person might make subtle mental connections that may be missed when reviewing other interviewers' notes. In fact, several other investigators listening to the interview noted this exposure—among hundreds of others—but thought little of it.

In this investigation, the finding of high strawberry and ice cream consumption among patients, coupled with the timing of the outbreak during a holiday period, helped make a sweet food (i.e., caramel apples) seem more plausible as the possible source.

To explore the caramel apple hypothesis, investigators asked five other patients about this exposure, and four reported having eaten them. On the basis of these initial results, investigators designed and administered a targeted questionnaire to patients involved in the outbreak, as well as to patients infected with unrelated strains of *L. monocytogenes* (i.e., a case–case study). This study, combined with testing of apples and the apple packing facility, confirmed that caramel apples were the source (2). Had a single interviewer performed multiple open-ended interviews to generate hypotheses before the shotgun questionnaire, the outbreak might have been solved sooner.

BOX 7.2
DEFINING EXPOSURE AND DISEASE

Because field analytic studies are used to quantify the association between exposure and disease, defining what is meant by *exposure* and *disease* is essential. *Exposure* is used broadly, meaning demographic characteristics, genetic or immunologic makeup, behaviors, environmental exposures, and other factors that might influence a person's risk for disease. Because precise information can help accurately estimate an exposure's effect on disease, exposure measures should be as objective and standard as possible. Developing a measure of exposure can be conceptually straightforward for an exposure that is a relatively discrete event or characteristic—for example, whether a person received a spinal injection with steroid medication compounded at a specific pharmacy or whether a person received a typhoid vaccination during the year before international travel. Although these exposures might be straightforward in theory, they can be subject to interpretation in practice. Should a patient injected with a medication from an unknown pharmacy be considered exposed? Whatever decision is made should be documented and applied consistently.

Additionally, exposures often are subject to the whims of memory. Memory aids (e.g., restaurant menus, vaccination cards, credit card receipts, and shopper cards) can be helpful. More than just a binary yes or no, the dose of an exposure can also be enlightening. For example, in an outbreak of fungal bloodstream infections linked to contaminated intravenous saline flushes administered at an oncology clinic, affected patients had received a greater number of flushes than unaffected patients (4). Similarly, in an outbreak of *Listeria monocytogenes* infections, the association with deli meat became apparent only when the exposure evaluated was consumption of deli meat more than twice a week (5).

Defining *disease* (e.g., does a person have botulism?) might sound simple, but often it is not; read more about making and applying disease case definitions in Chapter 3.

TYPES OF OBSERVATIONAL STUDIES FOR TESTING HYPOTHESES

Three types of observational studies are commonly used in the field. All are best performed by using a standard questionnaire specific for that investigation, developed on the basis of hypothesis-generating interviews.

Observational Study Type 1: Cohort

In concept, a cohort study, like an experimental study, begins with a group of persons without the disease under study, but with different exposure experiences, and follows them over time to find out whether they experience the disease or health condition of interest. However, in a cohort study, each person's exposure is merely recorded rather than assigned randomly by the investigator. Then the occurrence of disease among persons with different exposures is compared to assess whether the exposures are associated with increased risk for disease. Cohort studies can be prospective or retrospective.

Prospective Cohort Studies

A prospective cohort study enrolls participants before they experience the disease or condition of interest. The enrollees are then followed over time for occurrence of the disease or condition. The unexposed or lowest exposure group serves as the comparison group, providing an estimate of the baseline or expected amount of disease. An example of a prospective cohort study is the Framingham Heart Study. By assessing the exposures of an original cohort of more than 5,000 adults without cardiovascular disease (CVD), beginning in 1948 and following them over time, the study was the first to identify common CVD risk factors (6). Each case of CVD identified after enrollment was counted as an incident case. Incidence was then quantified as the number of cases divided by the sum of time that each person was followed (incidence rate) or as the number of cases divided by the number of participants being followed (attack rate or risk or incidence proportion). In field epidemiology, prospective cohort studies also often involve a group of persons who have had a known exposure (e.g., survived the World Trade Center attack on September 11, 2001 [7]) and who are then followed to examine the risk for subsequent illnesses with long incubation or latency periods.

Retrospective Cohort Studies

A retrospective cohort study enrolls a defined participant group after the disease or condition of interest has occurred. In field epidemiology, these studies are more common than prospective studies. The population affected is often well-defined (e.g., banquet attendees, a particular school's students, or workers in a certain industry). Investigators elicit exposure histories and compare disease incidence among persons with different exposures or exposure levels.

Observational Study Type 2: Case–Control

In a case–control study, the investigator must identify a comparison group of control persons who have had similar opportunities for exposure as the case-patients. Case–control studies are commonly performed in field epidemiology when a cohort study is impractical (e.g., no defined cohort or too many non-ill persons in the group to interview). Whereas a cohort study proceeds conceptually from exposure to disease or condition,

TABLE 7.1 Benefits and drawbacks of three observational study types commonly used in field investigations

Feature	Retrospective cohort study	Case–control study	Case–case study
Sample size	Larger	Smaller	Smaller
Costs	More (because of size)	Less	Less
Study time	Short	Short	Short
If disease is rare	Inefficient	Efficient	Efficient (if comparison cases already identified)
If exposure is rare	Efficient	Inefficient	Inefficient
If multiple exposures are relevant	Often can examine	Can examine	Can examine
If patients have multiple outcomes	Can examine	Cannot examine	Cannot examine
Natural history	Can ascertain	Cannot ascertain	Cannot ascertain
Disease risk	Can measure	Cannot measure	Cannot measure
Recall bias	Potential problem	Potential problem	Generally less of a problem
Selection bias	Potential problem	Potential problem	Potential problem
If population is not well-defined	Difficult	Advantageous	Advantageous

a case–control study begins conceptually with the disease or condition and looks backward at exposures. Excluding controls by symptoms alone might not guarantee that they do not have mild cases of the illness under investigation. Table 7.1 presents selected key differences between a case–control and retrospective cohort study.

Observational Study Type 3: Case–Case

In case–case studies, a group of patients with the same or similar disease serve as a comparison group (8). This method might require molecular subtyping of the suspected pathogen to distinguish outbreak-associated cases from other cases and is especially useful when relevant controls are difficult to identify. For example, controls for an investigation of *Listeria* illnesses typically are patients with immunocompromising conditions (e.g., cancer or corticosteroid use) who might be difficult to identify among the general population. Patients with *Listeria* isolates of a different subtype than the outbreak strain can serve as comparisons to help reduce bias when comparing food exposures. However, patients with similar illnesses can have similar exposures, which can introduce a bias, making identifying the source more difficult. Moreover, other considerations should influence the choice of a comparison group. If most outbreak-associated case-patients are from a single neighborhood or are of a certain race/ethnicity, other patients with listeriosis from across the country will serve as an inadequate comparison group.

SELECTION OF CONTROLS IN CASE–CONTROL STUDIES

Considerations for Selecting Controls

Selecting relevant controls is one of the most important considerations when designing a case–control study. Several key considerations are presented here; consult other resources for in-depth discussion (9,10). Ideally, controls should

- Thoroughly reflect the source population from which case-patients arose, and
- Provide a good estimate of the level of exposure one would expect from that population. Sometimes the source population is not so obvious, and a case–control study using controls from the general population might be needed to implicate a general exposure (e.g., visiting a specific clinic, restaurant, or fair). The investigation can then focus on specific exposures among persons with the general exposure (see also next section).

Controls should be chosen independently of any specific exposure under evaluation. If you select controls on the basis of lack of exposure, you are likely to find an association between illness and that exposure regardless of whether one exists. Also important is selecting controls from a source population in a way that minimizes confounding (see Chapter 8), which is the existence of a factor (e.g., annual income) that, by being associated with both exposure and disease, can affect the associations you are trying to examine.

When trying to enroll controls who reflect the source population, try to avoid overmatching (i.e., enrolling controls who are too similar to case-patients, resulting in fewer differences among case-patients and controls than ought to exist and decreased ability to identify exposure–disease associations). When conducting case–control studies in hospitals and other healthcare settings, ensure that controls do not have other diseases linked to the exposure under study.

Commonly Used Control Selection Methods

When an outbreak does not affect a defined population (e.g., potluck dinner attendees) but rather the community at large, a range of options can be used to determine how to select controls from a large group of persons.

- *Random-digit dialing.* This method, which involves selecting controls by using a system that randomly selects telephone numbers from a directory, has been a staple of US outbreak investigations. In recent years, however, declining response rates because of increasing use of caller identification and cellular phones and lack of readily available directory listings of cellular phone numbers by geographic area have made this method increasingly difficult. Even when this method was most useful, often 50 or more numbers needed to be dialed to reach one household or person who both answered and provided a usable match for the case-patient. Commercial databases that include cellular phone numbers have been used successfully to partially address this problem, but the method remains time-consuming (11).

- *Random or systematic sampling from a list.* For investigations in settings where a roster is available (e.g., attendees at a resort on certain dates), controls can be selected by either random or systematic sampling. Government records (e.g., motor vehicle, voter, or tax records) can provide lists of possible controls, but they might not be representative of the population being studied (11). For random sampling, a table or computer-generated list of random numbers can be used to select every *n*th persons to contact (e.g., every 12th or 13th).

- *Neighborhood.* Recruiting controls from the same neighborhood as case-patients (i.e., neighborhood matching) has commonly been used during case–control studies, particularly in low- and middle-income countries. For example, during an outbreak of typhoid fever in Tajikistan (12), investigators recruited controls by going door-to-door down a street, starting at a case-patient's house; a study of cholera in Haiti used a similar method (13). Typically, the immediately neighboring households are skipped to prevent overmatching.

- *Patients' friends or relatives.* Using friends and relatives as controls can be an effective technique when the characteristics of case-patients (e.g., very young children) make finding controls by a random method difficult. Typically, the investigator interviews a patient or his or her parent, then asks for the names and contact information for more friends or relatives who are needed as controls. One advantage is that the friends of an ill person are usually willing to participate, knowing their cooperation can help solve the puzzle. However, because they can have similar personal habits and preferences as patients, their exposures might be similar. Such overmatching can decrease the likelihood of finding the source of the illness or condition.

- *Databases of persons with exposure information.* Sources of data on persons with exposure information include survey data (e.g., FoodNet Population Survey [14]), public health databases of patients with other illnesses or a different subtype of the same illness, and previous studies. (Chapter 4 describes additional sources.)

When considering outside data sources, investigators must determine whether those data provide an appropriate comparison group. For example, persons in surveys might differ from case-patients in ways that are impossible to determine. Other patients might be so similar to case-patients that risky exposures are unidentifiable, or they might be so different that exposures identified as risks are not true risks.

MATCHING IN CASE–CONTROL STUDIES

To help control for confounding, controls can be matched to case-patients on characteristics specified by investigators, including age group, sex, race/ethnicity, and neighborhood. Such matching does not itself reduce confounding, but it enables greater efficiency when matched analyses are performed that do (15). When deciding to match, however, be judicious. Matching on too many characteristics can make controls difficult to find (making a tough process even harder). Imagine calling hundreds of random telephone numbers trying to find a man of a particular ethnicity aged 50–54 years who is then willing to answer your questions. Also, remember not to match on the exposure of interest or on any other characteristic you wish to examine. Matched case–control study data typically necessitate a matched analysis (e.g., conditional logistic regression) (15).

Matching Types

The two main types of matching are pair matching and frequency matching.

Pair Matching

In pair matching, each control is matched to a specific case-patient. This method can be helpful logistically because it allows matching by friends or relatives, neighborhood, or telephone exchange, but finding controls who meet specific criteria can be burdensome.

Frequency Matching

In frequency matching, also called *category matching*, controls are matched to case-patients in proportion to the distribution of a characteristic among case-patients. For example, if 20% of case-patients are children aged 5–18 years, 50% are adults aged 19–49 years, and 30% are adults 50 years or older, controls should be enrolled in similar proportions. This method works best when most case-patients have been identified before control selection begins. It is more efficient than pair matching because a person identified as a possible control who might not meet the criteria for matching a particular case-patient might meet criteria for one of the case-patient groups.

Number of Controls

Most field case–control studies use control-to-case-patient ratios of 1:1, 2:1, or 3:1. Enrolling more than one control per case-patient can increase study power, which might be needed to detect a statistically significant difference in exposure between case-patients and controls, particularly when an outbreak involves a limited number of cases. The incremental gain of adding more controls beyond three or four is small because study power begins to plateau. Note that not all case-patients need to have the same number of controls. Sample size calculations can help in estimating a target number of controls to enroll, although sample sizes in certain field investigations are limited more by time and resource constraints. Still, estimating study power under a range of scenarios is wise because an analytic study might not be worth doing if you have little chance of detecting a statistically significant association. Sample size calculators for unmatched case–control studies are available at http://www.openepi.com and in the StatCalc function of Epi Info (http://www.cdc.gov/epiinfo).

More than One Control Group

Sometimes the choice of a control group is so vexing that investigators decide to use more than one type of control group (e.g., a hospital-based group and a community group). If the two control groups provide similar results and conclusions about risk factors for disease, the credibility of the findings is increased. In contrast, if the two control groups yield conflicting results, interpretation becomes more difficult.

EXAMPLE: USING AN ANALYTIC STUDY TO SOLVE AN OUTBREAK AT A CHURCH POTLUCK DINNER (BUT NOT *THAT* CHURCH POTLUCK)

Since the 1940s, field epidemiology students have studied a classic outbreak of gastrointestinal illness at a church potluck dinner in Oswego, New York (16). However, the case study presented here, used to illustrate study designs, is a different potluck dinner.

In April 2015, an astute neurologist in Lancaster, Ohio, contacted the local health department about a patient in the emergency department with a suspected case of botulism. Within 2 hours, four more patients arrived with similar symptoms, including blurred vision and shortness of breath. Health officials immediately recognized this as a botulism outbreak.

- *Question*: What are some of the possible source populations (i.e., persons at risk) of this outbreak, given that botulinum toxin is usually spread through food but can be a bioterrorism agent? Think about how each of these possible scenarios for the toxin source might influence the population to study.
  - If the source is a widely distributed commercial product, then the population to study is persons across the United States and possibly abroad.
  - If the source is airborne, then the population to study is residents of a single city or area.
  - If the source is food from a restaurant, then the population to study is predominantly local residents and some travelers.
  - If the source is a meal at a workplace or social setting, then the population to study is meal attendees.
  - If the source is a meal at home, then the population to study is household members and any guests.

Descriptive epidemiology and questioning of the case-patients revealed that all had eaten at the same church potluck dinner and had no other common exposures, making the potluck the likely exposure site and attendees the likely source population. Thus, an analytic study would be targeted at potluck attendees, although investigators must remain alert to case-patients among nonattendees. As initial interviews were conducted, more cases of botulism were being diagnosed, quickly increasing to more than 25. The source of the outbreak needed to be identified rapidly to halt further exposure and illness.

- *Question*: What information would you need to design a study?
  - List of foods served at the potluck.
  - Approximate number of attendees.
  - A case definition.
  - Information from 5–10 hypothesis-generating interviews with a few case-patients or their family members.
- *Question*: What type of study might you conduct if an estimated 75 persons attended the potluck and nearly all guests were identifiable?

- A *cohort study* would be a reasonable option because a defined group exists (i.e., a cohort) of exposed persons who could be interviewed in a reasonable amount of time. The study would be retrospective because the outcome (i.e., botulism) has already occurred, and investigators could assess exposures retrospectively (i.e., foods eaten at the potluck) by interviewing attendees.
- In a cohort study, investigators can calculate the *attack rate* for botulism among potluck attendees who reported having eaten each food and for those who had not. For example, if 20 of the 30 attendees who had eaten a particular food (e.g., potato salad) had botulism, you would calculate the attack rate by dividing 20 (corresponding to cell a in Handout 7.1) by 30 (total exposed, or a + b), yielding approximately 67%. If 5 of the 45 attendees who had not eaten potato salad had botulism, the attack rate among the unexposed—5 / 45, corresponding to c / (c + d)—would be approximately 11%. The *risk ratio* would be 6, which is calculated by dividing the attack rate among the exposed (67%) by the attack rate among the unexposed (11%).
- *Question*: What type of study might you perform if more than 200 persons attended the potluck and investigators did not have a comprehensive attendee list?
  - A case–control study would be the most feasible option because the entire cohort could not be identified and because the large number of attendees could

---

HANDOUT 7.1

TWO-BY-TWO TABLE TO CALCULATE THE RELATIVE RISK, OR RISK RATIO, IN COHORT STUDIES

Two-by-two tables are covered in more detail in Chapter 8.

Cohort Study Approach

	Ill	Not Ill
Exposed	a	b
Unexposed	c	d

$$\text{Risk Ratio} = \frac{\text{Incidence in exposed}}{\text{Incidence in unexposed}} = \frac{\frac{a}{a+b}}{\frac{c}{c+d}}$$

make interviewing them all difficult. Rather than interview all non-ill persons, a subset could be interviewed as control subjects.

- The method of control subject selection should be considered carefully. If all attendees are not interviewed, determining the risk for botulism among the exposed and unexposed is impossible because investigators would not know the exposures for all non-ill attendees. Instead of risk, investigators calculate the *odds* of exposure, which can approximate risk. For example, if 20 (80%) of 25 case-patients had eaten potato salad, the odds of potato salad exposure among case-patients would be 20 / 5 = 4 (exposed / unexposed, or a / c in Handout 7.2). If 10 (20%) of 50 selected controls had eaten potato salad, the odds of exposure among control subjects would be 10 / 40 = 0.25 (or b / d in Handout 7.2). Dividing the odds of exposure among the case-patients (a / c) by the odds of exposure among control subjects (b / d) yields an *odds ratio* of 16 (4 / 0.25). The odds ratio is not a true measure of risk, but it can be used to implicate a food. An odds ratio can approximate a risk ratio when the outcome or disease is rare (e.g., roughly <5% of a population). In such cases, a / b is similar to a / (a + b). The odds ratio is typically higher than the risk ratio when >5% of exposed persons in the analysis have the illness.

HANDOUT 7.2
TWO-BY-TWO TABLE TO CALCULATE THE ODDS RATIO IN CASE–CONTROL STUDIES

A risk ratio cannot be calculated from a case–control study because true attack rates cannot be calculated.

Case-Control Study Approach

	III (Cases)	Not III (Controls)
Exposed	a	b
Unexposed	c	d

$$\text{Odds Ratio} = \frac{\text{Odds of exposure in cases}}{\text{Odds of exposure in controls}} = \frac{a/c}{b/d} = \frac{ad}{bc}$$

In the actual outbreak, 29 (38%) of 77 potluck attendees had botulism. The investigators performed a cohort study, interviewing 75 of the 77 attendees about 52 foods served (17). The attack rate among persons who had eaten potato salad was significantly and substantially higher than the attack rate among those who had not, with a risk ratio of 14 (95% confidence interval 5–42). One of the potato salads served was made with incorrectly home-canned potatoes (a known source of botulinum toxin), and samples of discarded potato salad tested positive for botulinum toxin, supporting the findings of the analytic study. (Of note, persons often blame potato salad for causing illness when, in fact, it rarely is a source. This outbreak was a notable exception.)

In field epidemiology, the link between exposure and illness is often so strong that it is evident despite such inherent study limitations as small sample size and exposure misclassification. In this outbreak, a few of the patients with botulism reported not having eaten potato salad, and some of the attendees without botulism reported having eaten it. In epidemiologic studies, you rarely find 100% concordance between exposure and outcome for various reasons, including incomplete or erroneous recall because remembering everything eaten is difficult. Here, cross-contamination of potato salad with other foods might have helped explain cases among patients who had not eaten potato salad because only a small amount of botulinum toxin is needed to produce illness.

OUTBREAKS WITH UNIVERSAL EXPOSURE

What kind of study would you design if your hypothesis-generating interviews lead you to believe that everyone, or nearly everyone, was exposed to the same suspected infection source? How would you test hypotheses if all barbecue attendees, ill and non-ill, had eaten the chicken or if all town residents had drunk municipal tap water, and no unexposed group exists for comparison? A few factors that might be of help are the exposure timing (e.g., a particularly undercooked batch of barbeque), the exposure place (e.g., a section of the water system more contaminated than others), and the exposure dose (e.g., number of chicken pieces eaten or glasses of water drunk). Including questions about the time, place, and frequency of highly suspected exposures in a questionnaire can improve the chances of detecting a difference (18).

CONCLUSION

Cohort, case–control, and case–case studies are the types of analytic studies that field epidemiologists use most often. They are best used as mechanisms for evaluating— quantifying and testing—hypotheses identified in earlier phases of the investigation.

Cohort studies, which are oriented conceptually from exposure to disease, are appropriate in settings in which an entire population is well-defined and available for enrollment (e.g., guests at a wedding reception). Cohort studies are also appropriate when well-defined groups can be enrolled by exposure status (e.g., employees working in different parts of a manufacturing plant). Case–control studies, in contrast, are useful when the population is less clearly defined. Case–control studies, oriented from disease to exposure, identify persons with disease and a comparable group of persons without disease (controls). Then the exposure experiences of the two groups are compared. Case–case studies are similar to case–control studies, except that controls have an illness not linked to the outbreak. Case–control studies are probably the type most often appropriate for field investigations. Although conceptually straightforward, the design of an effective epidemiologic study requires many careful decisions. Taking the time needed to develop good hypotheses can result in a questionnaire that is useful for identifying risk factors. The choice of an appropriate comparison group, how many controls per case-patient to enroll, whether to match, and how best to avoid potential biases are all crucial decisions for a successful study.

ACKNOWLEDGMENTS

This chapter relies heavily on the work of Richard C. Dicker, who authored this chapter in the previous edition.

REFERENCES

1. Gupta N, Hocevar SN, Moulton-Meissner HA, et al. Outbreak of *Serratia marcescens* bloodstream infections in patients receiving parenteral nutrition prepared by a compounding pharmacy. *Clin Infect Dis.* 2014;59:1–8.
2. Angelo K, Conrad A, Saupe A, et al. Multistate outbreak of *Listeria monocytogenes* infections linked to whole apples used in commercially produced, prepackaged caramel apples: United States, 2014–2015. *Epidemiol Infect.* 2017;145:848–56.
3. Neil KP, Biggerstaff G, MacDonald JK, et al. A novel vehicle for transmission of *Escherichia coli* O157: H7 to humans: multistate outbreak of *E. coli* O157: H7 infections associated with consumption of ready-to-bake commercial prepackaged cookie dough—United States, 2009. *Clin Infect Dis.* 2012;54:511–8.
4. Vasquez AM, Lake J, Ngai S, et al. Notes from the field: fungal bloodstream infections associated with a compounded intravenous medication at an outpatient oncology clinic—New York City, 2016. *MMWR.* 2016;65:1274–5.
5. Gottlieb SL, Newbern EC, Griffin PM, et al. Multistate outbreak of listeriosis linked to turkey deli meat and subsequent changes in US regulatory policy. *Clin Infect Dis.* 2006;42:29–36.
6. Framingham Heart Study: A Project of the National Heart, Lung, and Blood Institute and Boston University. Framingham, MA: Framingham Heart Study; 2017. https://www.framinghamheartstudy.org/

7. Jordan HT, Brackbill RM, Cone JE, et al. Mortality among survivors of the Sept 11, 2001, World Trade Center disaster: results from the World Trade Center Health Registry cohort. *Lancet.* 2011;378:879–87.

8. McCarthy N, Giesecke J. Case–case comparisons to study causation of common infectious diseases. *Int J Epidemiol.* 1999;28:764–8.

9. Rothman KJ, Greenland S. *Modern epidemiology.* 3rd ed. Philadelphia: Lippincott Williams & Wilkins; 2008.

10. Wacholder S, McLaughlin JK, Silverman DT, Mandel JS. Selection of controls in case–control studies. I. Principles. *Am J Epidemiol.* 1992;135:1019–28.

11. Chintapalli S, Goodman M, Allen M, et al. Assessment of a commercial searchable population directory as a means of selecting controls for case–control studies. *Public Health Rep.* 2009;124:378–83.

12. Centers for Disease Control and Prevention. Epidemiologic case studies: typhoid in Tajikistan. http://www.cdc.gov/epicasestudies/classroom_typhoid.html

13. Dunkle SE, Mba-Jonas A, Loharikar A, Fouche B, Peck M, Ayers T. Epidemic cholera in a crowded urban environment, Port-au-Prince, Haiti. *Emerg Infect Dis.* 2011;17:2143–6.

14. Centers for Disease Control and Prevention. Foodborne Diseases Active Surveillance Network (FoodNet): population survey. http://www.cdc.gov/foodnet/surveys/population.html

15. Pearce N. Analysis of matched case–control studies. *BMJ.* 2016;352:1969.

16. Centers for Disease Control and Prevention. Case studies in applied epidemiology: Oswego: an outbreak of gastrointestinal illness following a church supper. http://www.cdc.gov/eis/casestudies.html

17. McCarty CL, Angelo K, Beer KD, et al. Notes from the field.: large outbreak of botulism associated with a church potluck meal—Ohio, 2015. *MMWR.* 2015;64:802–3.

18. Tostmann A, Bousema JT, Oliver I. Investigation of outbreaks complicated by universal exposure. *Emerg Infect Dis.* 2012;18:1717–22.

/// 8 /// ANALYZING AND INTERPRETING DATA

RICHARD C. DICKER

INTRODUCTION

Field investigations are usually conducted to identify the factors that increased a person's risk for a disease or other health outcome. In certain field investigations, identifying the cause is sufficient; if the cause can be eliminated, the problem is solved. In other investigations, the goal is to quantify the association between exposure (or any population characteristic) and the health outcome to guide interventions or advance knowledge. Both types of field investigations require suitable, but not necessarily sophisticated, analytic methods. This chapter describes the strategy for planning an analysis, methods for conducting the analysis, and guidelines for interpreting the results.

PLANNING THE ANALYSIS

A thoughtfully planned and carefully executed analysis is as crucial for a field investigation as it is for a protocol-based study. Planning is necessary to ensure that the appropriate hypotheses will be considered and that the relevant data will be collected, recorded, managed, analyzed, and interpreted to address those hypotheses. Therefore, the time to decide what data to collect and how to analyze those data is before you design your questionnaire, *not* after you have collected the data.

An *analysis plan* is a document that guides how you progress from raw data to the final report. It describes where you are starting (data sources and data sets), how you will look at and analyze the data, and where you need to finish (final report). It lays out the key components of the analysis in a logical sequence and provides a guide to follow during the actual analysis.

An analysis plan includes some or most of the content listed in Box 8.1. Some of the listed elements are more likely to appear in an analysis plan for a protocol-based planned study, but even an outbreak investigation should include the key components in a more abbreviated analysis plan, or at least in a series of table shells.

- *Research question or hypotheses.* The analysis plan usually begins with the research questions or hypotheses you plan to address. Well-reasoned research questions or

---

BOX 8.1

COMPONENTS OF AN ANALYSIS PLAN

- List of the research questions or hypotheses
- Source(s) of data
  - Description of population or groups (inclusion or exclusion criteria)
  - Source of data or data sets, particularly for secondary data analysis or population denominators
  - Type of study
- How data will be manipulated
  - Data sets to be used or merged
  - New variables to be created
- Key variables (attach data dictionary of all variables)
  - Demographic and exposure variables
  - Outcome or endpoint variables
  - Stratification variables (e.g., potential confounders or effect modifiers)
- How variables will be analyzed (e.g., as a continuous variable or grouped in categories)
- How to deal with missing values
- Order of analysis (e.g., frequency distributions, two-way tables, stratified analysis, dose-response, or group analysis)
- Measures of occurrence, association, tests of significance, or confidence intervals to be used
- Table shells to be used in analysis
- Tables shells to be included in final report

---

hypotheses lead directly to the variables that need to be analyzed and the methods of analysis. For example, the question, "What caused the outbreak of gastroenteritis?" might be a suitable objective for a field investigation, but it is not a specific research question. A more specific question—for example, "Which foods were more likely to have been consumed by case-patients than by controls?"—indicates that key variables will be food items and case–control status and that the analysis method will be a two-by-two table for each food.

- *Analytic strategies.* Different types of studies (e.g., cohort, case–control, or cross-sectional) are analyzed with different measures and methods. Therefore, the analysis strategy must be consistent with how the data will be collected. For example, data from a simple retrospective cohort study should be analyzed by calculating and comparing attack rates among exposure groups. Data from a case–control study must be analyzed by comparing exposures among case-patients and controls, and the data must account for matching in the analysis if matching was used in the design. Data from a cross-sectional study or survey might need to incorporate weights or design effects in the analysis.

The analysis plan should specify which variables are most important— exposures and outcomes of interest, other known risk factors, study design factors (e.g., matching variables), potential confounders, and potential effect modifiers.

- *Data dictionary.* A data dictionary is a document that provides key information about each variable. Typically, a data dictionary lists each variable's name, a brief description, what type of variable it is (e.g., numeric, text, or date), allowable values, and an optional comment. Data dictionaries can be organized in different ways, but a tabular format with one row per variable, and columns for name, description, type, legal value, and comment is easy to organize (see example in Table 8.1 from an outbreak investigation of oropharyngeal tularemia [1]). A supplement to the data dictionary might include a copy of the questionnaire with the variable names written next to each question.

- *Get to know your data.* Plan to get to know your data by reviewing (1) the frequency of responses and descriptive statistics for each variable; (2) the minimum, maximum, and average values for each variable; (3) whether any variables have the same response for every record; and (4) whether any variables have many or all missing values. These patterns will influence how you analyze these variables or drop them from the analysis altogether.

- *Table shells.* The next step in developing the analysis plan is designing the table shells. A table shell, sometimes called a *dummy table*, is a table (e.g., frequency distribution or two-by-two table) that is titled and fully labeled but contains no data. The numbers will be filled in as the analysis progresses. Table shells provide a guide to the analysis, so their sequence should proceed in logical order from simple (e.g., descriptive epidemiology) to more complex (e.g., analytic epidemiology) (Box 8.2). Each table shell should indicate which measures (e.g., attack rates, risk ratios [RR] or odds ratios [ORs], 95% confidence intervals [CIs]) and statistics (e.g., chi-square and *p* value) should accompany the table. See Handout 8.1 for an example of a table shell created for the field investigation of oropharyngeal tularemia (1).

ANALYZING DATA FROM A FIELD INVESTIGATION

The first two tables usually generated as part of the analysis of data from a field investigation are those that describe clinical features of the case-patients and present the descriptive epidemiology. Because descriptive epidemiology is addressed in Chapter 6,

TABLE 8.1 Partial data dictionary from investigation of an outbreak of oropharyngeal tularemia (Sancaktepe Village, Bayburt Province, Turkey, July–August 2013)

Variable name	Description	Variable type	Legal value	Comment
ID	Participant identification number	Numeric		Assigned
HH_size	Number of persons living in the household	Numeric		
DOB	Date of birth	Date		dd/mm/yyyy
Lab_tularemia	Microagglutination test result	Numeric	1 = positive 2 = negative	
Age	Age (yrs)	Numeric		
Sex	Sex	Text	M = male F = female	
Fever	Fever	Numeric	1 = yes 2 = no	
Chills	Chills	Numeric	1 = yes 2 = no	
Sore throat	Sore throat	Numeric	1 = yes 2 = no	
Node_swollen	Swollen lymph node	Numeric	1 = yes 2 = no	
Node_where	Site of swollen lymph node	Text		
Case_susp	Meets definition of suspected case	Numeric	1 = yes 2 = no	Created variable: Swollen lymph node around neck or ears, sore throat, conjunctivitis, or ≥2 of fever, chills, myalgia, headache
Case_prob	Meets definition of probable case	Numeric	1 = yes 2 = no	Created variable: Swollen lymph node and (sore throat or fever)
Case_confirm	Meets definition of confirmed case	Numeric	1 = yes 2 = no	Created variable: Laboratory test-positive
Case_probconf	Meets definition of probable or confirmed case	Numeric	1 = yes 2 = no	Created variable: Case_prob = 1 or Case_confirm = 1
R_Tap_H2O	Drank tap water during Ramadan	Numeric	1 = yes 2 = no	

Source: Adapted from Reference 1.

BOX 8.2

SUGGESTED SEQUENCE OF DATA ANALYSES

Handout 8.2: Time, by date of illness onset (could be included in Table 1, but for outbreaks, better to display as an epidemic curve).

Table 1. Clinical features (e.g., signs and symptoms, percentage of laboratory-confirmed cases, percentage of hospitalized patients, and percentage of patients who died).

Table 2. Demographic (e.g., age and sex) and other key characteristics of study participants by case–control status if case–control study.

Place (geographic area of residence or occurrence in Table 2 or in a spot or shaded map).

Table 3. Primary tables of exposure-outcome association.

Table 4. Stratification (Table 3 with separate effects and assessment of confounding and effect modification).

Table 5. Refinements (Table 3 with, for example, dose-response, latency, and use of more sensitive or more specific case definition).

Table 6. Specific group analyses.

---

the remainder of this chapter addresses the analytic epidemiology tools used most commonly in field investigations.

Handout 8.2 depicts output from the Classic Analysis module of Epi Info 7 (Centers for Disease Control and Prevention, Atlanta, GA) (2). It demonstrates the output from the TABLES command for data from a typical field investigation. Note the key elements of the output: (1) a cross-tabulated table summarizing the results, (2) point estimates of measures of association, (3) 95% CIs for each point estimate, and (4) statistical test results. Each of these elements is discussed in the following sections.

Two-by-Two Tables

A *two-by-two table* is so named because it is a cross-tabulation of two variables—exposure and health outcome—that each have two categories, usually "yes" and "no" (Handout 8.3). The two-by-two table is the best way to summarize data that reflect the association between a particular exposure (e.g., consumption of a specific food) and the health outcome of interest (e.g., gastroenteritis). The association is usually quantified by calculating a measure of association (e.g., a risk ratio [RR] or OR) from the data in the two-by-two table (see the following section).

TABLE SHELL: ASSOCIATION BETWEEN DRINKING WATER FROM DIFFERENT SOURCES AND OROPHARYNGEAL TULAREMIA (SANCAKTEPE VILLAGE, BAYBURT PROVINCE, TURKEY, JULY–AUGUST 2013)

Exposure	No. exposed persons			No. unexposed persons			Risk ratio (95% CI)
	Ill	Well	Total	Attack rate (%)	Ill	Well	Total	Attack rate (%)	
Tap	—	—	—	—	—	—	—	—	(—)
Well	—	—	—	—	—	—	—	—	(—)
Spring	—	—	—	—	—	—	—	—	(—)
Bottle	—	—	—	—	—	—	—	—	(—)
Other	—	—	—	—	—	—	—	—	(—)

Abbreviation: CI, confidence interval.
Adapted from Reference 1.

TYPICAL OUTPUT FROM CLASSIC ANALYSIS MODULE, EPI INFO VERSION 7, USING THE TABLES COMMAND

TABLES VANILLA ILL

Vanilla Ice Cream	Ill? Yes	No	Total
Yes	43	11	54
Row%	79.63%	20.37%	100.00%
Col%	93.48%	37.93%	72.00%
No	3	18	21
Row%	14.29%	85.71%	100.00%
Col%	6.52%	62.07%	28.00%
Total	46	29	75
Row%	61.33%	38.67%	100.00%
Col%	100.00%	100.00%	100.00%

Single Table Analysis

	Point Estimate	95% Confidence Interval Lower	Upper
PARAMETERS: Odds-based			
Odds Ratio (cross product)	23.4545	5.8410	94.1811 (T)
Odds Ratio (MLE)	22.1490	5.9280	109.1473 (M)
		5.2153	138.3935 (F)
PARAMETERS: Risk-based			
Risk Ratio (RR)	5.5741	1.9383	16.0296 (T)
Risk Differences (RD%)	65.3439	46.9212	83.7666 (T)

(T=Taylor series; MLE= Maximum Likelihood Estimate; M=Mid–P; F=Fisher Exact)

STATISTICAL TESTS	Chi-square	1-tailed p	2-tailed p
Chi-square – uncorrected	27.2225		0.0000013505
Chi-square – Mantel-Haenszel	26.8596		0.0000013880
Chi-square – corrected (Yates)	24.5370		0.0000018982
Mid-p exact		0.0000001349	
Fisher exact		0.0000002597	0.0000002597

Source: Reference 2.

TABLE SHELL: ASSOCIATION BETWEEN DRINKING WATER FROM DIFFERENT SOURCES AND OROPHARYNGEAL TULAREMIA (SANCAKTEPE VILLAGE, BAYBURT PROVINCE, TURKEY, JULY–AUGUST 2013)

Exposure	No. exposed persons				No. unexposed persons				Risk ratio (95% CI)
	Ill	Well	Total	Attack rate (%)	Ill	Well	Total	Attack rate (%)	
Tap	—	—	—	—	—	—	—	—	— (—)
Well	—	—	—	—	—	—	—	—	— (—)
Spring	—	—	—	—	—	—	—	—	— (—)
Bottle	—	—	—	—	—	—	—	—	— (—)
Other	—	—	—	—	—	—	—	—	— (—)

Source: Adapted from Reference 1.

Abbreviation: CI, confidence interval.

- In a typical two-by-two table used in field epidemiology, disease status (e.g., ill or well, case or control) is represented along the top of the table, and exposure status (e.g., exposed or unexposed) along the side.

- Depending on the exposure being studied, the rows can be labeled as shown in Table 8.3, or for example, as *exposed* and *unexposed* or *ever* and *never*. By convention, the exposed group is placed on the top row.

- Depending on the disease or health outcome being studied, the columns can be labeled as shown in Handout 8.3, or for example, as *ill* and *well*, *case* and *control*, or *dead* and *alive*. By convention, the ill or case group is placed in the left column.

- The intersection of a row and a column in which a count is recorded is known as a *cell*. The letters *a, b, c,* and *d* within the four cells refer to the number of persons with the disease status indicated in the column heading at the top and the exposure status indicated in the row label to the left. For example, cell *c* contains the number of ill but unexposed persons. The row totals are labeled H_1 and H_0 (or H_2 [H for *horizontal*]) and the columns are labeled V_1 and V_0 (or V_2 [V for *vertical*]). The total number of persons included in the two-by-two table is written in the lower right corner and is represented by the letter T or N.

- If the data are from a cohort study, attack rates (i.e., the proportion of persons who become ill during the time period of interest) are sometimes provided to the right of the row totals. RRs or ORs, CIs, or *p* values are often provided to the right of or beneath the table.

The illustrative cross-tabulation of tap water consumption (exposure) and illness status (outcome) from the investigation of oropharyngeal tularemia is displayed in Table 8.2 (1).

TABLE 8.2 Consumption of tap water and risk for acquiring oropharyngeal tularemia (Sancaktepe Village, Turkey, July–August 2013)

		Ill	Well	Total	Attack rate (%)
Drank tap water	Yes	46	127	173	26.6
	No	9	76	85	10.6
	Total	55	203	258	21.3

Risk ratio = 26.59 / 10.59 = 2.5; 95% confidence interval = (1.3–4.9); chi-square (uncorrected) = 8.7 (*p* = 0.003).

Source: Adapted from Reference 1.

Measures of Association

A *measure of association* quantifies the strength or magnitude of the statistical association between an exposure and outcome. Measures of association are sometimes called *measures of effect* because if the exposure is causally related to the health outcome, the measure quantifies the effect of exposure on the probability that the health outcome will occur.

The measures of association most commonly used in field epidemiology are all ratios—RRs, ORs, prevalence ratios (PRs), and prevalence ORs (PORs). These ratios can be thought of as comparing the observed with the expected—that is, the observed amount of disease among persons exposed versus the expected (or baseline) amount of disease among persons unexposed. The measures clearly demonstrate whether the amount of disease among the exposed group is similar to, higher than, or lower than (and by how much) the amount of disease in the baseline group.

- The value of each measure of association equals 1.0 when the amount of disease is the same among the exposed and unexposed groups.
- The measure has a value greater than 1.0 when the amount of disease is greater among the exposed group than among the unexposed group, consistent with a harmful effect.
- The measure has a value less than 1.0 when the amount of disease among the exposed group is less than it is among the unexposed group, as when the exposure protects against occurrence of disease (e.g., vaccination).

Different measures of association are used with different types of studies. The most commonly used measure in a typical outbreak investigation retrospective cohort study is the *RR*, which is simply the ratio of attack rates. For most case–control studies, because attack rates cannot be calculated, the measure of choice is the *OR*.

Cross-sectional studies or surveys typically measure prevalence (existing cases) rather than incidence (new cases) of a health condition. Prevalence measures of association analogous to the RR and OR—the *PR* and *POR*, respectively—are commonly used.

Risk Ratio (Relative Risk)

The RR, the preferred measure for cohort studies, is calculated as the attack rate (risk) among the exposed group divided by the attack rate (risk) among the unexposed group. Using the notations in Handout 8.3,

$$RR = risk_{exposed} / risk_{unexposed} = (a/H_1)/(c/H_0)$$

From Table 8.2, the attack rate (i.e., risk) for acquiring oropharyngeal tularemia among persons who had drunk tap water at the banquet was 26.6%. The attack rate (i.e., risk) for those who had not drunk tap water was 10.6%. Thus, the RR is calculated as 0.266 / 0.106 = 2.5. That is, persons who had drunk tap water were 2.5 times as likely to become ill as those who had not drunk tap water (1).

Odds Ratio

The OR is the preferred measure of association for case–control data. Conceptually, it is calculated as the odds of exposure among case-patients divided by the odds of exposure among controls. However, in practice, it is calculated as the cross-product ratio. Using the notations in Handout 8.3,

$$OR = ad / bc$$

The illustrative data in Handout 8.4 are from a case–control study of acute renal failure in Panama in 2006 (3). Because the data are from a case–control study, neither attack rates (risks) nor an RR can be calculated. The OR—calculated as $37 \times 110 / (29 \times 4) = 35.1$—is exceptionally high, indicating a strong association between ingesting liquid cough syrup and acute renal failure.

HANDOUT 8.4

INGESTION OF PRESCRIPTION LIQUID COUGH SYRUP IN RESPONSE TO DIRECT QUESTIONING: ACUTE RENAL FAILURE CASE–CONTROL STUDY (PANAMA, 2006)

		Cases	Controls	Total
Used liquid cough syrup?	Yes	37	29	81
	No	4	110	35
	Total	41	139	116

Odds ratio = 35.1; 95% confidence interval = (11.6–106.4); chi-square (uncorrected) = 65.6 (p<0.001).

Source: Adapted from Reference 3.

The OR is a useful measure of association because it provides an estimate of the association between exposure and disease from case–control data when an RR cannot be calculated. Additionally, when the outcome is relatively uncommon among the population (e.g., <5%), the OR from a case–control study approximates the RR that would have been derived from a cohort study, had one been performed. However, when the outcome is more common, the OR overestimates the RR.

Prevalence Ratio and Prevalence Odds Ratio

Cross-sectional studies or surveys usually measure the prevalence rather than incidence of a health status (e.g., vaccination status) or condition (e.g., hypertension) among a population. The prevalence measures of association analogous to the RR and OR are, respectively, the *PR* and *POR*.

The PR is calculated as the prevalence among the index group divided by the prevalence among the comparison group. Using the notations in Handout 8.3,

$$PR = prevalence_{index} / prevalence_{comparison} = (a / H_1)/(c / H_0)$$

The POR is calculated like an OR.

$$POR = ad / bc$$

In a study of HIV seroprevalence among current users of crack cocaine versus never users, 165 of 780 current users were HIV-positive (prevalence = 21.2%), compared with 40 of 464 never users (prevalence = 8.6%) (4). The PR and POR were close (2.5 and 2.8, respectively), but the PR is easier to explain.

Measures of Public Health Impact

A *measure of public health impact* places the exposure–disease association in a public health perspective. The impact measure reflects the apparent contribution of the exposure to the health outcome among a population. For example, for an exposure associated with an increased risk for disease (e.g., smoking and lung cancer), the *attributable risk percent* represents the amount of lung cancer among smokers ascribed to smoking, which also can be regarded as the expected reduction in disease load if the exposure could be removed or had never existed.

For an exposure associated with a decreased risk for disease (e.g., vaccination), the *prevented fraction* represents the observed reduction in disease load attributable to the current level of exposure among the population. Note that the terms *attributable* and *prevented* convey more than mere statistical association. They imply a direct cause-and-effect relationship between exposure and disease. Therefore, these measures should be presented only after thoughtful inference of causality.

Attributable Risk Percent

The attributable risk percent (attributable fraction or proportion among the exposed, etiologic fraction) is the proportion of cases among the exposed group presumably attributable to the exposure. This measure assumes that the level of risk among the unexposed group (who are considered to have the baseline or background risk for disease) also applies to the exposed group, so that only the *excess* risk should be attributed to the exposure. The attributable risk percent can be calculated with either of the following algebraically equivalent formulas:

$$\text{Attributable risk percent} = \left(\text{risk}_{\text{exposed}} / \text{risk}_{\text{unexposed}}\right) / \text{risk}_{\text{exposed}} = (RR - 1)/RR$$

In a case–control study, if the OR is a reasonable approximation of the RR, an attributable risk percent can be calculated from the OR.

$$\text{Attributable risk percent} = (OR - 1)/OR$$

In the outbreak setting, attributable risk percent can be used to quantify how much of the disease burden can be ascribed to particular exposure.

Prevented Fraction Among the Exposed Group (Vaccine Efficacy)

The prevented fraction among the exposed group can be calculated when the RR or OR is less than 1.0. This measure is the proportion of potential cases prevented by a beneficial exposure (e.g., bed nets that prevent nighttime mosquito bites and, consequently, malaria). It can also be regarded as the proportion of new cases that would have occurred in the absence of the beneficial exposure. Algebraically, the prevented fraction among the exposed population is identical to vaccine efficacy.

$$\text{Prevented fraction among the exposed group} = \text{vaccine efficacy}$$
$$= \left(\text{risk}_{\text{unexposed}} / \text{risk}_{\text{exposed}}\right) / = \text{risk}_{\text{unexposed}} = 1 - RR$$

Handout 8.5 displays data from a varicella (chickenpox) outbreak at an elementary school in Nebraska in 2004 (5). The risk for varicella was 13.6% among vaccinated

HANDOUT 8.5

HANDOUT 8.5
VACCINATION STATUS AND OCCURRENCE OF VARICELLA: ELEMENTARY SCHOOL OUTBREAK (NEBRASKA, 2004)

	Ill	Well	Total	Risk for varicella
Vaccinated	15	100	115	13.0%
Unvaccinated	18	9	27	66.7%
Total	33	109	142	23.2%

Risk ratio = 13.0 / 66.7 = 0.195; vaccine efficacy = (66.7 – 13.0) / 66.7 = 80.5%.

Source: Adapted from Reference 5.

children and 66.7% among unvaccinated children. The vaccine efficacy based on these data was calculated as (0.667 – 0.130) / 0.667 = 0.805, or 80.5%. This vaccine efficacy of 80.5% indicates that vaccination prevented approximately 80% of the cases that would have otherwise occurred among vaccinated children had they not been vaccinated.

Tests of Statistical Significance

Tests of statistical significance are used to determine how likely the observed results would have occurred by chance alone if exposure was unrelated to the health outcome. This section describes the key factors to consider when applying statistical tests to data from two-by-two tables.

- Statistical testing begins with the assumption that, among the source population, exposure is unrelated to disease. This assumption is known as the *null hypothesis*. The *alternative hypothesis*, which will be adopted if the null hypothesis proves to be implausible, is that exposure *is* associated with disease.
- Next, compute a measure of association (e.g., an RR or OR).
- Then, choose and calculate the test of statistical significance (e.g., a chi-square). Epi Info and other computer programs perform these tests automatically. The test provides the probability of finding an association as strong as, or stronger than, the one observed if the null hypothesis were true. This probability is called the *p value*.

- A small *p* value means that you would be unlikely to observe such an association if the null hypothesis were true. In other words, a small *p* value indicates that the null hypothesis is implausible, given available data.
- If this *p* value is smaller than a predetermined cutoff, called *alpha* (usually 0.05 or 5%), you discard (reject) the null hypothesis in favor of the alternative hypothesis. The association is then said to be *statistically significant*.
- If the *p* value is larger than the cutoff (e.g., *p* value ≥0.06), do not reject the null hypothesis; the apparent association could be a chance finding.
- In reaching a decision about the null hypothesis, you might make one of two types of error.
  - In a *type I error* (also called *alpha error*), the null hypothesis is rejected when in fact it is true.
  - In a *type II error* (also called *beta error*), the null hypothesis is not rejected when in fact it is false.

Testing and Interpreting Data in a Two-by-Two Table

For data in a two-by-two table Epi Info reports the results from two different tests—chi-square test and Fisher exact test—each with variations (Handout 8.2). These tests are not specific to any particular measure of association. The same test can be used regardless of whether you are interested in RR, OR, or attributable risk percent.

- *Which test to use?*
  - *If the expected value in any cell is less than 5.* Fisher exact test is the commonly accepted standard when the expected value in any cell is less than 5. (Remember: The expected value for any cell can be determined by multiplying the row total by the column total and dividing by the table total.)
  - *If all expected values in the two-by-two table are 5 or greater.* Choose one of the chi-square tests. Fortunately, for most analyses, the three chi-square formulas provide *p* values sufficiently similar to make the same decision regarding the null hypothesis based on all three. However, when the different formulas point to different decisions (usually when all three *p* values are approximately 0.05), epidemiologic judgment is required. Some field epidemiologists prefer the Yates-corrected formula because they are least likely to make a type I error (but most likely to make a type II error). Others acknowledge that the Yates correction often overcompensates; therefore, they prefer the uncorrected formula. Epidemiologists who frequently perform stratified analyses are accustomed to

using the Mantel-Haenszel formula; therefore, they tend to use this formula even for simple two-by-two tables.

• *Measures of association versus test of significance.*

   • *Measure of association.* The measures of association (e.g., RRs and ORs) reflect the strength of the association between an exposure and a disease. These measures are usually independent of the size of the study and can be regarded as the best guess of the true degree of association among the source population. However, the measure gives no indication of its reliability (i.e., how much faith to put in it).

   • *Test of significance.* In contrast, a test of significance provides an indication of how likely it is that the observed association is the result of chance. Although the chi-square test statistic is influenced both by the magnitude of the association and the study size, it does not distinguish the contribution of each one. Thus, the measure of association and the test of significance (or a CI; see Confidence Intervals for Measures of Association) provide complementary information.

• *Interpreting statistical test results. Not significant* does not necessarily mean no association. The measures of association (RRs or ORs) indicate the direction and strength of the association. The statistical test indicates how likely it is that the observed association might have occurred by chance alone. Nonsignificance might reflect no association among the source population, but it might also reflect a study size too small to detect a true association among the source population.

   • *Role of statistical significance.* Statistical significance does not by itself indicate a cause-and-effect association. An observed association might indeed represent a causal connection, but it might also result from chance, selection bias, information bias, confounding, or other sources of error in the study's design, execution, or analysis. Statistical testing relates only to the role of chance in explaining an observed association, and statistical significance indicates only that chance is an unlikely, although not impossible, explanation of the association. Epidemiologic judgment is required when considering these and other criteria for inferring causation (e.g., consistency of the findings with those from other studies, the temporal association between exposure and disease, or biologic plausibility).

   • *Public health implications of statistical significance.* Finally, statistical significance does not necessarily mean public health significance. With a large study, a weak association with little public health or clinical relevance might nonetheless be statistically significant. More commonly, if a study is small, an association of public health or clinical importance might fail to reach statistically significance.

Confidence Intervals for Measures of Association

Many medical and public health journals now require that associations be described by measures of association and CIs rather than p values or other statistical tests. A measure of association such as an RR or OR provides a single value (point estimate) that best quantifies the association between an exposure and health outcome. A CI provides an interval estimate or range of values that acknowledge the uncertainty of the single number point estimate, particularly one that is based on a sample of the population.

The 95% Confidence Interval

Statisticians define a 95% CI as the interval that, given repeated sampling of the source population, will include, or cover, the true association value 95% of the time. The epidemiologic concept of a 95% CI is that it includes range of values consistent with the data in the study (6).

Relation Between Chi-Square Test and Confidence Interval

The chi-square test and the CI are closely related. The chi-square test uses the observed data to determine the probability (p value) under the null hypothesis, and one rejects the null hypothesis if the probability is less than alpha (e.g., 0.05). The CI uses a preselected probability value, alpha (e.g., 0.05), to determine the limits of the interval (1 − alpha = 0.95), and one rejects the null hypothesis if the interval does not include the null association value. Both indicate the precision of the observed association; both are influenced by the magnitude of the association and the size of the study group. Although both measure precision, neither addresses validity (lack of bias).

Interpreting the Confidence Interval

- *Meaning of a confidence interval.* A CI can be regarded as the range of values consistent with the data in a study. Suppose a study conducted locally yields an RR of 4.0 for the association between intravenous drug use and disease X; the 95% CI ranges from 3.0 to 5.3. From that study, the best estimate of the association between intravenous drug use and disease X among the general population is 4.0, but the data are consistent with values anywhere from 3.0 to 5.3. A study of the same association conducted elsewhere that yielded an RR of 3.2 or 5.2 would be considered compatible, but a study that yielded an RR of 1.2 or 6.2 would not be considered compatible. Now consider a different study that yields an RR of 1.0, a CI from 0.9 to 1.1, and a p value = 0.9. Rather than interpreting these results as nonsignificant and uninformative, you can conclude that the exposure neither increases nor decreases the risk for disease. That message can be reassuring if the exposure had been of concern to a worried public. Thus, the values that are included in the CI and values that are excluded by the CI both provide important information.

- *Width of the confidence interval.* The width of a CI (i.e., the included values) reflects the precision with which a study can pinpoint an association. A wide CI reflects a large amount of variability or imprecision. A narrow CI reflects less variability and higher precision. Usually, the larger the number of subjects or observations in a study, the greater the precision and the narrower the CI.

- *Relation of the confidence interval to the null hypothesis.* Because a CI reflects the range of values consistent with the data in a study, the CI can be used as a substitute for statistical testing (i.e., to determine whether the data are consistent with the null hypothesis). Remember: the null hypothesis specifies that the RR or OR equals 1.0; therefore, a CI that includes 1.0 is compatible with the null hypothesis. This is equivalent to concluding that the null hypothesis cannot be rejected. In contrast, a CI that does not include 1.0 indicates that the null hypothesis should be rejected because it is inconsistent with the study results. Thus, the CI can be used as a surrogate test of statistical significance.

Confidence Intervals in the Foodborne Outbreak Setting

In the setting of a foodborne outbreak, the goal is to identify the food or other vehicle that caused illness. In this setting, a measure of the association (e.g., an RR or OR) is calculated to identify the food(s) or other consumable(s) with high values that might have caused the outbreak. The investigator does not usually care if the RR for a specific food item is 5.7 or 9.3, just that the RR is high and unlikely to be caused by chance and, therefore, that the item should be further evaluated. For that purpose, the point estimate (RR or OR) plus a *p* value is adequate and a CI is unnecessary.

Summary Exposure Tables

For field investigations intended to identify one or more vehicles or risk factors for disease, consider constructing a single table that can summarize the associations for multiple exposures of interest. For foodborne outbreak investigations, the table typically includes one row for each food item and columns for the name of the food; numbers of ill and well persons, by food consumption history; food-specific attack rates (if a cohort study was

TABLE 8.3 Oropharyngeal tularemia attack rates and risk ratios by water source (Sancaktepe Village, Turkey, July–August 2013)

| | No. exposed persons | | | | No. unexposed persons | | | | Risk ratio |
Exposure	Ill	Well	Total	Attack rate (%)	Ill	Well	Total	Attack rate (%)	(95% CI)
Tap	46	127	173	27	9	76	85	11	2.5 (1.3–4.9)
Well	2	6	8	25	53	198	250	21	1.2 (0.4–4.0)
Spring	25	111	136	18	30	92	122	25	0.7 (0.5–1.2)
Bottle	5	26	31	16	50	177	227	22	0.7 (0.3–1.7)
Other	2	6	8	25	53	198	250	21	1.2 (0.4–4.0)

Abbreviation: CI, confidence interval.
Source: Adapted from Reference 1.

conducted); RR or OR; chi-square or *p* value; and, sometimes, a 95% CI. The food most likely to have caused illness will usually have both of the following characteristics:

1. An elevated RR, OR, or chi-square (small *p* value), reflecting a substantial difference in attack rates among those who consumed that food and those who did not.
2. The majority of the ill persons had consumed that food; therefore, the exposure can explain or account for most if not all of the cases.

In illustrative summary Table 8.3, tap water had the highest RR (and the only *p* value <0.05, based on the 95% CI excluding 1.0) and might account for 46 of 55 cases.

Stratified Analysis

Stratification is the examination of an exposure–disease association in two or more categories (strata) of a third variable (e.g., age). It is a useful tool for assessing whether *confounding* is present and, if it is, controlling for it. Stratification is also the best method for identifying *effect modification*. Both confounding and effect modification are addressed in following sections.

Stratification is also an effective method for examining the effects of two different exposures on a disease. For example, in a foodborne outbreak, two foods might seem to be associated with illness on the basis of elevated RRs or ORs. Possibly both foods were contaminated or included the same contaminated ingredient. Alternatively, the two foods might have been eaten together (e.g., peanut butter and jelly or doughnuts and milk), with only one being contaminated and the other guilty by association. Stratification is one way to tease apart the effects of the two foods.

Creating Strata of Two-by-Two Tables

- First, consider the categories of the third variable.
  - To stratify by sex, create a two-by-two table for males and another table for females.
  - To stratify by age, decide on age groupings, making certain not to have overlapping ages; then create a separate two-by-two table for each age group.
- For example, the data in Table 8.2 are stratified by sex in Handouts 8.6 and 8.7. The RR for drinking tap water and experiencing oropharyngeal tularemia is 2.3 among females and 3.6 among males, but stratification also allows you to see that women have a higher risk than men, regardless of tap water consumption.

The Two-by-Four Table

Stratified tables (e.g., Handouts 8.6 and 8.7) are useful when the stratification variable is not of primary interest (i.e., is not being examined as a cause of the outbreak). However, when each of the two exposures might be the cause, a two-by-four table is better for disentangling the effects of the two variables. Consider a case–control

---

HANDOUT 8.6

CONSUMPTION OF TAP WATER AND RISK FOR ACQUIRING OROPHARYNGEAL TULAREMIA AMONG WOMEN (SANCAKTEPE VILLAGE, TURKEY, JULY–AUGUST 2013)

Women		Ill	Well	Total	Attack rate (%)	Risk ratio
Drank tap water?	Yes	30	60	90	33.3	2.3
	No	7	41	48	14.6	
	Total	37	101	138	37.9	

Source: Adapted from Reference 1.

HANDOUT 8.7

CONSUMPTION OF TAP WATER AND RISK FOR ACQUIRING OROPHARYNGEAL TULAREMIA AMONG MEN (SANCAKTEPE VILLAGE, TURKEY, JULY–AUGUST 2013)

Men		Ill	Well	Total	Attack rate (%)	Risk ratio
Drank tap water?	Yes	16	67	83	19.3	3.6
	No	2	35	37	5.4	
	Total	18	102	120	15.0	

Source: Adapted from Reference 1.

---

study of a hypothetical hepatitis A outbreak that yielded elevated ORs both for doughnuts (OR = 6.0) and milk (OR = 3.9). The data organized in a two-by-four table (Handout 8.8) disentangle the effects of the two foods—exposure to doughnuts alone is strongly associated with illness (OR = 6.0), but exposure to milk alone is not (OR = 1.0).

HANDOUT 8.8

TWO-BY-FOUR TABLE DISPLAY OF THE ASSOCIATION BETWEEN HEPATITIS A AND CONSUMPTION OF DOUGHNUTS AND MILK: CASE–CONTROL STUDY FROM HYPOTHETICAL OUTBREAK

Doughnuts	Milk	Cases	Controls	Odds ratio
Yes	Yes	36	18	6.0
No	Yes	1	3	1.0
Yes	No	4	2	6.0
No	No	9	27	1.0 (Ref.)
	Total	50	50	

Crude odds ratio for doughnuts = 6.0; crude odds ratio for milk = 3.9.

When two foods cause illness—for example when they are both contaminated or have a common ingredient—the two-by-four table is the best way to see their individual and joint effects.

Confounding

Confounding is the distortion of an exposure–outcome association by the effect of a third factor (a *confounder*). A third factor might be a confounder if it is

- Associated with the outcome independent of the exposure—that is, it must be an independent risk factor; and,
- Associated with the exposure but is not a consequence of it.

Consider a hypothetical retrospective cohort study of mortality among manufacturing employees that determined that workers involved with the manufacturing process were substantially more likely to die during the follow-up period than office workers and salespersons in the same industry.

- The increase in mortality reflexively might be attributed to one or more exposures during the manufacturing process.
- If, however, the manufacturing workers' average age was 15 years older than the other workers, mortality reasonably could be expected to be higher among the older workers.
- In that situation, age likely is a confounder that could account for at least some of the increased mortality. (Note that age satisfies the two criteria described previously: increasing age is associated with increased mortality, regardless of occupation; and, in that industry, age was associated with job—specifically, manufacturing employees were older than the office workers).

Unfortunately, confounding is common. The first step in dealing with confounding is to look for it. If confounding is identified, the second step is to control for or adjust for its distorting effect by using available statistical methods.

Looking for Confounding

The most common method for looking for confounding is to stratify the exposure–outcome association of interest by the third variable suspected to be a confounder.

- To stratify (see previous section), create separate two-by-two tables for each category or stratum of the suspected confounder and consider the following when assessing suspected confounders:
  - Because one of the two criteria for a confounding variable is that it should be associated with the outcome, the list of potential confounders should include the known risk factors for the disease. The list also should include matching variables. Because age frequently is a confounder, it should be considered a potential confounder in any data set.
- For each stratum, compute a stratum-specific measure of association. If the stratification variable is sex, only women will be in one stratum and only men in the other. The exposure–outcome association is calculated separately for women and for men. Sex can no longer be a confounder in these strata because women are compared with women and men are compared with men.
- To look for confounding, first examine the smallest and largest values of the stratum-specific measures of association and compare them with the value of the combined table (called the *crude value*). Confounding is present if the crude value is outside the range between the smallest and largest stratum-specific values.
- Often, confounding is not that obvious. The more precise method for assessing confounding is to calculate a summary adjusted measure of association as a weighted average of the stratum-specific values (see the following section, Controlling for Confounding). After calculating a summary value, compare the summary value to the crude value to see if the two are appreciably different. Unfortunately, no universal rule or statistical test exists for determining what constitutes "appreciably different." In practice, assume that the summary adjusted value is more accurate. The question then becomes, "Does the crude value adequately approximate the adjusted value, or would the crude value be misleading to a reader?" If the crude and adjusted values are close, use the crude value because it is not misleading and is easier to explain. If the two values are appreciably different (some epidemiologists use 10% difference, others use 20%), use the adjusted value (Box 8.3).

BOX 8.3

METHODS FOR DETERMINING WHETHER CONFOUNDING IS PRESENT

1. If the crude risk ratio or odds ratio is outside the range of the stratum-specific ones.
2. If the crude risk ratio or odds ratio differs from the Mantel-Haenszel adjusted one by >10% or >20%.

Controlling for Confounding

- One method of controlling for confounding is by calculating a summary RR or OR based on a weighted average of the stratum-specific data. The Mantel-Haenszel technique (6) is a popular method for performing this task.
- A second method is by using a logistic regression model that includes the exposure of interest and one or more confounding variables. The model produces an estimate of the OR that controls for the effect of the confounding variable(s).

Effect Modification

Effect modification or *effect measure modification* means that the degree of association between an exposure and an outcome differs among different population groups. For example, measles vaccine is usually highly effective in preventing disease if administered to children aged 12 months or older but is less effective if administered before age 12 months. Similarly, tetracycline can cause tooth mottling among children, but not adults. In both examples, the association (or effect) of the exposure (measles vaccine or tetracycline) is a function of, or is modified by, a third variable (age in both examples).

Because effect modification means different effects among different groups, the first step in looking for effect modification is to stratify the exposure–outcome association of interest by the third variable suspected to be the effect modifier. Next, calculate the measure of association (e.g., RR or OR) for each stratum. Finally, assess whether the stratum-specific measures of association are substantially different by using one of two methods.

1. Examine the stratum-specific measures of association. Are they different enough to be of public health or scientific importance?
2. Determine whether the variation in magnitude of the association is statistically significant by using the Breslow-Day Test for homogeneity of odds ratios or by testing the interaction term in logistic regression.

If effect modification is present, present each stratum-specific result separately.

Dose-Response

In epidemiology, *dose-response* means increased risk for the health outcome with increasing (or, for a protective exposure, decreasing) amount of exposure. Amount of exposure reflects *quantity of exposure* (e.g., milligrams of folic acid or number of scoops of ice cream consumed), or *duration of exposure* (e.g., number of months or years of exposure), or both.

The presence of a dose-response effect is one of the well-recognized criteria for inferring causation. Therefore, when an association between an exposure and a health outcome has been identified based on an elevated RR or OR, consider assessing for a dose-response effect.

As always, the first step is to organize the data. One convenient format is a 2-by-H table, where H represents the categories or doses of exposure. An RR for a cohort study or an OR for a case–control study can be calculated for each dose relative to the lowest dose or the unexposed group (Handout 8.9). CIs can be calculated for each dose. Reviewing the data and the measures of association in this format and displaying the measures graphically can provide a sense of whether a dose-response association is present. Additionally, statistical techniques can be used to assess such associations, even when confounders must be considered.

Matching

The basic data layout for a matched-pair analysis is a two-by-two table that seems to resemble the simple unmatched two-by-two tables presented earlier in this chapter, but it is different (Handout 8.10). In the matched-pair two-by-two table, each cell represents the

---

HANDOUT 8.9
DATA LAYOUT AND NOTATION FOR DOSE-RESPONSE TABLE

Dose	Ill or case	Well or control	Total	Risk	Risk ratio	Odds ratio
Dose 3	a_3	b_3	H_3	a_3 / H_3	$Risk_3 / Risk_0$	$a_3 d / b_3 c$
Dose 2	a_2	b_2	H_2	a_2 / H_2	$Risk_2 / Risk_0$	$a_2 d / b_2 c$
Dose 1	a_1	b_1	H_1	a_1 / H_1	$Risk_1 / Risk_0$	$a_1 d / b_1 c$
Dose 0	c	d	H_0	c / H_0	1.0 (Ref.)	1.0 (Ref.)
Total	V_1	V_0				

HANDOUT 8.10

DATA LAYOUT AND NOTATION FOR MATCHED-PAIR TWO-BY-TWO TABLE

		Controls		Total
		Exposed	Unexposed	Total
Cases	Exposed	e	f	e + f
	Unexposed	g	h	g + h
	Total	e + g	f + h	e + f + g + h pairs

Odds ratio = f / g.

number of matched pairs that meet the row and column criteria. In the unmatched two-by-two table, each cell represents the number of persons who meet the criteria.

In Handout 8.10, cell *e* contains the number of pairs in which the case-patient is exposed and the control is exposed; cell *f* contains the number of pairs with an exposed case-patient and an unexposed control, cell *g* contains the number of pairs with an unexposed case-patient and an exposed control, and cell *h* contains the number of pairs in which neither the case-patient nor the matched control is exposed. Cells *e* and *h* are called *concordant pairs* because the case-patient and control are in the same exposure category. Cells *f* and *g* are called *discordant pairs*.

In a matched-pair analysis, only the discordant pairs are used to calculate the OR. The OR is computed as the ratio of the discordant pairs.

$$OR = f / g$$

The test of significance for a matched-pair analysis is the McNemar chi-square test.

Handout 8.11 displays data from the classic pair-matched case–control study conducted in 1980 to assess the association between tampon use and toxic shock syndrome (7).

- *Larger matched sets and variable matching.* In certain studies, two, three, four, or a variable number of controls are matched with case-patients. The best way to analyze these larger or variable matched sets is to consider each set (e.g., triplet or quadruplet) as a unique stratum and then analyze the data by using the Mantel-Haenszel

HANDOUT 8.11

CONTINUAL TAMPON USE DURING INDEX MENSTRUAL PERIOD: CENTERS FOR DISEASE CONTROL TOXIC SHOCK SYNDROME (MATCHED-PAIR) CASE–CONTROL STUDY, 1980

		Controls		Total
		Exposed	Unexposed	
Cases	Exposed	33	9	42
	Unexposed	1	1	2
	Total	34	10	44 pairs

Odds ratio = 9 / 1 = 9.0; uncorrected McNemar chi-square test = 6.40 (p = 0.01).

Source: Adapted from Reference 7.

methods or logistic regression to summarize the strata (see Controlling for Confounding).

- *Does a matched design require a matched analysis?* Usually, yes. In a pair-matched study, if the pairs are unique (e.g., siblings or friends), pair-matched analysis is needed. If the pairs are based on a nonunique characteristic (e.g., sex or grade in school), all of the case-patients and all of the controls from the same stratum (sex or grade) can be grouped together, and a stratified analysis can be performed.

In practice, some epidemiologists perform the matched analysis but then perform an unmatched analysis on the same data. If the results are similar, they might opt to present the data in unmatched fashion. In most instances, the unmatched OR will be closer to 1.0 than the matched OR (bias toward the null). This bias, which is related to confounding, might be either trivial or substantial. The chi-square test result from unmatched data can be particularly misleading because it is usually larger than the McNemar test result from the matched data. The decision to use a matched analysis or unmatched analysis is analogous to the decision to present crude or adjusted results; epidemiologic judgment must be used to avoid presenting unmatched results that are misleading.

Logistic Regression

In recent years, logistic regression has become a standard tool in the field epidemiologist's toolkit because user-friendly software has become widely available and its ability to assess effects of multiple variables has become appreciated. *Logistic regression* is a statistical modeling method analogous to linear regression but for a binary outcome (e.g., ill/well or case/control). As with other types of regression, the outcome (the dependent variable) is modeled as a function of one or more independent variables. The independent variables include the exposure(s) of interest and, often, confounders and interaction terms.

- The software package fits the data to the logistic model and provides output with beta coefficients for each independent term.
  - The exponentiation of a given beta coefficient (e^β) equals the OR for that variable while controlling for the effects of all of the other variables in the model.
  - If the model includes only the outcome variable and the primary exposure variable coded as $(0,1)$, e^β should equal the OR you can calculate from the two-by-two table. For example, a logistic regression model of the oropharyngeal tularemia data with tap water as the only independent variable yields an OR of 3.06, exactly the same value to the second decimal as the crude OR. Similarly, a model that includes both tap water and sex as independent variables yields an OR for tap water of 3.24, almost identical to the Mantel-Haenszel OR for tap water controlling for sex of 3.26. (Note that logistic regression provides ORs rather than RRs, which is not ideal for field epidemiology cohort studies.)
- Logistic regression also can be used to assess dose-response associations, effect modification, and more complex associations. A variant of logistic regression called *conditional logistic regression* is particularly appropriate for pair-matched data.

Sophisticated analytic techniques cannot atone for sloppy data! Analytic techniques such as those described in this chapter are only as good as the data to which they are applied. Analytic techniques—whether simple, stratified, or modeling—use the information at hand. They do not know or assess whether the correct comparison group was selected, the response rate was adequate, exposure and outcome were accurately defined, or the data coding and entry were free of errors. Analytic techniques are merely tools; the analyst is responsible for knowing the quality of the data and interpreting the results appropriately.

INTERPRETING DATA FROM A FIELD INVESTIGATION

A computer can crunch numbers more quickly and accurately than the investigator can by hand, but the computer cannot interpret the results. For a two-by-two table, Epi Info provides both an RR and an OR, but the investigator must choose which is best based on the type of study performed. For that table, the RR and the OR might be elevated; the *p* value might be less than 0.05; and the 95% CI might not include 1.0. However, do those statistical results guarantee that the exposure is a true cause of disease? Not necessarily. Although the association might be causal, flaws in study design, execution, and analysis can result in apparent associations that are actually artifacts. Chance, selection bias, information bias, confounding, and investigator error should all be evaluated as possible explanations for an observed association. The first step in evaluating whether an apparent association is real and causal is to review the list of factors that can cause a spurious association, as listed in Epidemiologic Interpretation Checklist 1 (Box 8.4).

Epidemiologic Interpretation Checklist 1

Chance is one possible explanation for an observed association between exposure and outcome. Under the null hypothesis, you assume that your study population is a sample from a source population in which that exposure is not associated with disease; that is, the RR and OR equal 1. Could an elevated (or lowered) OR be attributable simply to variation caused by chance? The role of chance is assessed by using tests of significance (or, as noted earlier, by interpreting CIs). Chance is an *unlikely* explanation if

- The *p* value is less than alpha (usually set at 0.05), or
- The CI for the RR or OR excludes 1.0.

BOX 8.4
EPIDEMIOLOGIC INTERPRETATION CHECKLIST 1

- Chance
- Selection bias
- Information bias
- Confounding
- Investigator error
- True association

However, chance can never be ruled out entirely. Even if the p value is as small as 0.01, that study might be the one study in 100 in which the null hypothesis *is* true and chance is the explanation. Note that tests of significance evaluate only the role of chance—they do not address the presence of selection bias, information bias, confounding, or investigator error.

Selection bias is a systematic error in the designation of the study groups or in the enrollment of study participants that results in a mistaken estimate of an exposure's effect on the risk for disease. Selection bias can be thought of as a problem resulting from who gets into the study or how. Selection bias can arise from the faulty design of a case–control study through, for example, use of an overly broad case definition (so that some persons in the case group do not actually have the disease being studied) or inappropriate control group, or when asymptomatic cases are undetected among the controls. In the execution phase, selection bias can result if eligible persons with certain exposure and disease characteristics choose not to participate or cannot be located. For example, if ill persons with the exposure of interest know the hypothesis of the study and are more willing to participate than other ill persons, cell a in the two-by-two table will be artificially inflated compared with cell c, and the OR also will be inflated. Evaluating the possible role of selection bias requires examining how case-patients and controls were specified and were enrolled.

Information bias is a systematic error in the data collection from or about the study participants that results in a mistaken estimate of an exposure's effect on the risk for disease. Information bias might arise by including poor wording or understanding of a question on a questionnaire; poor recall; inconsistent interviewing technique; or if a person knowingly provides false information, either to hide the truth or, as is common among certain cultures, in an attempt to please the interviewer.

Confounding is the distortion of an exposure–disease association by the effect of a third factor, as discussed earlier in this chapter. To evaluate the role of confounding, ensure that potential confounders have been identified, evaluated, and controlled for as necessary.

Investigator error can occur at any step of a field investigation, including design, conduct, analysis, and interpretation. In the analysis, a misplaced semicolon in a computer program, an erroneous transcription of a value, use of the wrong formula, or misreading of results can all yield artifactual associations. Preventing this type of error requires rigorous checking of work and asking colleagues to carefully review the work and conclusions.

To reemphasize, *before considering whether an association is causal, consider whether the association can be explained by chance, selection bias, information bias, confounding, or investigator error.* Now suppose that an elevated RR or OR has a small p value and narrow CI that does not include 1.0; therefore, chance is an unlikely explanation. Specification of

---

BOX 8.5

EPIDEMIOLOGIC INTERPRETATION CHECKLIST 2

- Strength of the association
- Biologic plausibility
- Consistency with other studies
- Exposure precedes disease
- Dose-response effect

---

case-patients and controls was reasonable and participation was good; therefore, selection bias is an unlikely explanation. Information was collected by using a standard questionnaire by an experienced and well-trained interviewer. Confounding by other risk factors was assessed and determined not to be present or to have been controlled for. Data entry and calculations were verified. However, before concluding that the association is causal, the strength of the association, its biologic plausibility, consistency with results from other studies, temporal sequence, and dose-response association, if any, need to be considered (Box 8.5).

Epidemiologic Interpretation Checklist 2

Strength of the association means that a stronger association has more causal credibility than a weak one. If the true RR is 1.0, subtle selection bias, information bias, or confounding can result in an RR of 1.5, but the bias would have to be dramatic and hopefully obvious to the investigator to account for an RR of 9.0.

Biological plausibility means an association has causal credibility if is consistent with the known pathophysiology, known vehicles, natural history of the health outcome, animal models, and other relevant biological factors. For an implicated food vehicle in an infectious disease outbreak, has the food been implicated in previous outbreaks, or—even better— has the agent been identified in the food? Although some outbreaks are caused by new or previously unrecognized pathogens, vehicles, or risk factors, most are caused by those that have been recognized previously.

Consider *consistency with other studies*. Are the results consistent with those from previous studies? A finding is more plausible if it has been replicated by different investigators using different methods for different populations.

Exposure precedes disease seems obvious, but in a retrospective cohort study, documenting that exposure precedes disease can be difficult. Suppose, for example, that persons with a particular type of leukemia are more likely than controls to have antibodies to a particular virus. It might be tempting to conclude that the virus caused the leukemia, but caution is required because viral infection might have occurred after the onset of leukemic changes.

Evidence of a *dose-response effect* adds weight to the evidence for causation. A dose-response effect is not a *necessary* feature for an association to be causal; some causal association might exhibit a threshold effect, for example. Nevertheless, it is usually thought to add credibility to the association.

In many field investigations, a likely culprit might not meet all the criteria discussed in this chapter. Perhaps the response rate was less than ideal, the etiologic agent could not be isolated from the implicated food, or no dose-response was identified. Nevertheless, if the public's health is at risk, failure to meet every criterion should not be used as an excuse for inaction. As George Comstock stated, "The art of epidemiologic reasoning is to draw sensible conclusions from imperfect data" (8). After all, field epidemiology is a tool for public health action to promote and protect the public's health on the basis of science (sound epidemiologic methods), causal reasoning, and a healthy dose of practical common sense.

All scientific work is incomplete—whether it be observational or experimental. All scientific work is liable to be upset or modified by advancing knowledge. That does not confer upon us a freedom to ignore the knowledge we already have, or to postpone the action it seems to demand at a given time (9).

—Sir Austin Bradford Hill (1897–1991), English Epidemiologist and Statistician

REFERENCES

1. Aktas D, Celebi B, Isik ME, et al. Oropharyngeal tularemia outbreak associated with drinking contaminated tap water, Turkey, July–September 2013. *Emerg Infect Dis.* 2015;21:2194–6.
2. Centers for Disease Control and Prevention. Epi Info. https://www.cdc.gov/epiinfo/index.html
3. Rentz ED, Lewis L, Mujica OJ, et al. Outbreak of acute renal failure in Panama in 2006: a case--control study. *Bull World Health Organ.* 2008;86:749–56.
4. Edlin BR, Irwin KL, Faruque S, et al. Intersecting epidemics—crack cocaine use and HIV infection among inner-city young adults. *N Eng J Med.* 1994;331:1422–7.
5. Centers for Disease Control and Prevention. Varicella outbreak among vaccinated children—Nebraska, 2004. *MMWR.* 2006;55;749–52.

6. Rothman KJ. *Epidemiology: an introduction.* New York: Oxford University Press; 2002: *p.* 113–29.

7. Shands KN, Schmid GP, Dan BB, et al. Toxic-shock syndrome in menstruating women: association with tampon use and *Staphylococcus aureus* and clinical features in 52 women. *N Engl J Med.* 1980;303:1436–42.

8. Comstock GW. Vaccine evaluation by case–control or prospective studies. *Am J Epidemiol.* 1990;131:205–7.

9. Hill AB. The environment and disease: association or causation? *Proc R Soc Med.* 1965;58:295–300.

///9/// OPTIMIZING EPIDEMIOLOGY–
LABORATORY
COLLABORATIONS

M. SHANNON KECKLER,
REYNOLDS M. SALERNO,
AND MICHAEL W. SHAW

Sans laboratoires les savants sont des soldats sans armes.

Without laboratories men of science are soldiers without arms.

—Louis Pasteur (1923)

> Alexander Langmuir was quoted in the early 1960s instructing incoming Epidemic Intelligence Service (EIS) officers that the only need for the laboratory in an outbreak investigation was to "prove their conclusions were right."
>
> —Walter R. Dowdle (2011)

INTRODUCTION

Although these isolated quotes make Louis Pasteur and Alexander Langmuir seem to have opposing ideas about the role of the laboratory in outbreak investigations, each quote has some validity. In the late nineteenth century, Pasteur's laboratory data supporting the "germ theory" of disease not only led to pasteurization and vaccination (1), but also provided the evidence that swayed the court of scientific opinion toward accepting the theory that microorganisms are a cause of disease. This shift in scientific focus shed light on the then relatively unknown work of Dr. James Lind, Dr. Ignaz Semmelweiss, and Dr. John Snow, whose elegant maps and statistics introduced epidemiology as a science. Nearly a century later, at the time of Dr. Langmuir's comment (2), a field investigation team, armed only with epidemiology tools, arrived in Pontiac, Michigan, and determined the chain of infection in a point-source outbreak associated with an unknown microbial agent growing in a new reservoir with a new mode of transmission (3). Importantly, the epidemiology results were used to halt the Pontiac fever outbreak—8 years *before* the laboratory of the Center for Disease Control (later Centers for Disease Control and Prevention [CDC]) identified *Legionella* spp. as the causative agent (4). These examples demonstrate that comparing the relative importance of epidemiology and laboratory science to a field investigation is similar to the age-old debate about the order of appearance of the chicken or the egg—it is circular and obscures more fundamental truths. What both Pasteur and Langmuir believed—and what history has shown—is that both epidemiologists and laboratory scientists can make independent discoveries that have significant scientific impact, but collaboration across these disciplines has a synergistic effect, yielding public health data that are stronger than either discipline can provide alone (2).

Modern Role of Public Health Laboratories in Field Investigations

During the early 1980s, revolutionary developments in molecular biology and computer science began to be reflected in technologic advances in laboratory science. As a result, investigators can now accomplish sample collection, electronic sample receipt and tracking, sample processing, patient diagnostics, chemical identification and quantification, microbial identification, and antimicrobial susceptibility testing more rapidly, safely, and accurately than ever before. Laboratory technology—including whole-genome sequencing, bioinformatics, and other technologies associated with advanced molecular detection—continues to develop at a phenomenal pace.

As laboratory technology has expanded over time, so has the laboratory role in field investigations. In addition to the traditional roles of providing causative agent and point-source identification and case confirmation, current laboratory results can be leveraged to inform *all* aspects of an outbreak investigation. Critical field investigation goals that have been informed by laboratory data include

- Etiologic agent identification and characterization (5,6).
- Case determination and detection (7,8).
- Point-source identification (9).
- Clinical care guidance and case management (10–12).
- Root cause analysis and intervention design (13).
- Outbreak control (14–16).
- Chain of infection definition (17,18).

Improving a multidisciplinary understanding of epidemiologic needs and requirements, as well as ways to best leverage advanced diagnostic laboratory capabilities, will continue to strengthen the performance of future outbreak investigation teams.

Chapter Goals

This chapter provides general guidance and recommendations for the field investigation team. While the chapter's primary focus is infectious disease outbreaks, laboratory-related information for nonbiological exposures also is included. These instructions, although not necessarily universal, are intended to help the team consider how to integrate local, state, regional, national, and international laboratory expertise and capacity throughout the outbreak investigation process. Online resource links for the specific laboratory-related tasks involved in a field investigation are included to provide access to the most recently updated information.

FIVE STEPS FOR EFFECTIVE EPIDEMIOLOGY–LABORATORY COLLABORATIONS

These recommendations represent a best-case scenario. Adjustments to laboratory-related plans often are required because of resource or time constraints, emergencies, and local considerations. Local considerations can include policies, regulations, environment, climate, culture, infrastructure, and socioeconomics. In many cases, the field investigation team needs to use judgment to adapt these recommendations to the unique local circumstances—but only after careful consideration of their effects on safety, patient care, and outbreak control. This analysis should involve collaboration with field epidemiologists, laboratory experts, and local stakeholders.

Step 1. Involve the Laboratory Early and Often

Because new technologies are regularly added to the arsenal of available laboratory tests, listing them is impractical. This evolving catalog of tests means that optimal sample types also can change, thus dictating changes in collection protocols. *Therefore, it is vital that outbreak investigators contact the relevant laboratories as soon as possible, preferably before deploying to the field investigation site.* Local health department, state public health, and contract laboratories can perform some testing, whereas CDC subject-matter experts and laboratories can support investigations as needed through consultation, testing, and collaboration.

The general types of laboratory activities performed by CDC include

- Outbreak investigation.
- Emergency response.
- Population health studies.
- Laboratory quality improvement.
- Culture-based pathogen detection and characterization.
- Molecular-based pathogen detection and characterization.
- Detection of high-consequence pathogens.
- Genetic studies.
- Biomonitoring.
- Vaccine development.
- Pathogen discovery.
- Newborn screening.
- Occupational health.
- Chemical exposure testing.
- Assessment of environmental exposure.

A public health professional conducting an outbreak investigation should use the following checklist to enhance the effectiveness of these early communications with the laboratory receiving samples. This early communication is especially important in outbreaks of unknown etiology to ensure that samples are collected in a manner that enables rapid laboratory testing of a variety of potential etiologic hypotheses. It is also important to remain aware that etiologic hypotheses based on clinical signs and symptoms should include consideration of multiple factors (both biological and abiological) (19).

- If the investigation involves a suspected pathogen (e.g., bacteria, viruses, parasites, fungi) or biological toxin as an etiologic agent, then consult local laboratory resources and appropriate clinical and laboratory guidance (20). Pathogen-specific tests and contacts for CDC resources also can be found in the CDC Laboratory Test Directory (http://www.cdc.gov/laboratory/specimen-submission/list.html).

- If the investigation involves a suspected chemical or radiologic agent as an etiologic agent or if the outbreak involves a noninfectious disease or if the event might have been caused by biological, chemical, or radiologic terrorism, then contact the local or state public health department. CDC's National Center for Environmental Health, Division of Laboratory Services (NCEH-DLS) (http://www.cdc.gov/nceh/dls/) also can offer guidance on options for testing and epidemiologic data, local laboratory resources, and relevant studies (21–25) and should guide testing during the investigation.

- Consult test descriptions relevant for the suspected agent and collaborate with the appropriate laboratory to determine the tests to perform based on the needs of the field investigation.

- Inform the laboratory of the purpose of the samples so that resources can be prioritized. The various purposes of sample submittal can include management of patient care, outbreak source identification, surveillance, research, law enforcement, and definition of cases.

- Gather information about the turnaround time for the selected test to manage expectations during the field investigation. Some tests can take up to 2 months to yield data.

Special Consideration: Test Selection

Test selection is one of the most important tasks to complete as early in the investigation as possible. A large number of tests are available to identify and characterize microorganisms, and serologic and antimicrobial susceptibility tests are available to provide a better understanding of potential exposures and inform treatment and infection control decisions. Local, state, and federal public health laboratories, as well as private hospital and contract laboratories, are available testing resources. However, it is important that the field investigator inquire about the accreditations or quality management programs of the laboratories to ensure use of the best resources for each field investigation. CDC laboratories can perform more than 300 infectious disease tests for a wide variety of microorganisms; the current list of available tests can be found at http://www.cdc.gov/laboratory/specimen-submission/list.html. This list can be used to select the appropriate tests for the suspected organism during a field investigation or to find CDC contact information for subject-matter experts on a particular organism.

Not all field investigations involve infectious microorganisms. For those investigations of noninfectious sources, some local and state health departments and NCEH-DLS perform testing in the areas of chronic disease markers, chemical and radiologic threat agents, environmental chemicals, newborn screening, and nutritional markers of disease. NCEH-DLS also can provide the field investigation team with appropriate sampling containers and protocols to minimize sample contamination from extraneous sources, as well as personnel to assist the field team. Contact NCEH-DLS directly through its website (http://www.cdc.gov/nceh/dls/).

To ensure the most rapid turnaround of accurate test samples, laboratories need lead time to order surge supplies, rearrange workloads, implement or modify protocols, and train additional staff. Laboratory experts can also help with some of the more difficult aspects of test selection. For example, specific symptoms (e.g., atypical pneumonia) can be associated with exposure to multiple biological and abiological etiologic agents; similar organisms (e.g., *Chlamydia* spp.) can cause different symptoms. In addition, multiple types of tests are available for most organisms, and not all of them give results that can be interpreted in the same way (i.e., a positive reverse-transcription polymerase chain reaction [RT-PCR] is not the same as a positive culture because RT-PCR tests for presence of nucleic acids and culture tests for viable organisms). Endemic diseases at the field investigation site also can affect testing for specific organisms (e.g., dengue, chikungunya, and Zika viruses), and some infections might require testing across multiple labs with different sample collection and submission requirements (e.g., healthcare-associated fungal infections might need testing by an environmental laboratory *and* a mycology laboratory). The setting (e.g., hospital), geography (e.g., Old World vs. New World hantaviruses), disease (e.g., genital ulcer disease), circumstances (e.g., biodefense), agent grouping (e.g., respiratory agents), sample type (e.g., whole blood), or purpose (e.g., surveillance) of the samples also can form the basis of test selection instead of, or in addition to, the suspected organism. Finally, some tests (especially chemical, radiologic, and molecular) are often exquisitely sensitive, and great care must be taken when selecting these tests to ensure appropriate sampling.

Special Consideration: Classic Versus Molecular Tests

Advanced molecular technologies backed by bioinformatics provide powerful new molecular detection systems that enable public health agencies to conduct surveillance, identify pathogens, recognize outbreaks, track transmission of a pathogen, detect antimicrobial resistance, and identify better ways to prevent disease. Genomics is central to many advanced molecular detection systems, and proteomics and transcriptomics are becoming important tools for public health. Molecular testing often can yield results more quickly than tests based on classical culture-based microbiology or serology/immunology, making them attractive alternatives during a field investigation. These tests play an increasingly important role in the general trend toward culture-independent diagnostic tests, which have the advantage of quickly and simultaneously testing for multiple pathogens within one sample. However, classical tests remain critical for completely characterizing disease-causing organisms and host responses and identifying new pathogens and new methods of antimicrobial resistance because detecting the presence of organism DNA/RNA by PCR is not the same as detecting a viable organism. Thus, investigation planning should include sample collection protocols suitable for the tests deemed most effective after consultation with the receiving laboratory.

Rapid molecular tests, such as real-time PCR, can yield definitive results within hours of sample receipt in the laboratory, but these use primers and probes designed to detect likely pathogens, which means these assays might miss an unsuspected or new pathogen. Technologies based on mass spectrometry (e.g., matrix-assisted laser desorption ionization–time of flight) are similarly limited in that the signal is compared with a reference library of likely pathogens. In contrast, untargeted nucleic acid sequencing (e.g., microbiome sequence analysis) can theoretically identify all organisms in a sample but present formidable analytic challenges because of the computational resources required to filter out irrelevant signals from host genome and benign commensal organisms. Even when a rapid molecular test identifies a pathogen, additional characterization using classical protocols often is needed to present a complete picture of the epidemiologic situation. For example, real-time PCR might identify the causative pathogen in an outbreak of meningitis as *Neisseria meningitides*, but the picture would be incomplete without also determining the serotype, which requires classical culture techniques.

Deciding on the tests to be performed on the samples before embarking on an investigation is necessary. The types of samples suitable for culture-independent diagnostic

tests, which focus on the genotype (sequencing or PCR methods) or physical characteristics (mass spectroscopy) of the organism, can be different from those sample types
needed for classical culture methods, which focus on the phenotype of the organism
through methods such as serotyping and antimicrobial susceptibility testing. Protocols
for culture-independent diagnostic tests often destroy the sample during nucleic acid
or other target extraction, leaving no viable organisms to culture. Ideally, multiple
samples should be collected, enabling both molecular and classical testing. However, if
samples are in short supply or packaging and shipping limitations are a factor, testing
and sample collection decisions should be made in advance in collaboration with the
laboratory to determine whether molecular or classic tests would generate the most
useful information.

For all tests, consult with the laboratory as early in the investigation as possible to address the following criteria for appropriate test selection:

- Preapproval.
- Supplemental information.
- Supplemental forms.
- Sample types.
- Acceptable samples.
- Minimum volumes required.
- Storage and preservation of samples.
- Sample transport medium.
- Sample labeling.
- Shipping instructions.
- Sample handling requirements.
- Testing methods.
- Testing turnaround time.
- Test interferences and limitations.
- Additional information.
- Laboratory points of contact.

Step 2. Collaborate on the Planning and Execution of Field Sample Collection

Collaborate with the laboratory before collecting samples to ensure samples are collected safely and are acceptable for the selected test. Accidental exposures during
sample collection could result in severe illness, and unacceptable sample collection
can result in missed opportunities for testing. For example, collecting blood from 20

people with potential exposures to an unknown pathogen and using the wrong anti-coagulant can result in delayed microbial identification and delayed treatment, which could have serious consequences. The laboratory scientist can also provide ecology, growth, transmission, and pathogenesis expertise about microorganisms, as well as chemical and radiologic expertise. This expertise can support the investigation in many ways, some of which include

- A risk assessment of the planned sampling activities to create a safe environment for the work. At a minimum, the risk assessment should identify the potential biological, chemical, radiologic, and physical hazards and plan appropriate mitigations, including the use of personal protective equipment (PPE), to minimize exposure to hazards.
- A sampling plan, which includes preliminary hypotheses and ways the laboratory can assist in testing those hypotheses through targeted sampling.
- Sample collection methods, which need to be appropriate and sufficient for the specific tests (e.g., immunologic assays require specific timing of sample collection for diagnostic testing to be performed).
- Sample collection training, including assessing whether all the field investigators have adequate sampling experience and training (including training in PPE use) or whether laboratory personnel should deploy to the field to collect samples.
- Sample transport. Ideally, sampling activities should be planned to ensure that shipments arrive at the receiving laboratory on a weekday. Some shipments cannot be accepted on weekends.

A public health professional conducting an outbreak investigation should follow these generalized recommendations during sampling:

- Identify and obtain appropriate PPE in sufficient quantities before deploying to the field and double-check it for completeness at the sample collection location. Ensure the team has been trained in donning, doffing, cleaning/disinfection, storage, and proper disposal of the designated PPE.
- Review all relevant safety, infection control, and patient management guidelines before, and adhere to them during, sample collection. For instance, identify and maintain a specific area for donning and doffing the designated PPE and have a plan for managing sample collection waste.
- Collect an appropriate volume of sample.

- Label each clinical sample with at least two identifiers that link the sample to the patient, with the expectation that personal identifying information will not be used.
- Label each nonclinical sample (e.g., environmental, animal) with at least two identifiers that enable linking of the sample with the most pertinent organism, place, or thing (e.g., OrganismID and LocationID, SampleTypeID and MedicalDeviceID).
- Coordinate with local and state labs and clinicians to obtain samples. Do not collect samples without specific training in the collection procedure because *the generalized guidance in this chapter might not be appropriate for a specific requested test.*
- Review the special considerations discussed later and contact the laboratory for specific guidance before sampling.

Special Consideration: Risk Assessment

A risk is the possibility that an undesired event will occur (i.e., a function of the likelihood and consequences of a particular undesired event). Before conducting a field investigation or any laboratory activity, assess the risks associated with that activity. The epidemiologists and the laboratory scientists should conduct the risk assessment for a field investigation jointly, with assistance from other subject-matter experts including local and state public health laboratory scientists and epidemiologists, clinicians, appropriate facility staff, and appropriate emergency response planners and responders. Share the results of the risk assessment among the investigation team members so that everyone understands the risks involved. Use the results of the risk assessment as the basis for determining how to mitigate those risks. During the investigation, routinely monitor and reassess operations to identify and mitigate additional risks and to account for any new information or circumstance associated with particular activities. After the field investigation, review operations to identify ways to improve future field investigation risk assessment.

The principles of risk governance (26,27) articulate that a risk assessment should follow three general steps:

1. *Define the situation*: What work will occur?
2. *Define the risks in that situation*: What can go wrong?
3. *Characterize each of the risks*: How likely is each risk to occur? What would be the consequences of each risk?

Start the risk assessment process by thoroughly defining the situation and the activity. Particularly important is where the work will take place, who will conduct it (including their knowledge, skills, and abilities), what equipment they will use (including sampling and PPE), and what hazards they will encounter. A *hazard* is something that has the potential to cause harm, such as a sharp object or a biological agent. Considerations of risk should address the most obvious agent-related hazards of a field investigation (e.g., unintended exposure, physical injury). However, risk assessments should also encompass the less obvious hazards that could result in negative consequences. For each field investigation, in addition to agent-related hazards, also consider any investigation activities–related hazards that might result in negative outcomes (e.g., poor sample collection yielding incorrect or ambiguous laboratory results; shipping hazard resulting in delayed or incorrect case management; data management issues with patient privacy or consent; inadvertent violation of facility rules or local, state, or federal regulations; miscommunications that might erode collaborative relationships).

In a field investigation, the hazards are multifactorial, diverse, unique, and potentially of major consequence. To mitigate the risks, everyone involved in an investigation must consider everything that might go wrong during the various stages of that activity and then evaluate each risk from the perspective of its likelihood of occurrence and the consequences. After prioritizing those risks from highest to lowest, review the use of specific mitigations measures to reduce those identified risks. Before work begins, agree that the mitigated risks are acceptable. *If the risks cannot be adequately mitigated and remain unacceptable, do not undertake the work.*

Special Consideration: Etiologic Agents of Disease Syndromes

The same disease syndrome (e.g., respiratory) can be caused by one or more of many pathogens (e.g., influenza virus, *Legionella spp.*, or hantaviruses) or by an abiological chemical or radiation exposure (e.g., chemical-induced acute respiratory distress syndrome). It is also possible for clinical presentations to be atypical, which can complicate field investigations (28–30). To maximize the effectiveness of investigations of outbreaks of unknown etiology, investigators need to collaborate with laboratory and epidemiology subject matter experts representing a diverse range of potential etiologic agents. Table 9.1 can be used as a tool in these larger discussions to help formulate hypotheses about the etiologic agents of various disease syndromes and to determine appropriate samples to collect for testing. Additional online resources for investigations of outbreaks of unknown etiology based on disease syndrome are also identified.

Special Consideration: Sample Collection

Table 9.2 shows sample collection supplies, a basic collection procedure, and sampling considerations for various clinical sample types for infectious disease testing. For

TABLE 9.1 Infectious disease[a] syndromes and types of clinical samples

Syndrome and online resource	Some possible etiologies	Sample type	Suspected agent
Dermatologic	Chickenpox, monkeypox, variola, vaccinia, measles, cutaneous anthrax, herpes,	Vesicular fluid, scab, serum, vesicular exudate	Viruses, bacteria,
Diarrheal (http://cifor.us/products/guidelines)	Watery (cholera), dysentery (shigellosis), febrile gastroenteritis (typhoid fever), vomiting (norovirus, bacterial intoxications)	Feces, blood, emesis	Bacteria, viruses, parasites, toxins, chemicals
Hemorrhagic fever	Arboviral (dengue fever), arenaviral (Lassa fever), filoviral (Ebola virus disease), malaria	Blood, blood smear, serum, postmortem tissue biopsy	Viruses, parasites
Jaundice	Hepatitis A–E, spirochetal (leptospirosis), yellow fever	Serum, postmortem liver biopsy, blood culture, urine	Viruses, bacteria
Neurologic	Guillain-Barré syndrome, polio, meningoencephalitis, rabies, meningitis	Stool, cerebrospinal fluid, blood, blood smear, serum, throat swab, postmortem samples	Viruses, bacteria
Ophthalmologic	Trachoma, keratoconjunctivitis, conjunctivitis	Conjunctival swab/smear, serum, throat swab	Viruses, bacteria
Respiratory (https://www.cdc.gov/urdo/index.html)	Influenza, hantavirus, pertussis, legionellosis, pneumonia, tuberculosis, severe acute respiratory syndrome coronavirus	Throat swab, serum, nasopharyngeal swab, blood, sputum, urine	Viruses, bacteria, toxins
Systemic	Varied and often caused by same agent as other syndromes	Postmortem tissue biopsy, serum, cerebrospinal fluid, urine, blood culture, aspirate, blood smear	Viruses, parasites, bacteria

[a]For definition and review of syndromes for chemical or radiologic agents, see the CDC Emergency Preparedness and Response website for chemical (https://emergency.cdc.gov/chemical/) and radiologic (https://emergency.cdc.gov/radiation/index.asp) emergencies. *Source*: Reference 38.

TABLE 9.2 Sample collection for suspected infectious agent exposures

Sample type	Supplies	Considerations
Blood	Sterile collection tubes	Patient age and other demographics may be useful for laboratory to select reference ranges.
	Needles and syringes	
	Tourniquet	Collect ~2.5 mL of blood for every 1 mL of serum needed.
	Skin antiseptic solution	Store blood immediately on ice unless given other instruction by the lab. Do not freeze.
	Gauze pads	
	Bandage	EDTA is the preferred anticoagulant.
	Labels	If collecting into a vacuum tube with additive, fill the tube until vacuum stops to maintain effective concentration of blood and additive, and mix by gently inverting tube 8–10 times.
	Necessary forms	
	Sharps container	
	Infectious waste bags	
	Hand hygiene supplies	Use plastic tubes whenever possible.
	Latex or nitrile gloves	Try to avoid hemolysis by consulting with the lab about sample collection location, method, and needle gauge.
	Lab coat	
	Face shield or goggles	Try to avoid hyperbilirubinemia and lipemia by consulting with the lab about fasting requirements.
	Mask, if respiratory symptoms	Obtain samples before treatment, if possible. If treatment has already started note the treatment information on the sample line list.
Sputum	Sterile wide-mouth container	Avoid collecting salvia or postnasal discharge.
	Latex or nitrile gloves	Viral and bacterial samples might have different storage and transport conditions.
	Laboratory coat	
	Labels	
	Necessary forms	
	Infectious waste bags	
	Hand hygiene supplies	
Feces	Sterile container	Obtain samples before treatment, if possible. If treatment has already started, note the treatment information on the sample line list.
	Latex or nitrile gloves	
	Lab coat	
	Labels	Collect as soon as possible after onset of diarrhea.
	Necessary forms	Keep at 4–8°C.
	Infectious waste bags	Parasitic tests might require a fixative.
	Hand hygiene supplies	

(continued)

TABLE 9.2 (Continued)

Sample type	Supplies	Considerations
Swabs	Sterile swabs Sterile saline Sterile transport tubes Latex or nitrile gloves Face shield or goggles Lab coat Labels Necessary forms Infectious waste bags Hand hygiene supplies	Premoisten swab with saline Use only sterile Dacron or Rayon swabs with plastic shafts or, if available, flocked swabs. Do NOT use calcium alginate swabs, cotton swabs, or swabs with wooden sticks. Place swabs in agent-specific media for transport.
Urine	Sterile container Antiseptic wipes Latex or nitrile gloves Lab coat Labels Any necessary forms Infectious waste bags Hand hygiene supplies Face shield or goggles	Obtain samples before treatment, if possible. If treatment has already started note the treatment information on the sample line list. If collecting from debilitated patients, assist in cleaning the external genitalia before collection If collecting from infants, use a urine collection bag if necessary. Chemical and biological tests might differ in collection, storage, and transport conditions. Keep samples at 4°C.
Vesicular fluid, scabs, aspirates	Sterile swabs Sterile saline Sterile transport tubes Sterile lancet or needle Syringe and wide-bore needle Sterile forceps Skin antiseptic solution Latex or nitrile gloves Face shield or goggles Lab coat Labels Necessary forms Infectious waste bags Hand hygiene supplies	A suspected case of smallpox must be immediately reported to the state public health lab and CDC. Viral and bacterial samples might have different storage and transport conditions.

TABLE 9.3 Sample collection for suspected environmental toxicant exposures

Suspected toxicant	Sample to collect in order of preference	Adults and children ≥10 years old	Children <10 years old/ babies
Organic	1. Serum 2. Urine 3. Whole blood (Heparin)	1. Two 10 mL tubes without anticoagulant 2. 50 mL 3. One 7 mL tube or three 4 mL tubes or four 3 mL tubes	1. One 5-mL tube without anticoagulant 2. 10–20 mL 3. Two 3 mL tubes
Inorganic	1. Urine 2. Whole blood (EDTA) 3. Serum	1. 50 mL 2. One 3 mL tube 3. One 7 mL trace metals-free tube	1. 10–20 mL 2. One 3 mL tube 3. One 7 mL trace metals-free tube
Unknown	1. Serum 2. Urine 3. Whole blood (EDTA) 4. Whole blood (Heparin)	1. Two 10 mL tubes without anticoagulant 2. 50 mL 3. One 2 mL tube 4. One 7 mL tube or three 4 mL tubes or four 3 mL tubes	1. One 5 mL tube without anticoagulant 2. 10–20 mL 3. One 2 mL tube 4. Two 3 mL tubes

similar information for environmental toxicant testing, see Table 9.3. These guidelines are presented to help in planning for sample collection in the field but should always be discussed with the laboratory before sample collection takes place.

Special Consideration: Potential Sampling Pitfalls

One reason it is important to contact the laboratory before sampling is because of sampling pitfalls. The pitfalls can include issues with sampling tools (e.g., inhibition of tests by certain swab materials), sample collection technique (e.g., hemolysis of blood samples), sample storage (e.g., degradation of RNA), or sample timing (e.g., matched sera). Table 9.4 describes some specific pitfalls to avoid, but it is not a comprehensive list, so consult with the laboratory prior to collecting samples.

Special Consideration: Personal Protective Equipment

PPE is specialized clothing or equipment used to protect against exposure to hazards that can cause serious injury or illness. Exposures can result from contact with chemical, radiologic, physical, electrical, mechanical, or other hazards. PPE may include items such as gloves, safety glasses and shoes, earplugs or muffs, hard hats, respirators, or coveralls, vests, and full-body suits. *PPE selection should be tailored to the specific risks associated with*

TABLE 9.4 Specific sampling pitfalls, by laboratory test type

Test type	Consideration
Antimicrobial susceptibility testing	Store at conditions best suited to maintaining viability of culture.
	Low viral loads and genetic variance can affect assays.
	Include treatment history of patient.
Culture	Therapeutic agents can affect the detection of organisms.
	Preservatives (formalin or alcohol) can affect organism viability.
	Disinfectants (chlorine, Lysol, alcohol) can affect tests.
	Cultures of some organisms might require stricter shipping rules.
	Storing blood at temperatures other than 2–8°C can affect tests.
	Multiple freezes–thaws (especially ≥3) can affect test performance.
Molecular	Hemolysis can affect test results.
	Heparin can interfere with molecular assays.
	Insufficient volume of sample can invalidate tests.
	Therapeutic agents can affect the detection of organisms.
	Co-infections or contaminations can affect test results.
	Calcium alginate swabs or swabs with wooden sticks can contain substances that inhibit some molecular assays.
	Not separating serum from cells in blood samples can result in RNA degradation.
	Multiple freezes–thaws (especially ≥3) can affect test performance.
Pathology	Prolonged fixation (>2 weeks) can interfere with some assays.
	Decomposition of tissues can affect test performance.
	Less than 1:10 ratio of tissue to 10% formalin can prevent fixation.
Serology	Failure to collect paired samples (acute and convalescent) can result in uninterpretable results
	Contamination can interfere with testing.
	Bilirubin, lipids, and hemoglobin can interfere with serologic assays.
	Not separating and freezing serum from cells in blood samples can result in antibody degradation.
	Failure to use plastic tubes can prevent shipment and may result in samples not being accepted at the lab.
	Pooled samples can cause difficulties in interpretation of lab results.

each individual field investigation. The Occupational Safety and Health Administration has created multiple online resources that can be used to help select appropriate PPE and identify additional safety-related information for specific hazards (https://www.osha.gov/dts/osta/oshasoft/index.html). Additional Occupational Safety and Health Administration (https://www.osha.gov/Publications/osha3151.pdf) and National Institute for Occupational Safety and Health (https://www.cdc.gov/niosh/docs/2005-100/pdfs/2005-100.pdf) guidance is also available.

In general, there are three major questions to consider when selecting PPE. First, what is the anticipated exposure type (splash, spill, spray), volume (large, small), and source (chemical, biological, or radiologic agent)? Second, what PPE is durable enough and appropriate for the task (protect against fluids, powders, gases)? Third, how will the PPE affect movement and work (appropriate size, not too hot)? Some PPE considerations are shown in Table 9.5, but investigation teams should consult with appropriate laboratory scientists on the types of PPE that are most effective for any particular field investigation as biological, chemical, and radiologic hazards each require specialized PPE.

Step 3. Collaborate with Laboratory for Storage and Shipment of Samples

The sender is responsible for ensuring that samples are stored and transported to the laboratory under appropriate conditions. Shipping requirements for infectious or potentially harmful samples submitted for diagnostic or investigational purposes must be packaged and shipped in compliance with appropriate regulations. Before shipping any samples from the field investigation, consult with the receiving laboratory and appropriate shipping experts to ensure adherence to relevant regulations and best practices. The information and links given here provide a starting point to navigating the storage, submission, and shipping requirements you may need to address.

- Samples to be sent to CDC for infectious disease testing:
  - *Storage requirements*: See the specific storage requirements for each test at https://www.cdc.gov/laboratory/specimen-submission/list.html
  - *Submission forms*: https://www.cdc.gov/laboratory/specimen-submission/form.html
  - *Shipping instructions*: http://www.cdc.gov/laboratory/specimen-submission/shipping-packing.html
- Samples to be sent to CDC for chemical or radiologic testing:
  - *Radiologic*: https://emergency.cdc.gov/radiation/labinfo.asp
  - *Chemical*: https://emergency.cdc.gov/chemical/lab.asp

TABLE 9.5 Personal protective equipment (PPE) considerations for collecting potentially infectious samples[a]

Examples of PPE	When to wear	Considerations
Apron, lab coat, gown, coveralls	To protect skin and clothing from splash hazards	Recommend clean, disposable, fluid-resistant isolation gown that covers torso, fits comfortably, and has long sleeves that are snug at wrists. Consider coverage (i.e., apron instead of gown for limited potential contamination), cleaning (i.e., laundering and reuse of gown), permeability to fluids, and patient risk (i.e., sterile gown for invasive procedure).
Latex or nitrile gloves	To protect hands from touch hazards	Recommend single pair of nonsterile, disposable vinyl, latex, or nitrile gloves changed between patients and samples or when torn or soiled. When selecting or using gloves, consider fit of gloves, duration of task, "wetness" of task, potential for transmission from gloves to patient, potential for touching environmental surfaces.
Surgical masks	To protect mouth and nose from splash, spray hazards	Recommend masks that cover nose and mouth and prevent fluid penetration with flexible nose piece and elastic straps to secure fit. If aerosols are a concern, wear a respirator instead.
N95 respirator, elastomeric respirator, PAPR	To protect respiratory tract from inhalable particulate hazards	Recommend N95 to protect from inhalable particles <5 μ in diameter. For an invasive procedure that might result in large droplets or copious aerosols, consider a higher level respirator (e.g., PAPR). Respirator use requires medical evaluation, fit testing, training, and fit checking before each use.
Goggles, safety glasses, face shield	To protect eyes from splash hazards	Recommend snug-fitting, antifog goggles or safety glasses or face shield that covers forehead and below chin and wraps around the side of the face. Personal glasses are not a substitute for goggles. Wear goggles that fit over prescription lenses.

[a]For definition and review of PPE for chemical or radiologic agents, please see the CDC Emergency Preparedness and Response website for chemical (https://emergency.cdc.gov/chemical/) and radiologic (https://emergency.cdc.gov/radiation/index.asp) emergencies. PAPR, powered air purifying respirator; PPE, personal protective equipment.

- Samples to be sent to a state, regional, or local laboratory
  - Work with the state, regional, local, or facility representative to contact the appropriate laboratory.
  - In the event of an emergency in the field, contact the state public health laboratory. A list of emergency contacts for state public health laboratories can be found at http://www.aphl.org/programs/preparedness/Crisis-Management/Pages/Emergency-Lab-Contacts.aspx

The following checklist provides some practical advice about packaging and shipping samples.

- Double-check that all sample containers are closed and intact.
- Disinfect the outside of the sample container before transport, storage, or shipment. Be sure to maintain the integrity of the labels.
- Transport samples in their primary container (e.g., tube, bottle, sample container) placed into a sealed and leak-proof secondary container (plastic bag, plastic container) prior to placing in the outer container (shipping envelope, shipping box).
- Ensure samples are cushioned to prevent breakage.
- Create a line-list of the samples with all appropriate information (e.g., sample site, sample type, patient identifier, device identifier, environment location, suspected source of sample).
- In some investigations (e.g., when criminal activity is suspected), a formal chain of custody form may be needed. Consult your local public health officials, shipping experts, and the receiving laboratory to obtain appropriate forms.
- Determine the specific shipping requirements of the samples (https://www.iata.org/whatwedo/cargo/dgr/Documents/infectious-substance-classification-DGR56-en.pdf).
- Provide the tracking number of the shipment to the laboratory.

Step 4. Collaborate on the Interpretation of Laboratory Test Results

Laboratory tests are more complicated than ever to interpret, and the subsequent conclusions from—and uses of—laboratory data from any field investigation are most effective and reliable when collaboration is strong among the following:

- Laboratory scientists, who can explain the language of the laboratory report and any specifics of the test or organism.
- Epidemiologists, who interpret the tests in the context of the field investigation.
- Clinicians, who interpret the tests in the context of patient management.

Because each of these specialties has different knowledge and serves different purposes, laboratory data are most effective when interpretation occurs in collaboration. This ensures that data limitations and strengths are understood and that the potential occurrence and consequences of false positives or negatives, undetermined results due to improper sample collection or insufficient sample volume, and nonreportable results due to values below the limit of detection or other confounders found during testing are minimized. Issues to consider when interpreting laboratory results may include the following:

- Laboratory tests for field investigations should be interpreted in the context of properly framed epidemiologic hypotheses. Investigators should always consider why the test was chosen and what was being asked.
- Interpretation of test results depends on sensitivity and specificity of the selected test. Consider how the prevalence of disease will affect the predictive value of the test.
- Consider what population the test characteristics are derived from and how that might differ from the population being tested.
- If a sample is negative on nonspecific media, the sample cannot be interpreted as negative unless it is also negative on a suspected agent-specific medium.
- In field investigations that involve emerging pathogens, Koch's postulates form the basis of proof that an emergent agent is the etiologic agent. Therefore, the interpretation should consider the successful fulfillment of each of Koch's postulates. Just because an agent is found does not necessarily mean it caused the disease.
- Consider the status of the patient because pathogens behave differently in different hosts. Patient factors to consider include immunologic status, treatments administered, age, physiologic status, sex, and race.
- Molecular typing and other relatedness studies can confirm the relatedness of isolates to support the epidemiologic hypotheses generated by the field investigation. Interpretation of relatedness is specific for the typing assay used.
- Reference ranges are not precise and can vary by laboratory, depend on the test, and are typically selected to contain 95% of healthy persons. However, correlation between out-of-range values and illness is not always clear. Consider the sample size used to collect the values that established the reference range, the demographics of the population, and the reference range sample population.

Interpreting test results in collaboration with the laboratory is a standard best practice. Table 9.6 shows some considerations for interpretation of laboratory results; these

TABLE 9.6 Interpretation guidelines for types of laboratory tests

Test type	True positive	False positive	True negative	False negative
Molecular	Presence of suspected organism in sample: "positive"	Nonspecific binding of primers or probe Cross-contamination of samples	Absence of suspected organism in sample: "negative"	Failure of amplification reaction Failure of primer or probe binding
Culture	Presence of suspected organism in sample: "positive"	Contamination during collection Cross-contamination with another sample in lab	Absence of suspected organism in sample: "negative"	Sample collected after antimicrobial treatment began Media used for growth does not support suspect organism Source of infection was removed
Serology (39)	Presence of antibodies specific for suspected agent: "exposure"	Cross-reactivity Nonspecific inhibitors and agglutinins	Absence of antibodies specific for suspected agent: "no exposure"	Tolerance Improper timing of sample Nonspecific inhibitors Toxic substances Antibiotic-induced suppression incomplete or blocking antibody
Antimicrobial resistance testing (40)	Microorganism is inhibited by normal doses of antimicrobial agent(s): "susceptible"	Wrong assay selected for organism or drug being tested Media not sufficient for growth of organism being tested Insufficient number of organisms added Wrong standard tables used	Microorganism is not inhibited by normal doses of antimicrobial agents: "resistant"	Wrong assay selected for organism or drug being tested Insufficient antimicrobial added Wrong standard tables used
Pathology (41)	Presence of suspected organism in pathology sample: "positive"	Cross-reactivity Nonspecific interactions	Absence of suspected organism in pathology sample: "negative"	Wrong assay selected for sample type or organism Failure of stain or specific antibodies Wrong sample type submitted

can be used as a guide to facilitate collaborations with clinicians, epidemiologists, and laboratory scientists.

Step 5. Continue Laboratory Collaboration Through Publication of Findings

Any field investigation could lead to discovery of a new pandemic pathogen (31), identification of a product or device hazard (32), discovery of an old pathogen in a new place (33), identification of a new risk to public health (34), or even arrest of a criminal (35). Given the significance of field investigations, accuracy and completeness are critical. History has shown that when public health recommendations must (for political reasons or in emergency situations) be based solely on epidemiologic data, unintended consequences can occur (36). Similarly, poor laboratory diagnostic capabilities also can create unnecessary difficulties in patient care (37). Therefore, the most effective and reliable field investigation teams are built on a strong collaboration between epidemiology and laboratory science. Sustaining that cooperation through all stages of the scientific process, including analysis of the data, formulation of conclusions, and presentation or publication of results, is also necessary. Several general considerations can help inform that collaboration:

- Investigators should understand the tests and how to interpret them, including knowing the test limitations and considering those limitations in the context of the hypotheses.
- Laboratory staff should conduct data analysis from laboratory samples using appropriate biostatistics and reference standards.
- Field investigators should collaborate with the laboratory staff to determine whether laboratory results support or refute the epidemiologic hypotheses.
- Field investigators (both epidemiologists and laboratory scientists) should collaborate to design laboratory or epidemiologic studies that can further develop the field investigation findings into public health guidance.
- Field investigators and laboratory staff should jointly pursue publication of results, as deemed appropriate by the investigation and in accordance with all appropriate author guidelines.

CONCLUSION

Epidemiology is the scientific foundation of public health. However, like any foundation, it must rest on solid ground—in this case, a composite of scientific disciplines. Local, state, and federal public health laboratories have experts in a wide variety of technical areas, including microbiology, parasitology, mycology, statistics, bioinformatics, molecular biology, toxicology, ecology, chemistry, occupational health, microbial ecology, laboratory science, environmental health, biosafety, biosecurity, clinical management, and medical technology. Therefore, creating stable and sustainable collaborations with the laboratory will improve the practice of epidemiology and, in turn, improve public health.

REFERENCES

1. Berche, P., Louis Pasteur, from crystals of life to vaccination. *Clin Microbiol Infect.* 2012;18 Suppl 5:1–6.
2. Dowdle WR, Mayer LW, Steinberg KK, Ghiya ND, Popovic T; CDC. Laboratory contributions to public health. *MMWR Suppl.* 2011;60:27–34.
3. Glick TH, Gregg MB, Berman B, Mallison G, Rhodes WW Jr, Kassanoff I. Pontiac fever. An epidemic of unknown etiology in a health department: I. Clinical and epidemiologic aspects. *Am J Epidemiol.* 1978;107:149–60.
4. Kaufmann AF, McDade JE, Patton CM, et al. Pontiac fever: isolation of the etiologic agent (*Legionella pneumophilia*) and demonstration of its mode of transmission. *Am J Epidemiol.* 1981;114:337–47.
5. Jernigan DB, Raghunathan PL, Bell BP, et al. Investigation of bioterrorism-related anthrax, United States, 2001: epidemiologic findings. *Emerg Infect Dis.* 2002;8:1019–28.
6. Gieraltowski L, Higa J, Peralta V, et al. National outbreak of multidrug resistant *Salmonella* Heidelberg infections linked to a single poultry company. *PLoS One.* 2016;11:e0162369.
7. CDC. Severe acute respiratory syndrome (SARS) and coronavirus testing—United States, 2003. *MMWR.* 2003;52:297–302.
8. Moturi E, Mahmud A, Kamadjeu R, et al. Contribution of contact sampling in increasing sensitivity of poliovirus detection during a polio outbreak—Somalia, 2013. *Open Forum Infect Dis.* 2016;3:ofw111.
9. Hoffmaster AR, Fitzgerald CC, Ribot E, Mayer LW. Molecular subtyping of *Bacillus anthracis* and the 2001 bioterrorism-associated anthrax outbreak, United States. *Emerg Infect Dis.* 2002;8:1111–6.
10. Nakao JH, Talkington D, Bopp CA, et al. Unusually high illness severity and short incubation periods in two foodborne outbreaks of *Salmonella* Heidelberg infections with potential coincident *Staphylococcus aureus* intoxication. *Epidemiol Infect.* 2018;146:19–27.
11. Folster JP, Grass JE, Bicknese A, Taylor J, Friedman CR, Whichard JM. Characterization of resistance genes and plasmids from outbreaks and illness clusters caused by *Salmonella* resistant to ceftriaxone in the United States, 2011–2012. *Microb Drug Resist.* 2017;23:188–93.
12. de Oliveira AM, Skarbinski J, Ouma PO, et al. Performance of malaria rapid diagnostic tests as part of routine malaria case management in Kenya. *Am J Trop Med Hyg.* 2009;80:470–4.
13. Tyndall JA, Gerona R, De Portu G, et al. An outbreak of acute delirium from exposure to the synthetic cannabinoid AB-CHMINACA. *Clin Toxicol (Phila).* 2015;53:950–6.
14. Flint M, Goodman CH, Bearden S, et al. Ebola virus diagnostics: the US Centers for Disease Control and Prevention laboratory in Sierra Leone, August 2014 to March 2015. *J Infect Dis.* 2015;212 Suppl 2:S350–8.
15. Jelden KC, Iwen PC, Herstein JJ, et al. U.S. Ebola treatment center clinical laboratory support. *J Clin Microbiol.* 2016;54:1031–5.
16. McCarty CL, Basler C, Karwowski M, et al. Response to importation of a case of Ebola virus disease—Ohio, October 2014. *MMWR.* 2014;63:1089–91.
17. CDC. Spinal and paraspinal infections associated with contaminated methylprednisolone acetate injections—Michigan, 2012–2013. *MMWR.* 2013;62:377–81.
18. Lockhart SR, Pham CD, Gade L, et al. Preliminary laboratory report of fungal infections associated with contaminated methylprednisolone injections. *J Clin Microbiol.* 2013;51:2654–61.

19. CDC. Recognition of illness associated with exposure to chemical agents—United States, 2003. *MMWR.* 2003;52:938–40.

20. Baron EJ, Miller JM, Weinstein MP, et al. A guide to utilization of the microbiology laboratory for diagnosis of infectious diseases: 2013 recommendations by the Infectious Diseases Society of America (IDSA) and the American Society for Microbiology (ASM)(a). *Clin Infect Dis.* 2013;57:e22–e121.

21. Chen L, Brueck SE, Niemeier MT. Evaluation of potential noise exposures in hospital operating rooms. *AORN J.* 2012;96:412–8.

22. Dickerson AS, Rahbar MH, Han I, et al. Autism spectrum disorder prevalence and proximity to industrial facilities releasing arsenic, lead or mercury. *Sci Total Environ.* 2015;536:245–51.

23. Erck Lambert AB, Parks SE, Camperlengo L, et al. Death scene investigation and autopsy practices in sudden unexpected infant deaths. *J Pediatr.* 2016;174:84–90 e1.

24. Kennedy C, Lordo R, Sucosky MS, Boehm R, Brown MJ. Evaluating the effectiveness of state specific lead-based paint hazard risk reduction laws in preventing recurring incidences of lead poisoning in children. *Int J Hyg Environ Health.* 2016;219:110–7.

25. Miller CW1, Ansari A, Martin C, Chang A, Buzzell J, Whitcomb RC Jr. Use of epidemiological data and direct bioassay for prioritization of affected populations in a large-scale radiation emergency. *Health Phys.* 2011;101:209–15.

26. Renn O, Graham P. *Risk governance: towards an integrative approach.* Geneva: International Risk Governance Council; 2005:157.

27. Salerno RM, Gaudioso J. *Laboratory biorisk management: biosafety and biosecurity.* Boca Raton, FL: CRC Press; 2015.

28. Sejvar J, Lutterloh E, Naiene J, et al. Neurologic manifestations associated with an outbreak of typhoid fever, Malawi–Mozambique, 2009: an epidemiologic investigation. *PLoS One.* 2012;7:e46099.

29. Balestri R, Bellino M, Landini L, et al. Atypical presentation of enterovirus infection in adults: outbreak of 'hand, foot, mouth and scalp disease' in northern Italy. *J Eur Acad Dermatol Venereol.* 2017;32:e60–e61.

30. Majumdar R, Jana CK, Ghosh S, Biswas U. Clinical spectrum of dengue fever in a tertiary care centre with particular reference to atypical presentation in the 2012 outbreak in Kolkata. *J Indian Med Assoc.* 2012;110:904–6.

31. CDC. Pneumocystis pneumonia—Los Angeles. *MMWR.* 1981;30:250–2.

32. Hawley B, Casey ML, Cox-Ganser JM, Edwards N, Fedan KB, Cummings KJ. Notes from the field: respiratory symptoms and skin irritation among hospital workers using a new disinfection product—Pennsylvania, 2015. *MMWR.* 2016;65:400–1.

33. Duffy MR, Chen TH, Hancock WT, et al. Zika virus outbreak on Yap Island, Federated States of Micronesia. *N Engl J Med.* 2009;360:2536–43.

34. Cherry C, Leong K, Wallen R, Buttke D. Notes from the field: injuries associated with bison encounters—Yellowstone National Park, 2015. *MMWR.* 2016;65:293–4.

35. Istre GR, Gustafson TL, Baron RC, Martin DL, Orlowski JP. A mysterious cluster of deaths and cardiopulmonary arrests in a pediatric intensive care unit. *N Engl J Med.* 1985;313:205–11.

36. Sencer D. How should the federal government respond to the influenza problem caused by a new virus? In: Neustadt RE, Fineberg HV. *The swine flu affair: decision-making on a slippery disease.* Washington, DC: National Academies Press; 1978. https://www.ncbi.nlm.nih.gov/books/NBK219607/

37. Moore A, Nelson C, Molins C, Mead P, Schriefer M. Current guidelines, common clinical pitfalls, and future directions for laboratory diagnosis of Lyme disease, United States. *Emerg Infect Dis.* 2016;22.

38. World Health Organization. *Guidelines for the collection of clinical specimens during field investigation of outbreaks.* Geneva: World Health Organization; 2000.

39. Crump JA1, Corder JR, Henshaw NG, Reller LB. Development, implementation, and impact of acceptability criteria for serologic tests for infectious diseases. *J Clin Microbiol.* 2004;42:881–3.

40. Jorgensen JH, Ferraro MJ. Antimicrobial susceptibility testing: a review of general principles and contemporary practices. *Clin Infect Dis.* 2009;49:1749–55.

41. Empson MB. Statistics in the pathology laboratory: diagnostic test interpretation. *Pathology.* 2002;34:365–9.

/// 10 /// COLLECTING AND ANALYZING QUALITATIVE DATA

BRENT WOLFF, FRANK MAHONEY, ANNA LEENA LOHINIVA, AND MELISSA CORKUM

INTRODUCTION

Qualitative research methods are a key component of field epidemiologic investigations because they can provide insight into the perceptions, values, opinions, and community norms where investigations are being conducted (1,2). Open-ended inquiry methods, the mainstay of qualitative interview techniques, are essential in formative research for exploring contextual factors and rationales for risk behaviors that do not fit neatly into predefined categories. For example, during the 2014–2015 Ebola virus disease outbreaks in parts of West Africa, understanding the cultural implications of burial practices within different communities was crucial to designing and monitoring interventions for safe burials (Box 10.1). In program evaluations, qualitative methods can assist the investigator in diagnosing what went right or wrong as part of a process evaluation or in troubleshooting why a program might not be working as well as expected. When designing an intervention, qualitative methods can be useful in exploring dimensions of acceptability to increase the chances of intervention acceptance and success. When performed

---

BOX 10.1
QUALITATIVE RESEARCH DURING THE EBOLA VIRUS DISEASE OUTBREAKS IN PARTS OF WEST AFRICA (2014)

Qualitative research was used extensively in response to the Ebola virus disease outbreaks in parts of West Africa to understand burial practices and to design culturally appropriate strategies to ensure safe burials. Qualitative studies were also used to monitor key aspects of the response.

In October 2014, Liberia experienced an abrupt and steady decrease in case counts and deaths in contrast with predicted disease models of an increased case count. At the time, communities were resistant to entering Ebola treatment centers, raising the possibility that patients were not being referred for care and communities might be conducting occult burials.

To assess what was happening at the community level, the Liberian Emergency Operations Center recruited epidemiologists from the US Department of Health and Human Services/Centers for Disease Control and Prevention and the African Union to investigate the problem.

Teams conducted in-depth interviews and focus group discussions with community leaders, local funeral directors, and coffin makers and learned that communities were not conducting occult burials and that the overall number of burials was less than what they had experienced in previous years. Other key findings included the willingness of funeral directors to cooperate with disease response efforts, the need for training of funeral home workers, and considerable community resistance to cremation practices. These findings prompted the Emergency Operations Center to open a burial ground for Ebola decedents, support enhanced testing of burials in the private sector, and train private-sector funeral workers regarding safe burial practices.

Source: Melissa Corkum, personal communication.

in conjunction with quantitative studies, qualitative methods can help the investigator confirm, challenge, or deepen the validity of conclusions than either component might have yielded alone (1,2).

CHOOSING WHEN TO APPLY QUALITATIVE METHODS

Similar to quantitative approaches, qualitative research seeks answers to specific questions by using rigorous approaches to collecting and compiling information and producing findings that can be applicable beyond the study population. The fundamental difference in approaches lies in how they translate real-life complexities of initial observations into units of analysis. Data collected in qualitative studies typically are in the form of text or visual images, which provide rich sources of insight but also tend to be bulky and time-consuming to code and analyze. Practically speaking, qualitative study designs tend to favor small, purposively selected samples ideal for case studies or in-depth analysis (1). The combination of purposive sampling and open-ended question formats deprive qualitative study designs of the power to quantify and generalize conclusions, one of the key limitations of this approach.

Qualitative scientists might argue, however, that the generalizability and precision possible through probabilistic sampling and categorical outcomes are achieved at the cost of enhanced validity, nuance, and naturalism that less structured approaches offer (3). Open-ended techniques are particularly useful for understanding subjective meanings and motivations underlying behavior. They enable investigators to be equally adept at exploring factors observed and unobserved, intentions as well as actions, internal meanings as well as external consequences, options considered but not taken, and unmeasurable as well as measurable outcomes. These methods are important when the source of or solution to a public health problem is rooted in local perceptions rather than objectively measurable characteristics selected by outside observers (3). Ultimately, such approaches have the ability to go beyond quantifying questions of *how much* or *how many* to take on questions of *how* or *why* from the perspective and in the words of the study subjects themselves (1,2).

Another key advantage of qualitative methods for field investigations is their flexibility (4). Qualitative designs not only enable but also encourage flexibility in the content and flow of questions to challenge and probe for deeper meanings or follow new leads if they lead to deeper understanding of an issue (5). It is not uncommon for topic guides to be adjusted in the course of fieldwork to investigate emerging themes relevant to answering the original study question. As discussed herein, qualitative study designs allow flexibility in sample size to accommodate the need for more or fewer interviews among particular groups to determine the root cause of an issue (see the section on Sampling and Recruitment in Qualitative Research). In the context of field investigations, such methods can be extremely useful for investigating complex or fast-moving situations where the dimensions of analysis cannot be fully anticipated.

Ultimately, the decision whether to include qualitative research in a particular field investigation depends mainly on the nature of the research question itself. Certain types of research topics lend themselves more naturally to qualitative rather than other approaches (Table 10.1). These include exploratory investigations when not enough is known about

TABLE 10.1 Examples of research topics for which qualitative methods should be considered for field investigations

Research topic	Use when	Examples
Exploratory research	The relevant questions or answer options are unknown in advance	In-depth case studies
		Situation analyses by viewing a problem from multiple perspectives
		Hypothesis generation
Understanding the role of context	Risk exposure or care-seeking behavior is embedded in particular social or physical environments	Key barriers or enablers to effective response
		Competing concerns that might interfere with each other
		Environmental behavioral interactions
Understanding the role of perceptions and subjective meaning	Different perception or meaning of the same observable facts influence risk exposure or behavioral response	Why or why not questions
		Understanding how persons make health decisions
		Exploring options considered but not taken
Understanding context and meaning of hidden, sensitive, or illegal behaviors	Legal barriers or social desirability biases prevent candid reporting by using conventional interviewing methods	Risky sexual or drug use behaviors
		Quality-of-care questions
		Questions that require a higher degree of trust between respondent and interviewer to obtain valid answers
Evaluating how interventions work in practice	Evaluating What went right or, more commonly, what went wrong with a public health response Process or outcome evaluations Who benefited in what way from what perceived change in practice	'How' questions
		Why interventions fail
		Unintended consequences of programs
		Patient–provider interactions

a problem to formulate a hypothesis or develop a fixed set of questions and answer codes. They include research questions where intentions matter as much as actions and "why?" or "why not?" questions matter as much as precise estimation of measured outcomes. Qualitative approaches also work well when contextual influences, subjective meanings, stigma, or strong social desirability biases lower faith in the validity of responses coming from a relatively impersonal survey questionnaire interview.

The availability of personnel with training and experience in qualitative interviewing or observation is critical for obtaining the best quality data but is not absolutely required for rapid assessment in field settings. Qualitative interviewing requires a broader set of skills than survey interviewing. It is not enough to follow a topic guide like a questionnaire, in order, from top to bottom. A qualitative interviewer must exercise judgment to decide when to probe and when to move on, when to encourage, challenge, or follow relevant leads even if they are not written in the topic guide. Ability to engage with informants, connect ideas during the interview, and think on one's feet are common characteristics of good qualitative interviewers. By far the most important qualification in conducting qualitative fieldwork is a firm grasp of the research objectives; with this qualification, a member of the research team armed with curiosity and a topic guide can learn on the job with successful results.

COMMONLY USED QUALITATIVE METHODS IN FIELD INVESTIGATIONS

Semi-Structured Interviews

Semi-structured interviews can be conducted with single participants (in-depth or individual key informants) or with groups (focus group discussions [FGDs] or key informant groups). These interviews follow a suggested topic guide rather than a fixed questionnaire format. Topic guides typically consist of a limited number (10–15) of broad, open-ended questions followed by bulleted points to facilitate optional probing. The conversational back-and-forth nature of a semi-structured format puts the researcher and researched (the interview participants) on more equal footing than allowed by more structured formats. *Respondents,* the term used in the case of quantitative questionnaire interviews, become *informants* in the case of individual semi-structured in-depth interviews (IDIs) or *participants* in the case of FGDs. Freedom to probe beyond initial responses enables interviewers to actively engage with the interviewee to seek clarity, openness, and depth by challenging informants to reach below layers of self-presentation and social desirability. In this respect, interviewing is sometimes compared with peeling an onion, with the first version of events accessible to the public, including survey interviewers, and deeper inner layers accessible to those who invest the time and effort to build rapport and gain trust. (The theory of the active interview suggests that all interviews involve staged social encounters where the interviewee is constantly assessing interviewer intentions and adjusting his or her responses accordingly [1]. Consequently good rapport is important for any type of interview. Survey formats give interviewers less freedom to divert from the preset script of questions and formal probes.)

Individual In-Depth Interviews and Key-Informant Interviews

The most common forms of individual semi-structured interviews are IDIs and key informant interviews (KIIs). IDIs are conducted among informants typically selected for first-hand experience (e.g., service users, participants, survivors) relevant to the research topic. These are typically conducted as one-on-one face-to-face interviews (two-on-one if translators are needed) to maximize rapport-building and confidentiality. KIIs are similar to IDIs but focus on individual persons with special knowledge or influence (e.g., community leaders or health authorities) that give them broader perspective or deeper insight into the topic area (Box 10.2). Whereas IDIs tend to focus on personal experiences, context, meaning, and implications for informants, KIIs tend to steer away from personal questions in favor of expert insights or community perspectives. IDIs enable flexible sampling strategies and represent the interviewing reference standard for confidentiality, rapport, richness, and contextual detail. However, IDIs are time- and labor-intensive to collect and analyze. Because confidentiality is not a concern in KIIs, these interviews might be conducted as individual or group interviews, as required for the topic area.

Focus Group Discussions and Group Key Informant Interviews

FGDs are semi-structured group interviews in which six to eight participants, homogeneous with respect to a shared experience, behavior, or demographic characteristic, are guided through a topic guide by a trained moderator (6). (Advice on ideal group interview size varies. The principle is to convene a group large enough to foster an open, lively discussion of the topic, and small enough to ensure all participants stay fully engaged in the process.) Over the course of discussion, the moderator is expected to pose questions, foster group participation, and probe for clarity and depth. Long a staple of market research, focus groups have become a widely used social science technique with broad applications in public health, and they are especially popular as a rapid method for assessing community norms and shared perceptions.

Focus groups have certain useful advantages during field investigations. They are highly adaptable, inexpensive to arrange and conduct, and often enjoyable for participants. Group dynamics effectively tap into collective knowledge and experience

---

BOX 10.2

IDENTIFYING BARRIERS AND SOLUTIONS TO IMPROVED HEALTHCARE WORKER PRACTICES IN EGYPT

Egypt's National Infection Prevention and Control (IPC) program undertook qualitative research to gain an understanding of the contextual behaviors and motivations of healthcare workers in complying with IPC guidelines. The study was undertaken to guide the development of effective behavior change interventions in healthcare settings to improve IPC compliance.

Key informant interviews and focus group discussions were conducted in two governorates among cleaning staff, nursing staff, and physicians in different types of healthcare facilities. The findings highlighted social and cultural barriers to IPC compliance, enabling the IPC program to design responses. For example,

- Informants expressed difficulty in complying with IPC measures that forced them to act outside their normal roles in an ingrained hospital culture.
  Response: Role models and champions were introduced to help catalyze change.
- Informants described fatalistic attitudes that undermined energy and interest in modifying behavior.
  Response: Accordingly, interventions affirming institutional commitment to change while challenging fatalistic assumptions were developed.
- Informants did not perceive IPC as effective.
  Response: Trainings were amended to include scientific evidence justifying IPC practices.
- Informants perceived hygiene as something they took pride in and were judged on.
  Response: Public recognition of optimal IPC practice was introduced to tap into positive social desirability and professional pride in maintaining hygiene in the work environment.

Qualitative research identified sources of resistance to quality clinical practice in Egypt's healthcare settings and culturally appropriate responses to overcome that resistance.

Source: Anna Leena Lohiniva, personal communication.

---

to serve as a proxy informant for the community as a whole. They are also capable of recreating a microcosm of social norms where social, moral, and emotional dimensions of topics are allowed to emerge. Skilled moderators can also exploit the tendency of small groups to seek consensus to bring out disagreements that the participants will work to resolve in a way that can lead to deeper understanding. There are also limitations on focus group methods. Lack of confidentiality during group interviews means they should not be used to explore personal experiences of a sensitive nature on ethical grounds. Participants may take it on themselves to volunteer such information, but moderators are generally encouraged to steer the conversation back to general observations to avoid putting pressure on other participants to disclose in a similar way. Similarly, FGDs are subject by design to strong social desirability biases. Qualitative study designs using focus groups sometimes add individual interviews precisely to enable participants to describe personal experiences or personal views that would be difficult or inappropriate to share in a group setting. Focus groups run the risk of producing broad but shallow analyses of issues if groups reach comfortable but superficial consensus around complex topics. This weakness can be countered by training moderators to probe effectively and challenge any consensus that sounds too simplistic or contradictory with prior knowledge. However, FGDs are surprisingly robust against the influence of strongly opinionated participants, highly adaptable, and well suited to application in study designs where systematic comparisons across different groups are called for.

Like FGDs, group KIIs rely on positive chemistry and the stimulating effects of group discussion but aim to gather expert knowledge or oversight on a particular topic rather than lived experience of embedded social actors. Group KIIs have no minimum size requirements and can involve as few as two or three participants.

Visualization Methods

Visualization methods have been developed as a way to enhance participation and empower interviewees relative to researchers during group data collection (7). Visualization methods involve asking participants to engage in collective problem-solving of challenges expressed through group production of maps, diagrams, or other images. For example, participants from the community might be asked to sketch a map of their community and to highlight features of relevance to the research topic (e.g., access to health facilities or sites of risk concentrations). Body diagramming is another visualization tool in which community members are asked to depict how and where a health threat affects the human body as a way of understanding folk conceptions of health, disease, treatment, and prevention. Ensuing debate and dialogue regarding construction of images can be recorded and analyzed in conjunction with the visual image itself. Visualization exercises were initially designed to accommodate groups the size of entire communities, but they can work equally well with smaller groups corresponding to the size of FGDs or group KIIs.

SAMPLING AND RECRUITMENT FOR QUALITATIVE RESEARCH

Selecting a Sample of Study Participants

Fundamental differences between qualitative and quantitative approaches to research emerge most clearly in the practice of sampling and recruitment of study participants. Qualitative samples are typically small and purposive. In-depth interview informants are usually selected on the basis of unique characteristics or personal experiences that make them exemplary for the study, if not typical in other respects. Key informants are selected for their unique knowledge or influence in the study domain. Focus group mobilization often seeks participants who are typical with respect to others in the community having similar exposure or shared characteristics. Often, however, participants in qualitative studies are selected because they are exceptional rather than simply representative. Their value lies not in their generalizability but in their ability to generate insight into the key questions driving the study.

Determining Sample Size

Sample size determination for qualitative studies also follows a different logic than that used for probability sample surveys. For example, whereas some qualitative methods specify ideal ranges of participants that constitute a valid observation (e.g., focus groups), there are no rules on how many observations it takes to attain valid results. In theory, sample size in qualitative designs should be determined by the *saturation principle*, where interviews are conducted until additional interviews yield no additional insights into the topic of research (8). Practically speaking, designing a study with a range in number of interviews is advisable for providing a level of flexibility if additional interviews are needed to reach clear conclusions.

Recruiting Study Participants

Recruitment strategies for qualitative studies typically involve some degree of participant self-selection (e.g., advertising in public spaces for interested participants) and purposive selection (e.g., identification of key informants). Purposive selection in community settings often requires authorization from local authorities and assistance from local mobilizers before the informed consent process can begin. Clearly specifying eligibility criteria is crucial for minimizing the tendency of study mobilizers to apply their own filters regarding who reflects the community in the best light. In addition to formal eligibility criteria, character traits (e.g., articulate and interested in participating) and convenience (e.g., not too far away) are legitimate considerations for whom to include in the sample. Accommodations to personality and convenience help to ensure the small number of interviews in a typical qualitative design yields maximum value for minimum investment. This is one reason why random sampling of qualitative informants is not only unnecessary but also potentially counterproductive.

MANAGING, CONDENSING, DISPLAYING, AND INTERPRETING QUALITATIVE DATA

Analysis of qualitative data can be divided into four stages: data management, data condensation, data display, and drawing and verifying conclusions (9).

Managing Qualitative Data

From the outset, developing a clear organization system for qualitative data is important. Ideally, naming conventions for original data files and subsequent analysis should be recorded in a data dictionary file that includes dates, locations, defining individual or group characteristics, interviewer characteristics, and other defining features. Digital recordings of interviews or visualization products should be reviewed to ensure fidelity of analyzed data to original observations. If ethics agreements require that no names or identifying characteristics be recorded, all individual names must be removed from final transcriptions before analysis begins. If data are analyzed by using textual data analysis software, maintaining careful version control over the data files is crucial, especially when multiple coders are involved.

Condensing Qualitative Data

Condensing refers to the process of selecting, focusing, simplifying, and abstracting the data available at the time of the original observation, then transforming the condensed data into a data set that can be analyzed. In qualitative research, most of the time investment required to complete a study comes *after* the fieldwork is complete. A single hour of taped individual interview can take a full day to transcribe and additional time to translate if necessary. Group interviews can take even longer because of the difficulty of transcribing active group input. Each stage of data condensation involves multiple decisions that require clear rules and close supervision. A typical challenge is finding the right balance between fidelity to the rhythm and texture of original language and clarity of the translated version in the language of analysis. For example, discussions among groups with little or no education should not emerge after the transcription (and translation) process sounding like university graduates. Judgment must be exercised about which terms should be translated and which terms should be kept in vernacular because there is no appropriate term in English to capture the richness of its meaning.

Displaying Qualitative Data

After the initial condensation, qualitative analysis depends on how the data are displayed. Decisions regarding how data are summarized and laid out to facilitate comparison influence the depth and detail of the investigation's conclusions. Displays might range from full verbatim transcripts of interviews to bulleted summaries or distilled summaries of interview notes. In a field setting, a useful and commonly used display format is an *overview chart* in which key themes or research questions are listed in rows in a word processer table or in a spreadsheet and individual informant or group entry characteristics are listed across columns. Overview charts are useful because they allow easy, systematic comparison of results.

Drawing and Verifying Conclusions

Analyzing qualitative data is an iterative and ideally interactive process that leads to rigorous and systematic interpretation of textual or visual data. At least four common steps are involved:

- *Reading and rereading.* The core of qualitative analysis is careful, systematic, and repeated reading of text to identify consistent themes and interconnections emerging from the data. The act of repeated reading inevitably yields new themes, connections, and deeper meanings from the first reading. Reading the full text of interviews multiple times before subdividing according to coded themes is key to appreciating the full context and flow of each interview before subdividing and extracting coded sections of text for separate analysis.
- *Coding.* A common technique in qualitative analysis involves developing codes for labeling sections of text for selective retrieval in later stages of analysis and verification. Different approaches can be used for textual coding. One approach, *structural coding,* follows the structure of the interview guide. Another approach, *thematic coding,* labels common themes that appear across interviews, whether by design of the topic guide or emerging themes assigned based on further analysis. To avoid

the problem of shift and drift in codes across time or multiple coders, qualitative investigators should develop a standard codebook with written definitions and rules about when codes should start and stop. Coding is also an iterative process in which new codes that emerge from repeated reading are layered on top of existing codes. Development and refinement of the codebook is inseparably part of the analysis.

- *Analyzing and writing memos.* As codes are being developed and refined, answers to the original research question should begin to emerge. Coding can facilitate that process through selective text retrieval during which similarities within and between coding categories can be extracted and compared systematically. Because no *p* values can be derived in qualitative analyses to mark the transition from tentative to firm conclusions, standard practice is to write memos to record evolving insights and emerging patterns in the data and how they relate to the original research questions. Writing memos is intended to catalyze further thinking about the data, thus initiating new connections that can lead to further coding and deeper understanding.

- *Verifying conclusions.* Analysis rigor depends as much on the thoroughness of the cross-examination and attempt to find alternative conclusions as on the quality of original conclusions. Cross-examining conclusions can occur in different ways. One way is encouraging regular interaction between analysts to challenge conclusions and pose alternative explanations for the same data. Another way is quizzing the data (i.e., retrieving coded segments by using Boolean logic to systematically compare code contents where they overlap with other codes or informant characteristics). If alternative explanations for initial conclusions are more difficult to justify, confidence in those conclusions is strengthened.

CODING AND ANALYSIS REQUIREMENTS

Above all, qualitative data analysis requires sufficient time and immersion in the data. Computer textual software programs can facilitate selective text retrieval and quizzing the data, but discerning patterns and arriving at conclusions can be done only by the analysts. This requirement involves intensive reading and rereading, developing codebooks and coding, discussing and debating, revising codebooks, and recoding as needed until clear patterns emerge from the data. Although quality and depth of analysis is usually proportional to the time invested, a number of techniques, including some mentioned earlier, can be used to expedite analysis under field conditions.

- *Detailed notes instead of full transcriptions.* Assigning one or two note-takers to an interview can be considered where the time needed for full transcription and translation is not feasible. Even if plans are in place for full transcriptions after fieldwork, asking note-takers to submit organized summary notes is a useful technique for getting real-time feedback on interview content and making adjustments to topic guides or interviewer training as needed.
- *Summary overview charts for thematic coding.* (See discussion under "Displaying Data.") If there is limited time for full transcription and/or systematic coding of text interviews using textual analysis software in the field, an overview chart is a useful technique for rapid manual coding.
- *Thematic extract files.* This is a slightly expanded version of manual thematic coding that is useful when full transcriptions of interviews are available. With use of a word processing program, files can be sectioned according to themes, or separate files can be created for each theme. Relevant extracts from transcripts or analyst notes can be copied and pasted into files or sections of files corresponding to each theme. This is particularly useful for storing appropriate quotes that can be used to illustrate thematic conclusions in final reports or manuscripts.
- *Teamwork.* Qualitative analysis can be performed by a single analyst, but it is usually beneficial to involve more than one. Qualitative conclusions involve subjective judgment calls. Having more than one coder or analyst working on a project enables more interactive discussion and debate before reaching consensus on conclusions.
- *Computer textual analysis software.* Computer-assisted analysis has a number of advantages for qualitative analysis (10). These include
  - Systematic coding.
  - Selective retrieval of coded segments.
  - Verifying conclusions ("quizzing the data").
  - Working on larger data sets with multiple separate files.
  - Working in teams with multiple coders to allow intercoder reliability to be measured and monitored.

The most widely used software packages (e.g., NVivo [QSR International Pty. Ltd., Melbourne, VIC, Australia] and ATLAS.ti [Scientific Software Development GmbH, Berlin, Germany]) evolved to include sophisticated analytic features covering a wide array of applications but are relatively expensive in terms of license cost and initial investment in time and training. A promising development is the advent of free or low-cost Web-based services (e.g., Dedoose [Sociocultural Research Consultants LLC, Manhattan

Beach, CA]) that have many of the same analytic features on a more affordable subscription basis and that enable local research counterparts to remain engaged through the analysis phase (see Teamwork criteria). The start-up costs of computer-assisted analysis need to be weighed against their analytic benefits, which tend to decline with the volume and complexity of data to be analyzed. For rapid situational analyses or small scale qualitative studies (e.g. fewer than 30 observations as an informal rule of thumb), manual coding and analysis using word processing or spreadsheet programs is faster and sufficient to enable rigorous analysis and verification of conclusions.

CONCLUSION

Qualitative methods belong to a branch of social science inquiry that emphasizes the importance of context, subjective meanings, and motivations in understanding human behavior patterns. Qualitative approaches definitionally rely on open-ended, semistructured, non-numeric strategies for asking questions and recording responses. Conclusions are drawn from systematic visual or textual analysis involving repeated reading, coding, and organizing information into structured and emerging themes. Because textual analysis is relatively time- and skill-intensive, qualitative samples tend to be small and purposively selected to yield the maximum amount of information from the minimum amount of data collection. Although qualitative approaches cannot provide representative or generalizable findings in a statistical sense, they can offer an unparalleled level of detail, nuance, and naturalistic insight into the chosen subject of study. Qualitative methods enable investigators to "hear the voice" of the researched in a way that questionnaire methods, even with the occasional open-ended response option, cannot.

Whether or when to use qualitative methods in field epidemiology studies ultimately depends on the nature of the public health question to be answered. Qualitative approaches make sense when a study question about behavior patterns or program performance leads with *why, why not,* or *how*. Similarly, they are appropriate when the answer to the study question depends on understanding the problem from the perspective of social actors in real-life settings or when the object of study cannot be adequately captured, quantified, or categorized through a battery of closed-ended survey questions (e.g., stigma or the foundation of health beliefs). Another justification for qualitative methods occurs when the topic is especially sensitive or subject to strong social desirability biases that require developing trust with the informant and persistent probing to reach the truth. Finally, qualitative methods make sense when the study question is exploratory in nature, where this approach enables the investigator the freedom and flexibility to adjust topic guides and probe beyond the original topic guides.

Given that the conditions just described probably apply more often than not in everyday field epidemiology, it might be surprising that such approaches are not incorporated more routinely into standard epidemiologic training. Part of the answer might have to do with the subjective element in qualitative sampling and analysis that seems at odds with core scientific values of objectivity. Part of it might have to do with the skill requirements for good qualitative interviewing, which are generally more difficult to find than those required for routine survey interviewing.

For the field epidemiologist unfamiliar with qualitative study design, it is important to emphasize that obtaining important insights from applying basic approaches is possible, even without a seasoned team of qualitative researchers on hand to do the work. The flexibility of qualitative methods also tends to make them forgiving with practice and persistence. Beyond the required study approvals and ethical clearances, the basic essential requirements for collecting qualitative data in field settings start with an interviewer having a strong command of the research question, basic interactive and language skills, and a healthy sense of curiosity, armed with a simple open-ended topic guide and a tape recorder or note-taker to capture the key points of the discussion. Readily available manuals on qualitative study design, methods, and analysis can provide additional guidance to improve the quality of data collection and analysis.

REFERENCES

1. Patton MQ. *Qualitative research and evaluation methods: integrating theory and practice*. 4th ed. Thousand Oaks, CA: Sage; 2015.
2. Hennink M, Hutter I, Bailey A. *Qualitative research methods*. Thousand Oaks, CA: Sage; 2010.
3. Lincoln YS, Guba EG. *The constructivist credo*. Walnut Creek, CA: Left Coast Press; 2013.
4. Mack N, Woodsong C, MacQueen KM, Guest G, Namey E. Qualitative research methods: a data collectors field guide. https://www.fhi360.org/sites/default/files/media/documents/Qualitative%20Research%20Methods%20-%20A%20Data%20Collector%27s%20Field%20Guide.pdf
5. Kvale S, Brinkmann S. *Interviews: learning the craft of qualitative research*. Thousand Oaks, CA: Sage; 2009:230–43.
6. Krueger RA, Casey MA. *Focus groups: a practical guide for applied research*. Thousand Oaks, CA: Sage; 2014.
7. Margolis E, Pauwels L. *The Sage handbook of visual research methods*. Thousand Oaks, CA: Sage; 2011.
8. Mason M. Sample size and saturation in PhD studies using qualitative interviews. *Forum*: *Qualitative Social Research/Sozialforschung*. 2010;11(3).
9. Miles MB, Huberman AM, Saldana J. *Qualitative data analysis: a methods sourcebook*. 3rd ed. Thousand Oaks, CA: Sage; 2014.
10. Silver C, Lewins A. *Using software in qualitative research: a step-by-step guide*. Thousand Oaks, CA; Sage: 2014.

/// 11 /// DEVELOPING INTERVENTIONS

JAMES L. HADLER, JAY K. VARMA, DUC J. VUGIA, AND RICHARD A. GOODMAN

> *All scientific work is incomplete—whether it be observational or experimental. All scientific work is liable to be upset or modified by advancing knowledge. That does not confer upon us a freedom to ignore the knowledge we already have, or to postpone the action that it appears to demand at a given time.*
>
> —Sir Austin Bradford Hill, British Epidemiologist (1897–1991) (1)

GUIDING PRINCIPLES FOR INTERVENTIONS

Public health officials who have responsibility and legal authority for making decisions about interventions should consider certain key principles: selecting the appropriate intervention, facilitating implementation of the intervention, and assessing the effectiveness of the intervention (Box 11.1).

BOX 11.1

GUIDING PRINCIPLES FOR INTERVENTIONS USED DURING EPIDEMIOLOGIC FIELD INVESTIGATIONS OF ACUTE PUBLIC HEALTH PROBLEMS

- As soon as an acute public health problem is detected, a public health responsibility and societal expectation exist to intervene as soon as possible to minimize preventable morbidity and mortality.
- Public health interventions should be scientifically driven on the basis of established facts and data, current investigation findings, and knowledge from previous investigations and studies. Although salient sociopolitical forces (e.g., public fear or political outcry) might create pressures for rapid public health interventions, the interventions must be based on evidence. However, adapting certain intervention components might be necessary to make them more acceptable and responsive to the needs of the affected community, potentially affected persons, elected officials, and the media.
- For any given problem, the type(s) and number of interventions to be implemented will vary, depending on the nature of the acute problem, including its cause, mode of spread, and other factors.
- The type(s) and number of interventions used might evolve as a function of incremental gains in information developed during the investigation.
- Most public health interventions demand—and even might be potentiated by—open, two-way communication between involved government agencies and the public.

DETERMINANTS FOR EMPLOYING INTERVENTIONS

Field epidemiologists must consider multiple crucial determinants during the course of making a decision about whether a scientifically rational basis exists for employing an intervention and when selecting one or more specific interventions optimally matched to the public health problem. These determinants, which might be both interrelated and not mutually exclusive, encompass a constellation of factors (e.g., specific knowledge of causative etiologic agent[s] and of reservoirs or mode[s] of acquisition or spread) and recognition of other causal determinants as reflected, in part, by assessing the investigation's ability to address the causation criteria (see the following section). This section examines three highly interrelated key determinants: severity of the problem, levels of certainty about key epidemiologic factors, and causation criteria. Additionally, it considers the sociopolitical context and its possible role in determining interventions.

Severity of the Problem

The severity of a specific problem is a principal determinant of the urgency and course of a field investigation and of any early intervention. The greater the severity, the sooner a public health intervention is expected. The primary determinants of severity are the consequences of the event and the probability of the event occurring. Consequences to consider include the most common symptoms and syndrome caused, duration of illness, complications including hospitalization and case-fatality rates, need for treatment, and economic impact. The consequences, even more than the probability, tend to drive perception of the importance of intervening.

One example is botulism, which is a low-probability but high-consequence event. Virtually all US cases trigger extensive epidemiologic investigations because identifying the food or beverage source can prevent additional intoxications, and identifying exposed or ill persons enables administration of life-saving antitoxin. Similarly, clusters of a healthcare-associated infection—especially among postsurgical or immunocompromised patients—are often investigated because of the potential for serious complications and greatly prolonged hospitalization, the possibility of iatrogenic illness as an avoidable medical event, and the immediate need to resolve questions about the safety of continuing to admit patients to the hospital (2).

Levels of Certainty About Agents, Sources, and Modes of Spread

In addition to severity, a spectrum of other factors influences the aggressiveness, extent, and scientific rigor of an epidemiologic field investigation. In the prototypic investigation, control measures are formulated only after other steps have been implemented (see Chapter 3). In practice, however, control measures might be appropriate or warranted at any step in the sequence. For most outbreaks of acute disease, the scope of an investigation is dictated by the levels of certainty about (1) the etiology of the problem (e.g., the specific pathogen or toxic agent) and (2) the source or mode of spread (e.g., waterborne, airborne, or vectorborne) (3). When the problem is identified initially, the levels of certainty about the etiology, source, and mode of spread can range from known to unknown (Figure 11.1). These basic dichotomies are illustrated in Figure 11.1 by four examples that represent the extremes. In certain situations, control measures follow policy or practice guidelines; in others, interventions are appropriate only after exhaustive epidemiologic investigation. Preliminary control measures often can start on the basis of limited initial information and then be modified as investigations proceed.

Source/Transmission

	Known	Unknown
Etiology — Known	Investigation + Control +++ Example: Suspected norovirus in restaurants and other food establishments (4)	Investigation +++ Control + Example: *Salmonella enteritica* serovar Typhimuruim in peanuts (6)
Etiology — Unknown	Investigation +++ Control +++ Example: Eosinophilia myalgia syndrome (7, 8)	Investigation +++ Control + Example: Legionnaires' disease (9)

FIGURE 11.1 Relative emphasis of investigative and control efforts (intervention options) in disease outbreaks as influenced by levels of certainty about etiology and source or mode of transmission. Investigation means extent of the investigation; control means the basis for rapid implementation of control or intervention measures at the time the problem is initially identified. Plus signs indicate the level of response indicated, ranging from + (low) to +++ (high).

For example, a suspected norovirus outbreak associated with a restaurant or food preparation establishment might warrant a spectrum of interventions, including

- Promptly excluding food service employees symptomatic with vomiting or diarrhea;
- Temporarily closing the restaurant;
- Replacing all food items;
- Sanitizing all surfaces and equipment;
- Monitoring food-handling practices until more specific information is available from the epidemiologic investigation;
- Educating food handlers about norovirus containment; and
- Providing training and education about health codes for restaurant owners (4).

In such an instance, the response will be based on knowledge of possible continuing sources of norovirus or some other enteric pathogen, exposure in a restaurant, and removal of those sources. Although this sort of prompt and appropriate response addresses the possibility of continued transmission on the basis of known agent-specific facts and experience, epidemiologists sometimes need to extend the investigation, depending on the circumstances and needs (e.g., when a trace-back is indicated to identify a continuing primary source for a restaurant-associated outbreak, such as shellfish or lettuce that was contaminated before being harvested) (5).

More commonly, a degree of uncertainty exists about the etiology or sources and the mode of spread (Figure 11.1). For most gastrointestinal outbreaks, selecting control measures depends on knowing whether transmission has resulted from person-to-person, foodborne, or waterborne spread and, if either of the two latter modes, on identifying the source. For example, an outbreak of *Salmonella enterica* serovar Typhimurium across multiple states during 2008 required extensive multipronged epidemiologic field investigations and analytic (case–control) studies before peanut butter and peanut butter–containing products were identified as the transmission vehicles (6). The converse situation—involving a presumed source but unknown etiology—is illustrated by the nationwide outbreak of eosinophilia myalgia syndrome in the United States in 1989 (7,8). During that outbreak, L-tryptophan, a nonprescription dietary supplement, initially was implicated as the source of the exposure, and contaminants in specific brands were eventually implicated through laboratory analysis. In the interim, epidemiologists issued recommendations preventing further exposures and cases. Finally, as illustrated by the Legionnaires' disease outbreak in 1976, an extensive field investigation can fail to identify the cause, the source, and mode of spread in time to control the acute problem but still can enable advances in knowledge that ultimately lead to preventive measures (9).

Causation and the Field Investigation

In his seminal article on criteria for assessing causal associations in epidemiology, Austin Bradford Hill concluded with a call for basing action on weighing the strength of the epidemiologic evidence against the severity of the consequences of delaying action and of taking premature action (1). These same concerns commonly confront epidemiologists during field investigations. The criteria specified by Hill—temporality, strength of association, biologic gradient, consistency, plausibility, coherence, experiment, and analogy—provide a useful framework for assessing the strength of epidemiologic evidence developed during a field investigation. *Assessing causality at each step in an investigation is important not only for assessing the strength of evidence developed up to that point, but also in helping to identify what evidence is missing or requires further attention and for planning additional approaches (e.g., data gathering and analysis) essential for supporting decisions regarding interventions.*

Such criteria as strength of association, dose-response, and temporality can increase confidence in initiating actions. Moreover, at any step in the investigation, evidence that satisfies a specific criterion might be unavailable. Nonetheless, field investigators should try to collect data for examining causality by using as many criteria as is feasible. Although a single criterion might not be convincing in a given context or fully accepted on the basis of the interpreter's viewpoint, a combination of well-assessed criteria pointing to a common exposure can strengthen confidence and facilitate support for directed interventions.

Epidemiology, in particular field epidemiology, is a relatively young scientific discipline in the medical world, acquiring academic, and then public, acceptance only gradually over the past five to six decades. Among certain sectors—for example, the legal profession, private enterprise, and even regulatory agencies—acceptance of epidemiologic conclusions has been slower, in part because of the nature of causation in epidemiology: epidemiologic evidence establishes associations, not hard, irrefutable proof. Meanwhile, epidemiologic evidence often is the first basis for implicating a causative agent or mode of spread before the results of more in-depth and lengthier scientific investigations become available to support decision-making about interventions. Moreover, and lamentably, epidemiologic evidence that compels epidemiologists to take prompt action might not readily convince others whose cooperation is necessary for initiating action. For example, years elapsed after field studies had clearly implicated antecedent aspirin use as a risk factor for Reye syndrome (10) before industry and the Food and Drug Administration accepted the association and issued warnings to that effect. The story of toxic shock syndrome further illustrates the reluctance of some to accept epidemiologic evidence in the face of an acute public health problem on the scale of a nationwide epidemic (11). These examples underscore the practical challenges in balancing the need to assess causality through the process of scientific inquiry with the potentially conflicting need to intervene quickly to protect the public's health.

During any outbreak, multiple groups of persons might be exposed, affected, or involved in some respect. Because of differences in knowledge, beliefs, and perceived impact of the outbreak, each group might draw different conclusions about causality from the same information. For example, in a suspected restaurant-associated foodborne illness outbreak, restaurant patrons, the public, owners and management, media, attorneys, and public health officials are each likely to have a different threshold for judging the degree of association between eating food from the restaurant and illness. In this situation, the public health field epidemiologist's concerns might focus especially on the criteria of strength of association and dose-response effect between exposure to a certain food item and illness, whereas a restaurant patron's primary concern is simply plausibility. In contrast, attorneys—who either are representing plaintiff-patrons who putatively acquired their illnesses as a result of restaurant exposure or are defending a restaurant epidemiologically associated with a foodborne illness epidemic—will approach such a problem by using a legal framework for causation, which varies from epidemiologic causation (12). In civil cases, the plaintiff's attorney in particular must meet a preponderance-of-evidence standard of proof, which means that the factfinder (i.e., the judge or jury) must believe that the plaintiff's version of events is more probable than not for the plaintiff to prevail (13); this standard also has been analogized to a probability of 0.51 or greater (14).

Sociopolitical Context

Field investigations often occur in the public limelight, whether intentionally or not. When a problem is perceived as severe (e.g., a death has occurred) and possibly ongoing, the public might demand information and action. In addition, when interest is intense among politicians, including executive branch leaders (e.g., governors and mayors), such leaders might wish to be visible and demonstrate their interest in protecting the public. For example, a schoolchild's death from meningitis might lead to political pressure to close the school. A hospital patient's death from Legionnaires' disease might lead to political pressure to consider closing the hospital.

As part of the deliberation about when and how to intervene, effective and continuous communication with all concerned entities is essential. These entities need to be aware of the possibilities, the ongoing risks (if any), and how best to address them given the level of information available. An essential component of any intervention is effective communication with political leaders and the public. Such communication will assist in enabling use of scientific factors as the determinants for selecting the intervention(s) to protect the public against disease and should help minimize the potential for unnecessary, costly, and misleading interventions. Nonetheless, the evidence-based perspective might not be the only one eventually considered in the choice of interventions. During the 2014–2015 Ebola virus disease epidemic in parts of West Africa, many US jurisdictions, often for political reasons, implemented strict quarantine and health monitoring for persons who had traveled to an affected country, despite these persons having no history of exposure to anyone with Ebola virus infection (15).

INTERVENTION OPTIONS

Interventions for preventing and controlling public health problems—including infectious disease outbreaks and noninfectious diseases, injuries, and disabilities—can be approached through different classification schemes. Examples of these approaches include

- Interventions targeting specific aspects of the relation between the host, environment, and disease- or injury-causing agent;
- Primary, secondary, and tertiary prevention options; and
- Haddon's injury prevention model, which keys on intervention strategies at the preevent, event, and postevent phases (16–18).

In addition to the specific nature of the etiologic agent, decision-makers might need to consider other factors, including

- The agent's reservoir or source;
- The mode of spread or transmission;
- Host-related risk factors;
- Environmental and other mediating factors;
- A priori evidence of effectiveness of the intervention;
- Operational and logistical feasibility; and
- Legal authority necessary to support implementing the measure.

In this chapter, the model used to systematically identify and characterize the spectrum of intervention options for outbreaks and other acute health threats focuses on two basic biologic and environmental dimensions: (1) interventions that can be directed at the source(s) of most infectious and other disease-causing agents and (2) interventions that can be directed at persons susceptible to such agents (Box 11.2). The first category— interventions directed at the source—includes measures that would eliminate the disease-causing agent's presence as a risk factor for susceptible populations (e.g., seizing and destroying contaminated foods or temporarily barring an infected person from preparing or serving food). Both categories encompass some of the same options and thus are not completely mutually exclusive. For example, during the 2016–2017 Zika virus infection outbreak, men returning from travel to epidemic areas were advised to use condoms when having sex with susceptible pregnant or potentially pregnant women, as well as for pregnant or potentially pregnant susceptible women to use condoms with any male partner who might have been exposed to the virus to decrease the women's risk for exposure (19).

During the Ebola virus disease epidemic in 2014–2015, public health officials in the United States used a combination of intervention measures directed at persons in whom

BOX 11.2
SELECTED PUBLIC HEALTH INTERVENTION OPTIONS FOR OUTBREAKS AND OTHER ACUTE HEALTH THREATS

These interventions are grouped according to those that can be directed at the source(s) of most infectious and other disease-causing agents and those that can be directed at persons susceptible to such agents.

INTERVENTIONS DIRECTED AT THE SOURCE
- Treat infected or affected persons and animals.
- Isolate infected persons, including cohorting, if needed.
- Use barrier methods (e.g., face masks, condoms).
- Monitor exposed persons for signs of illness.
- Quarantine contaminated sites or sources.
- Implement *cordon sanitaire*, close public places, and prevent gatherings to freeze or limit movement and minimize likelihood of mixing groups by exposure or infection status.
- Use contact tracing, partner notification, and treatment.
- Seize or destroy contaminated food, property, animals, or other sources.
- Clean and disinfect contaminated surfaces and other environmental repositories.
- Modify the affected environment through vector control.
- Modify the affected environment by restricting or controlling dangerous drugs or contaminants.
- Modify behavior to reduce risks to self or others.
- Deter through civil suits or criminal prosecution.

INTERVENTIONS DIRECTED AT SUSCEPTIBLE PERSONS OR ANIMALS
- Administer postexposure prophylaxis.
- Immunize or vaccinate in advance.
- Exclude unvaccinated persons from cohorts of vaccinated persons.
- Use barrier methods (e.g., face masks, condoms).
- Implement *cordon sanitaire*, close public places, and prevent gatherings to freeze or limit movement and minimize likelihood of mixing groups by exposure or infection status.
- Modify behavior to reduce risks to self or others.
- Use shelter-in-place (i.e., reverse quarantine).
- Issue press releases, health alerts, and other information about risk reduction.

Ebola virus disease was diagnosed (isolation), at their close contacts (active monitoring, quarantine, or restrictions on travel), at those providing healthcare to them (training in correct use of special protective gear and active monitoring), and at those arriving from selected countries (screening or active monitoring) (20).

Selection from measures listed in Box 11.2 and other alternatives might be considered at any stage of a field investigation. During early stages, interventions based on established guidelines for disease control can be applied. For example, as indicated earlier in this chapter, excluding symptomatic employees and removing all possible existing sources of an enteric pathogen such as norovirus from a food preparation facility can be done regardless of the actual source of the outbreak (4). If, at a subsequent point, the nature of the risk for infection is more sharply defined, then additional, tailored corrective measures can be directed at the source and/or mode of spread.

CHALLENGES AND EVOLVING APPROACHES IN INTERVENTIONS

Although this chapter has explored a science-based foundation for identifying, selecting, and implementing public health interventions, field investigators also must contend with a spectrum of new and evolving concerns that challenge decision-making about interventions. This section briefly addresses three such concerns.

1. *The dilemma public health officials face in selecting and implementing interventions when science-based information might be limited regarding their appropriateness or effectiveness.* For certain infectious diseases and other public health problems, recent efforts to plan for selecting and using different interventions have encountered controversy or other challenges because of limitations in the availability of science-based information about their benefits versus their societal costs. For example, during deliberations about what measures might be most effective for responding to an influenza A(H5N1) pandemic, many persons have questioned whether sufficient science-based evidence exists to support widespread use of some relatively draconian social distancing measures (21).

2. *The paramount importance of increasing an affected community's understanding of the nature of the public health problem and the rationale for the recommended intervention(s).* An influential trend in selecting and implementing interventions is the increasing role of community involvement. For example, for the past several decades, public health agencies have had to innovatively modify their responses to such problems as outbreaks of multidrug-resistant tuberculosis,

clusters of cases of human immunodeficiency virus infection, resurgent and antibiotic-resistant sexually transmitted diseases, and meningococcal disease among men who have sex with men (22–25). For some public health problems, traditional methods for investigation and contact evaluation have been supplanted by newer social network approaches—interventions that require increased involvement of community representatives. In such settings, community support is essential for the success of the investigation and longer term prevention and control measures; conversely, failure to obtain community trust and support can disable or constrain the impact of an investigation. This can be especially true when problems disproportionately affect groups who are marginalized and who otherwise might be initially reluctant to work with public health officials. The need for obtaining community trust also implicates the important role of health and risk communications, as well as the importance of explaining to the community both the rationale for and potential limitations of an intervention (e.g., why the intervention might not work or be 100% effective). Community representatives can also help disseminate information to persons most at risk through blogs, social media, mobile phone applications, or other nontraditional communication channels. The increasing role of community involvement in and support for public health interventions applies not only to infectious diseases but also to preventing and controlling environmental hazards, including substance abuse, injuries, and other noninfectious disease problems.

3. *The sometimes complex nature of making a decision about when to terminate an acute intervention or how to institutionalize or to sustain it for a longer period.* This final challenge encompasses the need to assess the effectiveness of each intervention and make decisions about whether and when to terminate or sustain it. At the earliest possible moment, data being generated by the epidemiologic investigation should be used to assess the effectiveness of each intervention. Such information also guides decision-making regarding modification or termination of already implemented interventions and selection and use of additional or new measures. A decision to leave an intervention in place long term or permanently might be made in situations where the public health risk cannot be eliminated and remains an ongoing threat (e.g., ban on use of lead-based paint or sustaining a recommendation to vaccinate men who have sex with men against meningococcal disease after an outbreak is over because of sustained higher risk [25]).

CONCLUSION

Epidemiologic field investigations usually are initiated in response to epidemics or the occurrence of other acute disease, injury, or environmental health problems. Under such circumstances, the primary objective of the field investigation is to use the scientific principles of epidemiology to determine a rational and appropriate response for ending or controlling the problem. Key factors that influence decisions about the timing and choice of public health interventions include a carefully crafted balance among

- The severity of the problem,
- The levels of scientific certainty of the findings,
- The extent to which causal criteria have been established,
- The intervention's operational and logistical feasibility,
- The public and political perceptions of what is the best course of action, and
- Legal considerations.

This chapter has examined essential factors epidemiologists and other public health officials must consider when making decisions about selecting and implementing public health interventions during epidemiologic field investigations. Taking these factors into account, the following actions should be reconsidered at each progressive stage of the field investigation:

- Define the scope of the public health problem with available information by assessing
  - The severity of the illness, injury, or environmental hazard;
  - The nature of the suspected etiologic agent;
  - The number of possible susceptible persons and the extent of their exposure; and
  - Possible reasons for the outbreak.
- Determine whether possible reasons for the outbreak might be ongoing, and, for all potentially ongoing reasons and exposures for which intervention(s) might be offered, consider what empiric interventions can be used to reduce or eliminate any ongoing risk for exposure or illness.
- For each potential intervention, consider the costs and benefits of implementing the intervention at that stage of the investigation in the absence of additional information.
- Implement all reasonable empiric interventions.

- Communicate the rationale for implementing or not implementing interventions at any point to persons within the community who have been exposed or affected, as well as others who might need to know.
- Continuously assess the effectiveness of and modify the interventions as new investigation information becomes available.

Adherence to these and other steps during epidemiologic field investigations can be integral to helping attain and optimize a scientifically rational basis for selecting and implementing public health interventions for controlling or terminating a problem.

NOTE

Portions of this chapter as incorporated within previous editions of this book were adapted from Goodman RA, Buehler JW, Koplan JP. The epidemiologic field investigation: science and judgment in public health practice. *Am J Epidemiol.* 1990;132:91–96.

ACKNOWLEDGMENTS

We acknowledge James W. Buehler and Jeffrey P. Koplan, whose work on Chapter 9, "Developing Interventions," in the first and second editions of this manual contributed in part to this chapter.

REFERENCES

1. Hill AB. The environment and disease: association or causation? *Proc R Soc Med.* 1965;58:295–300.
2. Gaynes R, Richards C, Edwards J, et al. Feeding back surveillance data to prevent hospital-acquired infections. *Emerg Infect Dis.* 2001;7:295–8.
3. Goodman RA, Buehler JW, Koplan JP. The epidemiologic field investigation: science and judgment in public health practice. *Am J Epidemiol.* 1990;132:91–6.
4. Centers for Disease Control and Prevention. Vital signs: foodborne norovirus outbreaks—United States, 2009–2012. *MMWR.* 2014;63:491–5.
5. Dowell SF, Groves C, Kirkland KB, et al. A multistate outbreak of oyster-associated gastroenteritis: implications for interstate tracing of contaminated shellfish. *J Infect Dis.* 1995;171:1497–503.
6. Centers for Disease Control and Prevention. Multistate outbreak of *Salmonella* infections associated with peanut butter and peanut butter–containing products—United States, 2008–2009. *MMWR.* 2009;58:85–90.
7. Centers for Disease Control and Prevention. Eosinophilia-myalgia syndrome—New Mexico. *MMWR.* 1989;38:765–7.
8. Centers for Disease Control and Prevention. Eosinophilia-myalgia syndrome and L-tryptophan-containing products—New Mexico, Minnesota, Oregon, and New York, 1989. *MMWR.* 1989;38:785–8.
9. Fraser DW, Tsai TR, Orenstein W, et al. Legionnaires' disease: description of an epidemic of pneumonia. *N Engl J Med.* 1977;297:1189–97.

10. Hurwitz ES, Schonberger LB. Reye syndrome—Ohio, Michigan. *MMWR*. 1997;46:750–5.

11. Osterholm MT, Davis JP, Gibson RW, et al. Tri-state toxic-shock syndrome study. I. Epidemiologic findings. *J Infect Dis*. 1982;145:431–40.

12. Goodman RA, Loue S, Shaw FE. Law in epidemiology. In: Bownson R, Petiti D, eds. *Applied epidemiology*. 2nd ed. New York: Oxford University Press; 2006:289–326.

13. Freer RD, Perdue WC, eds. *Civil procedure: cases, materials, and questions*. 2nd ed. Cincinnati, OH: Anderson Publishing Co.; 1997.

14. Lazzarini Z, Goodman RA, Dammers K. Criminal law and public health practice. In: Goodman RA, Hoffman RE, Lopez W, Matthews GW, Rothstein MA, Foster KL, eds. *Law in public health practice*. 2nd ed. New York: Oxford University Press; 2007:136–67.

15. American Civil Liberties Union and Yale Global Health Justice Partnership. Fear, politics, and Ebola: how quarantines hurt the fight against Ebola and violate the Constitution. https://www.law.yale.edu/system/files/documents/pdf/Intellectual_Life/aclu_yale_ghjp_-_fear_politics_and_ebola-december_2015.pdf

16. Wenzel RP. Overview: control of communicable diseases. In: Wallace RB, Kohatsu N, Brownson R, Schecter AJ, Scutchfield FD, eds. *Maxcy-Rosenau-Last public health & preventive medicine*. 15th ed. New York: McGraw-Hill Education; 2008:77–100.

17. Kim-Farley RJ. Global strategies for control of communicable diseases. In: Detels R, McEwen J, Beaglehole R, Tanaka H, eds. *Oxford textbook of public health*. 4th ed. New York: Oxford University Press; 2002:839–59.

18. Olsen J. Disease prevention and control of non-communicable diseases. In: Detels R, McEwen J, Beaglehole R, Tanaka H, eds. *Oxford textbook of public health*. 4th ed. New York: Oxford University Press; 2002:1811–22.

19. Oster AM, Russell K, Stryker JE, et al. Update: interim guidance for prevention of sexual transmission of Zika virus—United States, 2016. *MMWR*. 2016;65:323–5.

20. Centers for Disease Control and Prevention. Interim U.S. guidance for monitoring and movement of persons with potential Ebola virus exposure. http://www.cdc.gov/vhf/ebola/exposure/monitoring-and-movement-of-persons-with-exposure.html

21. Ferguson NM, Cummings DAT, Fraser C, Cajka JC, Cooley PC, Burke DS. Strategies for mitigating an influenza pandemic. *Nature*. 2006;442:448–52.

22. Centers for Disease Control and Prevention. Outbreak of syphilis among men who have sex with men—southern California, 2000. *MMWR*. 2001;50:117–20.

23. Centers for Disease Control and Prevention. HIV-related tuberculosis in a transgender network—Baltimore, Maryland, and New York City area, 1998–2000. *MMWR*. 2000;49:317–20.

24. Conrad C, Bradley HM, Boiz D, et al. Community outbreak of HIV infection linked to injection drug use of oxymorphone—Indiana, 2015. *MMWR*. 2015;64:443–4.

25. Kratz MM, Weiss D, Ridpath A, et al. Community-based outbreak of *Neisseria meningitidis* serogroup C infection in men who have sex with men, New York City, New York, USA, 2010–2013. *Emerg Infect Dis*. 2015;21:1379–86.

/// 12 /// # COMMUNICATING DURING AN OUTBREAK OR PUBLIC HEALTH INVESTIGATION

ABBIGAIL J. TUMPEY, DAVID DAIGLE, AND GLEN NOWAK

BACKGROUND

Evolving Outbreaks and Evolving Communication

Before an outbreak is recognized and an investigation begins, limited numbers of persons might be exposed to health risks without experiencing illness. As increasing numbers of persons are exposed to the risk or become ill, healthcare providers and others might become aware of the higher than expected number of illnesses and begin reporting the unusually high occurrences to local and state health authorities. This situation is often what prompts an outbreak investigation, and as that outbreak evolves, communications about it must evolve as well (1,2).

In today's 24-hour news and digital media environment, people constantly receive information from many sources, ranging from print media to television to alerts and social media on mobile devices. Immediately after the news media or community learns of a public health–related outbreak investigation, they want to know what is happening and who is affected. When the cause is rare but might cause substantial harm, news outlets often treat the event as breaking news and begin sustained coverage. From the beginning of an event to its resolution and follow-up, public health authorities are expected to provide the news media with timely, accurate information and answers about the outbreak's effects.

Because the ways in which receipt of news is evolving, the ways in which public health authorities communicate with the media and public needs to adapt in similar ways. In 2016, the Pew Research Center reported that approximately 4 in 10 US residents received their news from online sources, and 6 in 10 received their news through social media channels (3). Today, communications strategies during an outbreak response should include a mix of media outreach, partner and stakeholder outreach, and social media engagement (2).

Risk Perception and Communication

Knowing how the public or members of affected groups perceive a risk affects what you, as a field investigator, might communicate and how you frame the key messages. Many times, persons most affected by a disease outbreak or health threat perceive the risk differently from the experts who mitigate or prevent the risk. Additionally, persons perceive their own risks differently, depending on how likely they think the actual hazard will affect them personally and their beliefs about how severe the harm might be. Perceptions of health risks also are tied to the degree to which persons feel alarmed or outraged—when the event causes a high level of worry or anxiety, the risk is perceived to be at a similarly high level (4). Persons are usually more accepting of risks or feel less outrage when the risks are voluntary, under their control, have clear benefits, are naturally occurring, are generated from a trusted source, or are familiar (Table 12.1). Conversely, persons are less accepting of risks or have greater concern or anxiety when risks are imposed or created by others, controlled by others, have no clear benefit, are human-made, come from an untrusted source, or seem exotic. For example, many persons are more worried about flying in an airplane than driving a car, despite the fact that more car crashes than airplane crashes occur each year in the United States. Flying in an airplane is an event controlled by others and aligns with a risk perceived as less acceptable. The same is true

TABLE 12.1 Factors influencing risk perception

More acceptable risks are those perceived as	Less acceptable risks are those perceived as
Being voluntary or involving choice	Being imposed on the affected population or not allowing choice
Being under a person's control	Being controlled by others
Having clear benefits	Having intangible or deferred benefits
Naturally occurring	Human-made
Generated by a trusted source	Generated by an untrusted source
Being familiar	Being or seeming new or exotic
Affecting adults primarily	Affecting children primarily

Source: Adapted from References 4, 5.

for outbreaks and public health crises. Before communicating during an outbreak, think through how risk perceptions might influence the affected populations and, therefore, how you communicate about those risks. Also, keep in mind that persons will view public health recommendations and advice through a risk–benefit lens, with the same factors affecting whether they adopt a public health recommendation.

TRUST AND CREDIBILITY

Trust and credibility can greatly influence your ability to persuade affected persons to follow public health authorities' recommendations during an outbreak or public health response. The ability to contain and stop the outbreak might hinge on established relationships and coordination with key partners and stakeholders.

Risk communication literature identifies four factors that determine whether an audience, including journalists, will perceive a messenger as trusted and credible, including

- Empathy and caring,
- Honesty and openness,
- Dedication and commitment, and
- Competence and expertise (6,7).

Organizations and spokespersons who issue messages and information that convey these four factors are more likely to maintain and even build trust during a crisis. Examples of messages used in outbreak responses or public health investigations are provided in Box 12.1. These quotations encompass the four factors that foster trust and credibility.

EXAMPLES OF MESSAGES USED TO FACILITATE TRUST DURING OUTBREAK RESPONSES

We realize that you turn to our medical facility to get better. This event is intolerable to us as well, and we want to work with you to resolve the situation and ensure your safety and well-being. We are taking steps to ensure that this event never occurs again in our facility.

—Broward Health Medical Center Patient Notification Letter (October 2009) (8)

We want to ensure that every patient who might be at risk is tested. Thanks to the diligent work of our team [. . . .], we are confident that we are at a point where we've identified the vast majority of patients who were put at risk. Mayo Clinic will do whatever is necessary to support the needs of its patients. Patient safety is central to the trust the organization shares with its patients. Mayo Clinic is working to ensure that this doesn't happen again.

—Media quotation from Mayo Clinic's chief executive officer
(Jacksonville, FL, September 2010) (9)

I want to acknowledge the importance of uncertainty. At the early stages of an outbreak, there's much uncertainty, and probably more than everyone would like. Our guidelines and advice are likely to be interim and fluid, subject to change as we learn more. We're moving quickly to learn as much as possible and working with many local, state, and international partners to do so.

I want to recognize that while we're moving fast, it's very likely that this will be more of a marathon than a sprint. I want to acknowledge change. Our recommendations, advice, and approaches will likely change as we learn more about the virus and we learn more about its transmission.

I want to acknowledge that we're likely to see local approaches to controlling the spread of this virus, and that's important; that can be beneficial; that can teach us things that we want to use in other parts of the country and that other people in other places may find useful. Because things are changing, because flu viruses are unpredictable, and because there will be local adaptation, it's likely that [at] any given moment there will be confusing—or may be confusing or conflicting information available. We are very committed to minimizing where we find that, clearing up any of that misconception.

—Press briefing by the Centers for Disease Control and Prevention's Acting Director Richard
Besser, MD, during the early stages of the influenza A(H1N1) outbreak (April 2009) (10)

BEGINNING AN OUTBREAK RESPONSE

The early stages of an outbreak investigation can be a seemingly overwhelming challenge of tasks, long hours, and concerns. Will the situation evolve into a broader public health crisis? Will the outbreak be short or long term? Which population groups will be most at risk? To communicate effectively in this time of uncertainty, multiple components need to be in place.

Determining Roles and Responsibilities

Early in a public health investigation, the roles and responsibilities of the persons and organizations involved should be defined clearly; it is particularly important to determine who has primary responsibility and authority for communicating each aspect of the investigation to healthcare providers, the media, and the general public. Each entity's domain of expertise should be stipulated, including who will speak with the public and news media about each topic. If the outbreak response is domestic, the roles and responsibilities among the entities involved (e.g., federal, state, or local) should be clarified. If the response is international, that country's ministry of health will determine communication plans and responsibilities and serve as the communication lead within that country. The field investigator and, if part of the investigation team, the health communication specialist should foster effective collaboration and coordination among all of the agencies and organizations involved.

Situational Awareness

At the start of an investigation, you will need to assess the situation (11). The following steps will help you perform this task quickly:

- *Identify affected or potentially affected populations (i.e., target audiences).* Ask yourself, "Who is most at risk by the outbreak or public health threat?" "What populations are most vulnerable or at highest risk and need to be reached first?"
- *Identify behavioral factors that might place persons at risk.* Ask yourself, "Are behavioral factors placing persons at risk?" If so, "What are they?" Can you recommend actions that persons and healthcare providers can take to confront these behavioral factors and thus reduce their risk (e.g., get vaccinated or wash their hands frequently)? If the risk is unknown, can you provide information to the public and media about what is being done in the investigation to identify what places persons at risk?

- *Identify partners who might be able to reach affected persons or populations.* In an ideal situation, strong relationships will exist. However, if such relationships do not yet exist, quickly identify what relationships are crucial for containing and stopping the outbreak. Ask yourself, "Are healthcare providers available who might reach the affected persons or populations quickly?" "Who are the community leaders who can help reach the affected persons or populations?" "Will the public look to specific partners or persons for advice or direction (e.g., religious leaders or local thought leaders)?" Decide who should talk with those influential persons and what the timing should be for doing so.

- *Identify perceptions in the community that might affect communications.* Listen to community members. Work to get a better understanding of how local authorities, affected persons, and community leaders perceive the situation (7). Listen to concerns, critiques, and fears. When possible, have a discussion before issuing directives. Gain an understanding of what community members might know and believe about the illness and potential cause. Also work to understand the language, culture, and socioeconomic factors in the community that should be considered. Use this information to refine your communication efforts.

  - *Tailor health-related recommendations or guidance* and ensure that it is written in plain language to be more easily adopted or adhered to by the affected population and public health or healthcare entities.

  - *Build strong relationships with key persons in the community* who can help you contain or stop the outbreak and can provide ongoing insights.

  - *Ensure that messages to the media and public resonate.* The communications team will want to identify reliable information sources that can provide an ongoing assessment of current perceptions in the community (e.g., social media monitoring) (12). When you have this feedback loop in place, work to integrate the findings into ongoing decision making.

Solidifying the Communications Strategy

During an outbreak response, you might work with a team of communications experts, possibly including public affairs (media) specialists, risk communication experts, digital or social media experts, and other health communication staff. The communications team will solidify the communications strategy and develop communication resources aimed at reaching the affected (target) populations and partners who might influence them (e.g., healthcare providers or community leaders). These health-related messages should focus on behaviors that can contain or stop the outbreak. Box 12.2 lists communication

COMMUNICATION RESOURCES AND TOOLS OFTEN USED
FOR OUTBREAK RESPONSES

- *Internet site.* The response effort might need an Internet site to convey relevant and rapidly changing information about the outbreak. The site should be the main repository of scientific facts, data, and resources. All other communications should be based on the content of that site. Key information for the site might include the following:
  - Data or case counts;
  - Maps of the affected area;
  - Guidance for affected populations, the public, travelers to or from the region, and healthcare providers who are caring for the affected persons;
  - A section highlighting the newest information; and
  - A multimedia section for the media and the general public.
- *Call center.* The response effort might benefit from having a call center equipped to answer inquiries from the affected population, the worried well, and healthcare providers seeking information. Guidance is available for entities who are establishing a call center during an outbreak response.
- *Social media messages.* Create social media messages from the Internet site content. Communications staff should monitor social media regularly to identify and dispel myths and misperceptions.
- *Clinician outreach resources.* The response might require substantial communications with healthcare providers. Webinars, conference calls with partner organizations, videos for online clinical communities, or other forums might be considered to allow healthcare providers to access up-to-date information, ask questions, and obtain advice from other clinicians associated with the response.
- *Digital press kit for the news media.* A digital press kit with photos, videos, quotations from spokespersons, the latest data or information (e.g., graphics, charts, or maps), and information about how to obtain an interview is always helpful for reporters during an outbreak investigation.
- *Tailor communication resources.* The response might require translation for specific audiences, and communication materials might need to be tailored for reaching affected populations. Some responses use photo novellas, simple line art, text messaging, or community events to convey important information for specific audiences.

Source: Adapted from Reference 13.

resources often used during outbreak responses. Depending on where the outbreak is located and what populations are affected, the communications team might tailor additional resources to the investigation needs (e.g., posters for low-literacy readers or text-messaging alerts). The communication strategy most likely will evolve and adapt as the situation evolves and more is learned about the perceptions of your targeted audience and scope of the outbreak (1).

EFFECTIVE MESSAGING DURING OUTBREAK RESPONSES

Messages must resonate with affected populations before those persons will follow prevention recommendations. Box 12.3 outlines these key messaging development components in seven steps.

1. *Start with empathy.* Whether you are speaking to affected persons, community groups, or the media, start by expressing empathy. Acknowledge concerns and express understanding of how those affected by the illnesses or injuries are probably feeling. Recognize orally and in written materials that persons are anxious or worried and that you, too, have concerns. Demonstrate that you care and are working to understand their perspective.

2. *Identify and explain the public health threat.* Detail what you know about the situation (e.g., what is causing the harm, who is at risk, and what causes someone to be

---

BOX 12.3
WHAT TO INCLUDE WHEN DEVELOPING OUTBREAK-RELATED MESSAGES

- An expression of empathy.
- What's known and a call for action, including Who? What? When? Where? Why? How?
- What's known and what's not known, and how answers will be obtained for what's not yet known
- Explanations of what public health actions are being taken and why.
- A statement of commitment.
- When additional information will be provided.
- Where to find more information in the meantime.

Source: Adapted from Reference 14.

at risk). Provide advice that includes action steps for preventing harm or getting help. Persons affected by the situation might feel fear, loss of trust, and lack of control. Acknowledge uncertainties and do not over-reassure or overpromise.

3. *Explain what is currently known and unknown.* Provide specific details and timelines. Admit when information is not yet known. Explain what you are doing to learn more, and provide a timeframe for checking back in or when confirmed results are expected. During the early stages of an outbreak or investigation, you might have limited information to provide, which can be acknowledged by saying, for example, "We do not have sufficient information to share with you yet, but we are working to find the answers you need." Explain what is being done to minimize risks and harm to affected or potentially affected populations.

4. *Explain what public health actions are being taken and why.* Be prepared to describe which agencies are involved in the response, their roles, and their responsibilities. Also identify the investigative steps, actions being taken, or actions that are not being taken and why not. Say, for example, "We are not evacuating the area because people can safely shelter in place." When discussing public health actions, share dilemmas in the decision-making and foreshadow possibilities that can occur during the outbreak.

   a. *Share dilemmas.* Express that, in certain instances, public health decisions can have undesired consequences, involve tradeoffs, or require overcoming barriers to implementing the recommendations effectively. Be open about making decisions with incomplete or imperfect information.

   b. *Foreshadow possibilities.* Let the public and media know the assumptions, factors, and considerations that have gone into the decision-making thus far, including the possibility of changes in recommendations and actions, especially as more is learned. Let the audience know public health actions and recommendations might change during the coming days and weeks.

5. *Emphasize a commitment to the situation.* Convey a sense of urgency for bringing the situation under control. Let the audience know where it can access more information (e.g., an Internet site or call center) and when more information will be provided; for example, "Our next update will be tomorrow at noon."

Remember to follow risk communication best practices as outlined previously (e.g., recognize the affected populations are worried, concerned, and seeking guidance). Box 12.4 provides examples of how to convey risk communications messaging when speaking with an audience about an outbreak.

> **BOX 12.4**
> ## RISK COMMUNICATION MESSAGING TIPS AND EXAMPLES
>
> - Express empathy and understanding: "We know this situation is scary."
> - Do not over-reassure: "Let me make myself clear. This is a challenging situation."
> - Acknowledge uncertainty: "Here is what we do not know yet."
> - Share dilemmas: "We can do [X] or [Y]. If we do [X], here are the advantages and disadvantages. If we do [Y], the advantages and disadvantages are . . ."
> - Foreshadow possibilities: "Over the next several days, we might see more cases because . . . "
> - Express a desire to find the answers for what is not yet known: "We wish we had answers to . . ."
> - Explain the process in place for finding those answers: "Here is what we are doing to learn more."
> - Give the audience some things to do: "Here is what we need you to do."
>
> ---
> *Source: Adapted from Reference 14.*

WORKING WITH THE NEWS MEDIA

Preparing for a Media Interview or Public Appearance

Being a spokesperson is challenging, especially during investigations or a response that involves considerable media attention. If you are asked to be a spokesperson, take time to prepare and practice. Media interviews are the principal way in which reporters obtain their information from subject-matter experts and other sources. Learning how to navigate an interview is crucial.

You often can determine the overall communication objectives by answering the following two questions:

1. "What do we want the headlines to be?" Make two short lists, one that includes the desired headlines and one that includes headlines to avoid in the messaging. Think about the supporting messages that will help prompt the desired headlines.
2. "What is the most important information for the affected population to know immediately?" Identify the action steps you want the affected population to take and weave that messaging throughout the interview or public appearance.

For most news reports, you will have only one direct quotation; therefore, make it count. Write down your primary message point, often called the Single Overriding Health Communication Objective, or SOHCO (pronounced sock-O). You want your audience to remember this one key point because it is the most important message about the topic. A communications expert can help you refine the SOHCO and make sure it resonates. Say the SOHCO at the beginning of the interview. At the end of the interview, the reporter most likely will ask you if you have anything else that you have not covered. Take that opportunity to repeat the SOHCO; say, for example, "Thank you for your interest in this topic. The most important thing for your audience to remember is [repeat the SOHCO]."

Never provide an interview when first contacted by the media. When a reporter calls you directly, ask him or her for five pieces of information—name, contact information, a list of topics planned for discussion, how the interview will be conducted, and the deadline. Tell the reporter you will call back within a specific timeframe. Even if the reporter says the information is needed urgently, tell him or her you will call back promptly (e.g., in 5–10 minutes). A 5- or 10-minute delay will give you time to gather your thoughts, locate helpful or needed information, and identify key messages. Reviewing the common questions asked during a media interview will help you prepare your response (14,15).

You will need permission from the health authorities in the jurisdiction where the outbreak is occurring before you speak directly with any media. Unless you have that permission, you should direct anyone requesting an interview to the health authority in charge. Also, ensure you know your organization's policies regarding communications with the media (e.g., how to frame statements related to your organization's policies or official recommendations) and stay within the scope of your responsibilities when talking with reporters. Consult a communications expert assigned to the outbreak investigation about policies and prior clearances needed. Know your boundaries. If questions come up during an interview that fall under the purview or responsibility of other agencies or authorities, refer reporters to those entities or their spokespersons. Including a member of the communications team during the interview can help with obtaining follow-up information for the media.

Avoiding Communication Traps

Challenging situations and questions often occur during interactions with the news media or the public about an outbreak response or a public health investigation. Table 12.2 provides Do's and Don'ts for being a media spokesperson and avoiding possible communication traps.

TABLE 12.2 Do's and don'ts of being a spokesperson

Topic	Do . . .	Don't . . .
Expectations	Guide and help set realistic expectations about what is known, what is being done, and the effectiveness of efforts.	Overpromise or foster unrealistic expectations, particularly about certainty of the situation or a resolution.
Scientific terms and acronyms	Use clear communication; define technical terms in plain language; and use acronyms sparingly; if an acronym is necessary, define it at first use.	Use language that might not be understood by even a portion of the audience.
Negative allegations	Refute the allegation without repeating it.	Repeat or refer to the negative allegation.
Temperament	Remain calm; use a question or allegation as a springboard for saying something positive.	Let emotions interfere with your ability to communicate a positive message.
Clarity	Ask whether you have made the information clear.	Assume you have been understood.
Abstractions	Use examples or analogies to establish a common understanding.	Assume the audience understands the complexity of the situation.
Hypothetical traps	Focus on the facts at hand.	Speculate on hypothetical situations.
Promises	Promise only what you can deliver; set and follow strict deadlines.	Make promises you cannot keep or fail to follow through on promises made.
Risk	Give the best estimation, on the basis of the science, of the risk.	State absolutes or expect the general public to understand risk numbers.
Blame	Take responsibility for your organization's share of the problem; use empathy.	Try to shift blame or responsibility to others.
Data	Emphasize performance, trends, and achievements; explain what you are going to do to improve, especially if the numbers are frightening.	Place blame elsewhere or turn the conversation into an attack on the accuracy of the numbers or the system.

Source: Adapted from References 1, 6.

Multiple techniques can help you handle difficult questions. The two that most likely will be most helpful are *bridging* and *hooking and flagging*.

- *Bridging.* In this situation, you should acknowledge the reporter's question and then use a bridging phrase to transition to the crucial information you need to convey. For example,
  - *Redirect the reporter*: "What I think you are asking is . . ."
  - *Acknowledge concerns, and promote what public health personnel are doing*: "We have heard this concern, and we are taking the following steps to address it."
  - *Contradict and redirect*: "Not exactly; let me clarify . . ."
  - *Time*: "Historically, that was the case, but this is how we are addressing the problem today because now we know that . . ."
  - *When you do not have the answer*: "Because this is an ongoing investigation, I do not have all the answers, but what I can tell you is . . ."
- *Hooking and flagging.* These techniques can help drive home key public health information (or the SOHCO) in a soundbite format. When you *hook*, you provide the messaging in bite-sized chunks that help the audience retain more information. An example of this is providing the messaging in the form of steps; for example,
  - "We want people to remember three things. One, [public health recommendation 1]. Two, [public health recommendation 2]. And three, [public health recommendation 3]."

When you *flag* messaging, you verbally cue the reporter and audience to the key public health information they need to remember; for example,

- "I've talked about a lot of things today, but this is the most important thing people need to remember . . ."
- "The overall concern is . . ."
- "What is most important to remember is . . ."

Additional tips are included here for managing media interviews; these tips can vary on the basis of the type of media and format of the interview (Table 12.3).

TABLE 12.3 Tips for mastering media interviews

Media type	Interview format	
Print (e.g., newspaper or magazine)	By telephone	In person
On the record	Consider everything on the record. Even if a reporter promises you the information is off the record, consider every telephone call or email message to be on-the-record.	Consider everything on the record. Reporters will often be in an agency's or health department's emergency operations center during an outbreak or staying in the same hotel as you during field investigations; consider any passing comment as an on-the-record quotation, even after the "Thank you" and the pen is put away.
Tone and body language	Watch your tone and vocal inflections. Standing during a telephone interview will enable you to walk around and use hand gestures, which might make you feel more relaxed and make your tone more natural.	Watch your body language. If you are sitting in front of the reporter, be aware of what your body language is conveying; if you are talking about something sad, ensure your face and body language reflect the seriousness of the situation.
Silence during an interview	Do not try to fill the silence. Reporters are probably going to be typing during the interview; pause regularly to let them catch up; do not think you need to fill every silent moment.	Do not try to fill the silence. One savvy reporter often fills space during in-person interviews with a "Hmmm!" that demonstrates interest and can result in the interviewee continuing to talk on and on; however, wandering in the conversation during an interview will take you off-message.
Radio	Taped radio interview	Live radio interview (with call-in questions)
Word choice	Use shorter words that are easier for you to pronounce and easier for listeners to understand. If some words are hard for you to say, stay away from those or others that might be difficult for the audience to understand; ask someone in advance to listen to you talk through the information you intend to present.	
Vocal inflections	Be acutely aware of your vocal inflections; control your pitch, volume, and pace. Use a charismatic and empathetic tone; do not be energetic while conveying a sad situation. Be memorable; try to use the reporter's name or repeat the name of the caller when answering the question; for example, "Good question, Nancy."	

TABLE 12.3 Continued

Media type	Interview format	
Strategies to remember	Do not try to fill the space during a taped radio interview. You will probably provide a few quotations during the segment; write down the top three to five SOHCOs and repeat these key messages multiple times. If you do not like what you have said, ask the reporter if you can restate your answer in a tighter soundbite. Say, for example, "Let me see if I can say that more clearly."	Fill the space during a live radio interview. Prioritize your messaging, and try to use as many of the messages as possible in the segment. Use bridging or hooking and flagging techniques.[a]
TV interview	Taped interview	Live broadcast
Appearance	Appearances are important. Be likeable; smile, but only when appropriate. Be calm, and guard your facial expressions; you do not want to look shocked when the reporter asks a difficult question. Dress professionally; solid colors are best.	
Messaging	Soundbites are crucial. You will probably provide a few quotations in the segment; write down your top three to five SOHCOs and repeat them multiple times. If you do not like what you have said, ask the reporter if you can restate your answer in a tighter soundbite. Say, for example, "Let me see if I can say that more clearly."	Soundbites are crucial. Make sure your SOHCOs are utmost in mind. Use bridging or hooking and flagging techniques.[a]

[a] *Bridging*: Acknowledge the reporter's question and then use a bridging phrase to transition to the crucial information you need to convey. *Hooking and flagging*: A hook provides the messaging in bite-sized chunks that help the audience retain more information, and a flag verbally cues the reporter and audience to the key public health information they need to remember.

SOHCO, Single Overriding Health Communication Objective.

Source: Adapted from References 1, 6.

After the Interview

To the extent possible, try to assess the effectiveness of media interactions. Review news stories and media coverage to learn how reporters are using the information you provided. Assess whether the key messages (SOHCO) are being used and how—and whether the headlines approximate the ones that you were striving to convey. Each interview is an opportunity to learn and improve.

If a reporter publishes inaccurate information, or the information you provided to reporters changes, work with a communications or media specialist to call the reporters back and update them with the new or corrected information. In an ideal situation, the story will be published, and you will be satisfied with the headline and messages conveyed.

CONCLUSION

As technology and media evolve, the public will continue to adapt and get information in new ways. Public health officials communicating about risks must evolve as well so that they can reach target audiences with important and timely health-related information by using the audience's preferred communication mechanisms. The communication strategies outlined in this chapter have proved effective during outbreak responses and risk communication events and can be tailored and adapted to fit any public health event. During an outbreak, public health officials must quickly determine the communication purpose, the persons and populations most in need of information and guidance, ways to engage with news media and the public, and ways to gauge the effects of messages and materials. Knowledge of how the news media and journalists operate, as well as the ability to use risk communication principles and best practices, increases the likelihood of success during public health events.

ACKNOWLEDGMENTS

Katherine Lyon-Daniel and Sue Swenson, Centers for Disease Control and Prevention, provided assistance and technical review of the chapter.

REFERENCES

1. Reynolds B, Seeger, M. Crisis and emergency risk communications manual. 2014 edition. https://emergency.cdc.gov/cerc/manual/index.asp

2. World Health Organization. Communicating risk in public health emergencies: a WHO guideline for emergency risk communication (ERC) policy and practice. http://www.who.int/risk-communication/guidance/download/en/

3. Mitchell A, Gottfried J, Barthel M, Shearer E. *The modern news consumer: news attitudes and practices in the digital era.* Washington, DC: The Pew Research Center; 2016. http://www.journalism.org/2016/07/07/the-modern-news-consumer/

4. Sandman P. Hazard versus outrage in the public perception of risk. In: Covello VT, McCallum DB, Pavlova MT, eds. *Effective risk communications.* Vol. 4, Contemporary issues in risk analysis. New York: Plenum Press; 1989:45–9.

5. Covello V. Communicating radiation risks: crisis communications for emergency responders. https://go.usa.gov/xnM8X

6. Agency for Toxic Substances and Disease Registry. A primer on health risk communication principles and practices. http://www.atsdr.cdc.gov/risk/riskprimer/index.html

7. Reynolds B, Quinn Crouse S. Effective communication during an influenza pandemic: the value of using a crisis and emergency risk communication framework. *Health Promot Pract.* 2008;9(4 Suppl):13S–17S.

8. Centers for Disease Control and Prevention. Safe healthcare blog. What to tell patients when things go wrong (Part 2 of 2). https://blogs.cdc.gov/safehealthcare/what-to-tell-patients-when-things-go-wrong-part-2-of-2/

9. The Legal Examiner. New York City, New York. 5,000 Mayo Clinic and St. Luke's patients at risk for hepatitis C from hospital employee. http://newyorkcity.legalexaminer.com/miscellaneous/5000-mayo-clinic-and-st-lukes-patients-at-risk-for-hepatitis-c-from-hospital-employee/

10. Centers for Disease Control and Prevention. Press briefing transcripts: CDC briefing on public health investigation of human cases of swine influenza. https://www.cdc.gov/media/transcripts/2009/t090424.htm

11. World Health Organization. Outbreak communication planning guide. 2008 ed. http://www.who.int/ihr/elibrary/WHOOutbreakCommsPlanngGuide.pdf

12. Vijaykumar S, Nowak G, Himelboim I, Jin Y. Virtual Zika transmission after the first U.S. case: who said what and how it spread on Twitter. *Am J Infect Control.* 2018;pii:S0196–6553(17)31211–7.

13. Centers for Disease Control and Prevention. Injection safety: patient notification toolkit. https://www.cdc.gov/injectionsafety/pntoolkit/section3.html

14. Centers for Disease Control and Prevention. Emergency preparedness and response: manual and tools. http://emergency.cdc.gov/cerc/resources/index.asp

15. Covello V. *Risk and crisis communication: 77 questions commonly asked by journalists during a crisis.* New York: Center for Risk Communication; 2002. http://www.nwcphp.org/docs/pdf/journalist.pdf

Special Considerations

/// 13 /// LEGAL CONSIDERATIONS

JAMES D. HOLT, SUDEVI NAVALKAR GHOSH,
AND JENNIFER R. BLACK

INTRODUCTION

A core duty and primary function of any government is protection of the public's health and safety. Field epidemiology—including investigation of disease outbreaks and clusters—is a critical, basic government function conducted by public health agencies at the state and federal levels. The federal government's authority to protect public health and safety is found in the US Constitution. And while states address the protection of public health and safety in their individual constitutions, each state is also vested with "police powers," that is, inherent authority to impose restrictions on private rights for the sake of public welfare, order, and security. Both federal and state authorities are subject to the limitations and restraints of the US Constitution. These legal authorities enable public health officials to take certain actions during epidemiologic investigations, such as obtaining clinical specimens and data from persons affected by an outbreak; obtaining data from healthcare facilities; collecting environmental samples; protecting the privacy of personal information; and implementing and enforcing control measures, such as vaccination, chemoprophylaxis, quarantine, or even seizure or destruction of private property.[a]

This chapter provides an overview of legal considerations relating to field epidemiology and, more specifically, epidemiologic investigations. It discusses the interplay of federal and state laws; legal issues related to data collection, analysis, and dissemination, including health information privacy; special or unique jurisdictions; and state and federal cooperation in emergency responses, including investigations of disease outbreaks that may be terrorism-related.

GENERAL LEGAL AUTHORITIES

Article 1, Section 8, of the US Constitution authorizes Congress to impose taxes to provide for "the general Welfare of the United States"[b] and to regulate interstate commerce.[c] The epidemiologic investigations conducted by the Centers for Disease Control and Prevention (CDC) and members of the US Public Health Service are examples of federal activities that are generally supported by these authorities. Under the authority of the US Constitution's Commerce Clause, the federal government also oversees such health-related activities as the inspection of meat, poultry, and other foods; the regulation of drugs, biological products, and medical devices; and the regulation of biological agents that have the potential to pose a severe threat to public health and safety. Although the provisions in the US Constitution are broad, the activities of the federal government relating to health and welfare nonetheless must fit within these enumerated powers. Additionally, the Bill of Rights[d] can restrain the exercise of federal authority.

By contrast, a state's authority to protect public health—often included in the authorities referred to as "police powers"—is extensive (1). "The police power is the natural authority of sovereign governments to regulate private interests. We define police power as the inherent authority of the state (and, through delegation, local government) to enact laws and promulgate regulations to protect, preserve, and promote the health, safety, morals, and general welfare of the people. To achieve these communal benefits, the state retains the power to restrict, within federal and state constitutional limits, private interests; personal interests in autonomy, privacy, association, and liberty as well as economic interests in freedom to contract and uses of property" (2). "A state's police power . . . may be lawfully resorted to for the purpose of preserving the public health, safety or morals, or the abatement of public nuisances, and a large discretion is necessarily vested in the legislature to determine not only what the interests of the public require, but what measures are necessary for the protection of such interests" (notes omitted) (3). In many instances, a state has delegated its public health authority to county, parish, or municipal governments to examine, treat, and, in the event of certain contagious diseases, even quarantine citizens to protect the public health.

The authority of federal and state governments to enact laws protecting public health extends to the promulgation of regulations, the issuance of executive orders, and the publication of directives from health authorities that may have the force and effect of law (Box 13.1).

The exercise of a state's public health police powers has limitations. The US Constitution provides safeguards to ensure that the exercise of these powers is not excessive or unrestrained. For example, the Fourth Amendment protects citizens from unreasonable searches and seizures. Whereas the Fifth Amendment prohibits the federal government from depriving any person of life, liberty, or property without due process of law, the Fourteenth Amendment imposes similar due process protection on the individual states. "The guaranty of due process . . . demands only that the law shall not be unreasonable, arbitrary or capricious, and that the means selected shall have a real and substantial relation to the object sought to be attained" (4). The basic elements of due process include notice to the person involved and opportunity for a hearing or similar proceeding.

In the exercise of its public health police powers, a state must use the least restrictive alternative that will achieve the state's interest, particularly when the exercise involves

---

BOX 13.1

HEALTH AUTHORITIES

- A *statute* (or law) is an act of Congress (signed by the President) or a state legislature (signed by a governor).
- A *regulation* (or rule) is promulgated under the authority of a statute, has legal force, and is usually issued by an administrative agency.
- An *executive order* is generally a directive from the President or a governor to members of his or her executive branch but also may have legal force if used to meet a statutory prerequisite for the expansion of emergency response powers.

limitation of an individual's liberty. The standard used to determine that a government's exercise of its public health police powers is appropriate is whether the government action is necessary, uses reasonable means, is proportional, and avoids harm (5).

STATE AND FEDERAL LEGAL AUTHORITIES

Field epidemiology is defined generally as the application of epidemiologic methods to unexpected health problems when an epidemiologic investigation is needed (6). As field epidemiologists conduct such investigations, they should be cognizant of the legal authorities and potential legal parameters around their work to maximize the benefit of the work and minimize possible legal risks.

State Legal Authorities

A state's inherent "police powers" provide state and local health officials broad authority to conduct field epidemiology.[e] As a practical matter, institutions and individuals generally voluntarily cooperate in epidemiologic investigations. However, just as many field investigations require support from competent laboratory staff, a field investigation also may require support from competent legal staff when voluntary cooperation is not forthcoming. If an investigator meets with resistance, state and local public health officials may need the assistance of their general counsel or their state's attorney general for such actions as applying for a court order to compel an entity (or individual) to grant investigators access to premises or records.[f] Although assistance from legal counsel might never be needed, it is a good idea nonetheless to identify the attorney or legal office that can supply legal advice and support before the epidemiologic investigation begins.

In addition to the legal authorities that enable health agencies to undertake epidemiologic investigations, myriad related considerations exist regarding responsibilities and authorities for the individual elements of an investigation. Such considerations encompass the authorities necessary to

- Obtain microbiological and other laboratory specimens from hospitals and private laboratories;
- Review patients' medical records kept in the offices of physicians, dentists, and other healthcare providers;
- Administer questionnaires to and collect specimens from persons affected in the outbreak;

- Administer questionnaires to unaffected persons who might serve as controls in analytic studies and/or as important sources of information;
- Retain information about medical histories and laboratory results;
- Protect confidentiality;
- Implement a variety of measures intended to control the immediate problem, prevent recurrences, and evaluate the effectiveness of interventions;
- Collect additional data on an ongoing basis;
- Recall an implicated product;
- Close a business or otherwise restrict activities relating to the source of an outbreak;
- Use isolation or other forms of restrictions of activities of affected persons;
- Quarantine exposed persons;
- Vaccinate or administer antibiotics to exposed groups.

Public health surveillance systems in the United States are established as an exercise of the states' police powers. These state-based systems are designed for reporting of diseases and conditions of public health interest by healthcare professionals and laboratories. All states have laws and regulations that mandate the reporting of a list of diseases and conditions, as well as prescribing the timing and nature of information to be reported and the penalties for noncompliance with the reporting laws (7). Required disease reporting varies greatly among states and territories. Some states have general statutes that empower the health commissioner or state boards of health to create, monitor, and revise the list of reportable diseases and conditions (8). Some states require reports under both statutes and health department regulations (9). Reporting may be required of a variety of professionals and organizational entities, including physicians and other healthcare providers, diagnostic laboratories, clinical facilities, and schools and daycare centers (7,10,11).

The scope and nature of reporting requirements vary considerably by state, differing, for example, by the number of conditions required for reporting, time periods within which conditions must be reported, agencies to which reports must be submitted, and persons or sources required to report. Moreover, despite the legal requirements for reporting, adherence to and completeness of reporting also vary substantially by infectious disease agent, ranging from 6% to 90% for different common infectious conditions (12). The deficiencies in reporting by physicians are accounted for, in part, by limitations in physicians' knowledge of reporting requirements and procedures, as well as the assumption that laboratories have reported cases of infectious diseases (7,13).

Federal Legal Authorities

Federal public health officials have limited statutory authorities to initiate independent epidemiologic investigations. One general statutory authority that applies to federal epidemiologic investigations is section 301(a) of the Public Health Service Act (PHSA) (42 USC § 241(a)) (14), which provides

> The Secretary [of the US Department of Health and Human Services (HHS)] shall conduct in the [Public Health] Service, and encourage, cooperate with, and render assistance to the other appropriate public authorities, scientific institutions, and scientists in the conduct of, and promote the coordination of, research, investigations, experiments, demonstrations, and studies relating to the causes, diagnosis, treatment, control, and prevention of physical and mental diseases and impairments of man.

In addition, subsection 6 of section 301(a) of the PHSA authorizes the HHS Secretary to "make available to health officials, scientists, and appropriate public health and other nonprofit institutions and organizations, technical advice and assistance on the application of statistical methods to experiments, studies, and surveys in health and medical fields." Although these provisions are broadly worded and are permissive rather than compulsory, they nonetheless provide legal authority for assistance by federal epidemiologists in disease outbreaks and other instances in which such assistance is requested. In practice, local and state public health officials often request federal assistance in epidemiologic investigations. Federal public health employees who collaborate with state and local public health authorities in such investigations generally are assisting the state or local investigation under the state's authority.

LEGAL ISSUES RELATED TO PUBLIC HEALTH DATA COLLECTION, ANALYSIS, AND DISSEMINATION

Before undertaking epidemiologic field investigations, investigators should be aware of particular legal issues related to data collection, analysis, and dissemination that their investigatory work might implicate. Some important questions to consider are

- Who is asking for these data to be collected, analyzed, and/or disseminated?
- Why are these data being collected, analyzed, and/or disseminated?

- What type of data (e.g., state, county, geographic codes, individual names, social security numbers, or other personally identifiable codes) are being collected, analyzed, and/or disseminated?
- Under what legal authority are the data being collected, analyzed, and/or disseminated?
- How will the data be stored, secured, and maintained?
- Who will have access to the data and for what purposes?

Answers to these questions can identify which laws—federal and/or state—might apply to the field investigator undertaking the work, to the data being collected, and to any resultant response. For example, when a state public health official requests assistance from a CDC field investigator about an outbreak within a state, both federal and state laws could apply to various aspects of the investigation. At times, those laws may appear to conflict, especially where each respective jurisdiction has coordinated but separate roles and responsibilities. Each party (federal and state) in the investigation must ensure compliance with all laws that apply to it or its actions in the given circumstances. The remainder of this section addresses some of the primary legal issues and laws relevant to data collected as part of a field investigation.

Concepts Related to Public Health Data Collection, Protection, and Dissemination

- "Health information privacy" broadly refers to the rights of individuals to control the acquisition, uses, or disclosures of their identifiable health data.
- The closely related concept of "confidentiality" refers to the obligations of persons who receive information to respect the privacy interest of individuals who are the subjects of the data.
- "Security" refers to technologic or administrative safeguards or tools to protect identifiable health data from unauthorized or unwarranted access or disclosure.

Federal Laws Related to Public Health Data Collection, Protection, and Dissemination

Federal officials have limited authority to initiate epidemiologic investigations. In fact, many CDC authorities are permissive rather than compulsory; thus, CDC's involvement in state and local public health investigations usually is intended to assist the state or local investigator rather than exercise a specific federal authority. Field investigators need to be aware of the following laws, regulations, and legal provisions:

- The regulations found in part 46 of title 45 of the Code of Federal Regulations (CFR) (15) require that data collections deemed to be research require approval by an institutional review board and informed consent by research participants. These regulations protect the rights, welfare, and well-being of research participants. However, most epidemiologic investigations generally fall outside the scope of these regulations.

- The Paperwork Reduction Act of 1995 (16) and its implementing regulations (17) (PRA) may apply if a federal agency, including CDC, conducts or sponsors a data collection involving 10 or more respondents during a 12-month period. The purpose of the PRA is to ensure that federal agencies do not overburden the public with federally sponsored data collections, with duplicate data collections, and/ or with data collections that are not necessary to conduct government business. Data collections subject to the PRA require approval by the White House Office of Management and Budget.

- The Privacy Act of 1974 (18) is the federal law that protects the confidentiality of individually identifiable information when records are maintained by a federal agency in a system of records in which the information is retrieved by a person's name, identification number, or other unique identifier. The Privacy Act has four basic policy objectives:
  - To restrict disclosure of personally identifiable records maintained by agencies;
  - To grant individuals increased right of access to agency records maintained on themselves;
  - To grant individuals the right to seek amendment of agency records maintained on themselves upon showing that the records are not accurate, timely, or complete; and
  - To establish a code of "fair information practices" that requires agencies to comply with statutory norms for collection, maintenance, and dissemination of records.

- The Freedom of Information Act (19) (FOIA) "provides that any person has a right, enforceable in court, to obtain access to federal agency records, except to the extent that such records (or portions of them) are protected from public disclosure by one of nine exemptions or by one of three special law enforcement record exclusions. The FOIA thus established a statutory right of public access to Executive Branch information in the federal government" (20).
  - o FOIA exemption 3 protects information prohibited from disclosure by another federal statute provided that the statute either requires that the matters be withheld from the public in such a manner as to leave no discretion on the

issue or establishes particular criteria for withholding or refers to particular types of matters to be withheld. Examples are found in the Trade Secrets Act, PHSA section 308(d), and newly amended PHSA section 301(d).

- FOIA exemption 5 protects inter- or intra-agency memoranda or letters that would not be available by law to a party other than an agency in litigation with the agency. Courts have construed this language to exempt those documents, and only those documents, that are normally privileged from discovery in civil litigation (21).

- FOIA exemption 6 protects personal privacy interests by exempting records in personnel and medical files and similar files when the disclosure of such information would constitute a clearly unwarranted invasion of personal privacy.

- The Federal Records Act of 1950 (22–25) requires all federal agencies to make and preserve records containing adequate and proper documentation of their organization, function, policies, decisions, procedures, and essential transactions.

- The Health Insurance Portability and Accountability Act of 1996 (HIPAA) (26) was enacted in part to provide legal privacy protections for certain individually identifiable health information called protected health information (PHI). Specifically, HIPAA set out Standards for Privacy of Individually Identifiable Health Information, commonly known as the HIPAA Privacy Rule (27,28). The HIPAA Privacy Rule provides national standards for protecting the privacy of health information and regulate how certain "covered entities" (health plans, healthcare clearinghouses, and healthcare providers who engage in certain electronic transactions) use and disclose protected health information (29). Pursuant to the HIPAA Privacy Rule, these covered entities must provide certain assurances to patients and safeguards for securing patient records. However, appreciating the critical need for public health to use PHI to identify, address, and monitor the public's health, the HIPAA Privacy Rule expressly permits PHI to be shared for specified public health purposes. For example, covered entities may disclose PHI, without individual authorization, to a public health authority legally authorized to collect or receive the information for the purpose of preventing or controlling disease, injury, or disability. See 45 CFR § 164.512(b). Further, the HIPAA Privacy Rule permits covered entities to make disclosures that are required by other laws, including laws that require disclosures for public health purposes (30).

- HIPAA also enacted Security Standards for Protection of Electronic Protected Health Information, commonly known as the HIPAA Security Rule (31,32). The HIPAA Security Rule sets technical standards for ensuring proper access to electronic protected health information by authorized users and provides comprehensive security implementation requirements and specifications. Entities that transmit HIPAA-covered data need to ensure that methods of transmission, storage, and disposition comply with the Security Rule.

- Section 301(d) of the PHSA provides that persons engaged in certain research where identifiable, sensitive information is collected shall receive a certificate of confidentiality from HHS to protect the privacy of individual subjects of such research if the research is funded in whole or in part by the US government or may receive such a certificate from HHS where the research is funded by other parties. The use of this provision may require consultation with the appropriate offices within the respective HHS agency providing funding for the research.

- Sections 308(d) and 924(c) of the PHSA (33,34) provide protection for identifiable information collected respectively by CDC and the HHS' Agency for Healthcare Research and Quality (35,36). "Assurances of Confidentiality" under section 308(d) can be used to protect individuals and institutions providing information, and provides that "No [identifiable] information . . . may be used for any purpose other than the purpose for which it was supplied unless such establishment or person has consented." The use of this provision may require consultation with appropriate offices within the respective HHS agency.

- The E-Government Act of 2002 (37) in part protects the confidentiality of federal government statistical collections of identifiable information, including health information. The Act restricts the use of information gathered for statistical uses to the purposes for which it is gathered and penalizes unauthorized disclosures. It also requires federal agencies to conduct "privacy assessments" before developing or procuring information technology that collects, maintains, or disseminates identifiable information.

- Titles II and III of the E-Government Act of 2002 require that agencies evaluate systems that collect personally identifiable information to determine that the privacy of this information is adequately protected. Office of Management and Budget Memorandum M-07-16 (38) is guidance to the federal Executive Branch that defines personally identifiable information as "information which can be used to distinguish or trace an individual's identity, such as their name, social security number, biometric records, etc. alone, or when combined with other personal or identifying information which is linked or linkable to a specific individual, such as date and place of birth, mother's maiden name, etc." Each federal agency will have an established policy to identify, manage, and respond to suspected or confirmed breaches of personally identifiable information.

- The regulations found at 42 CFR Part 2 (39) implement section 543 of the PHSA (42 USC §290dd-2) (40) and provide for confidentiality of alcohol and drug abuse patient records regulations, more specifically, the confidentiality of the identity, diagnosis, prognosis, or treatment of any patient records maintained in connection with the performance of any federally assisted program or activity relating to substance abuse education, prevention, training, treatment, rehabilitation, or research.

- The Genetic Information Nondiscrimination Act of 2008 (Pub. L. 110-233, 122 Stat. 881) (41) is a federal law that protects individuals against discrimination based on their genetic information in health coverage (Title I) and in employment (Title II). Various regulatory provisions implement the Genetic Information Nondiscrimination Act: for the Department of Labor (29 CFR Part 2590) (42), for Department of the Treasury (26 CFR Part 54) (43), for HHS/Centers for Medicare and Medicaid (45 CFR Parts 144, 146, and 148) (44–46), for HHS/Office of Civil Rights (45 CFR Parts 160 and 164) (47,48) and for the Equal Employment Opportunity Commission (29 CFR Part 1635) (49).

State Laws Related to Public Health Data Collection, Protection, and Dissemination

State officials generally have broader authorities than federal officials with respect to the conduct of epidemiologic investigations within their jurisdiction, in particular regarding the roles and responsibilities of respective state and local officials and the rights and protections afforded to citizens within the jurisdiction. These authorities vary, however, from state to state, and sometimes even within a state, and find their basis in a range of federal, state, and local laws, regulations, and policies. For example, although many states have statutory laws similar to the federal Privacy Act and FOIA, and a few have passed additional privacy protections, most do not have comprehensive statutes regulating the acquisition, use, and disclosure of individual health data. Rather, state privacy laws tend to regulate specific data recipients (e.g., public health agencies, health insurers); certain medical tests, diseases, or conditions (e.g., genetic tests, HIV status, mental disorders); or particular data sources (e.g., nursing or healthcare facilities).

In addition, many healthcare organizations and entities that may contribute data or otherwise be engaged in an outbreak investigation may be considered "covered entities" subject to the HIPAA Privacy Rule. Although the HIPAA Privacy Rule expressly permits the disclosure without individual authorization of protected health information to public health authorities authorized by law to receive such information in the performance of their public health activities,[g] this disclosure is permissive and not mandatory. In addition, as covered entities, and depending on the level of data to be shared, with whom the data may be shared, and any relevant state laws, these entities may have to enter into data-sharing or other types of agreements to be able to provide the data, even for the investigation.

CONSIDERATIONS FOR SPECIAL JURISDICTIONS

An important step in investigating disease outbreaks is obtaining permission and co-operation from the appropriate authorities to conduct the investigation. In addition to identifying local, state, federal, and/or international health agencies involved, epidemiologists should also consider agencies with special jurisdiction (50). Although the following government entities each have special jurisdiction, agencies' jurisdictions often overlap and create complex cases. These special jurisdictions have autonomy and maintain their own public health programs that can address outbreaks. However, they also can request assistance from other health agencies to increase resources and decrease the time to contain an outbreak.

- *US Department of Defense (DoD).* Military commanders have jurisdiction over their bases and facilities. Public health responsibilities are vested in the DoD and the branch of the military (e.g., Department of the Army) affected by an outbreak. During an outbreak investigation at a military base, the field investigator must communicate and cooperate with the military base commander (51). The DoD has established the position of the Public Health Emergency Officer (PHEO). The PHEO is a uniformed services officer or a DoD civilian who is a member of a military service medical department and must be a clinician. The PHEO has relevant training in emergency management and experience in public health. In addition to being the advisor to the commander, the PHEO works with the installation and medical treatment facility emergency managers on all phases of public health emergency management. These personnel communicate with local and state health departments. The PHEO is the advisor to the installation/regional/geographic combatant commander on public health emergencies (52).
- *Tribal governments.* Tribal governments generally have complete sovereignty and autonomy over reservation lands. Nontribal groups can join an investigation only at the tribe's request. Investigations of outbreaks are led by tribal health staff, Indian Health Service (IHS),[h] or state health departments. The IHS can implement investigation measures and control but only with the authorization of the tribal government.

- *State and federal departments of correction.* State and federal prison systems have health policies and health departments with the responsibility to maintain prisoner health. Prison systems are insular, and their individual department of corrections may request public health assistance in an outbreak investigation (53).[i] Some prisons are run by the prison system of the state, but the Federal Bureau of Prisons has jurisdiction over federal correctional facilities and employs a Health Services Division (54).

- *US Department of the Interior (Interior Department).* The Interior Department has jurisdiction over federal lands and natural resources. It employs scientists in its Office of Public Health, and members of the Public Health Service are assigned to the National Park Service for investigations. These staff are knowledgeable about their jurisdictions and should be collaborated with when federal lands are involved in the outbreak investigation.

TERRORISM-RELATED INVESTIGATION

During the course of several weeks beginning September 18, 2001, letters containing live anthrax spores were mailed to several news media offices and to two US Senators. Five people died and 17 others were infected. These anthrax attacks increased recognition of the potential for criminal behavior and other deliberate actions to cause disease outbreaks and crystalized the concept of "forensic epidemiology." Forensic epidemiology has been characterized as "the use of epidemiologic methods as part of an ongoing investigation of a health problem for which there is suspicion or evidence of possible intentional acts or criminal behavior as factors contributing to the health problem" (55). The operational challenges during concurrent public health and law enforcement investigations have stimulated interdisciplinary collaboration that has resulted in the creation of joint agreements between law enforcement and public health authorities and publication of the Federal Bureau of Investigation's (FBI) *Joint Criminal and Epidemiological Investigations Handbook* (56). To assist in the development of local joint agreements, CDC's Public Health Law Program makes available two model memoranda of understanding (MOU) (57). One such MOU is the Model MOU for Joint Public Health/Law Enforcement Investigations (2008), which is designed as a starting point in setting forth the major gaps and problems in cross-sectoral and cross-jurisdictional emergency preparedness planning, as well as identifying some key opportunities for addressing them. A copy of the MOU can be obtained by contacting state and local public health officials or FBI Weapons of Mass Destruction coordinators in FBI field offices or by sending an email request to phlawprogram@cdc.gov. Another is the *Framework for Improving Cross Sector Coordination*. This document outlines the major gaps and problems in cross-sectoral and cross-jurisdictional emergency preparedness planning, as well as key opportunities for addressing them.

Officials conducting public health investigations also need to be aware that the possession of certain biological agents and toxins determined by the HHS Secretary to have the potential to pose a severe threat to public health and safety is regulated under part 73 of title 42 Code of Federal Regulations (58). A list of these "biological select agents and toxins" (BSAT) is found at 42 CFR §§ 73.3, 73.4 (59). Anyone in possession of or having access to BSAT is required to be registered with the federal government and undergo an FBI security risk assessment. Unregistered or nonapproved persons in possession of BSAT could be subject to civil monetary penalties (60) and/or criminal prosecution (61). However, exemptions exist for clinical or diagnostic laboratories and other entities that possess a BSAT contained in a specimen presented for diagnosis or verification provided that certain regulatory conditions are met (62). The HHS Secretary can temporarily exempt an individual or entity from the BSAT regulations on the basis of a determination that the exemption is necessary to provide for the timely participation of the individual or entity in response to a domestic or foreign public health emergency. In addition, BSAT seized by a federal law enforcement agency is excluded from the BSAT regulations provided that certain conditions are met (59). Information about the Federal Select Agent Program is available at http://www.selectagents.gov/.

CONCLUSION

Epidemiologists engaged in field work need to understand the scope of the legal authority of public health officials to investigate diseases. Federal and state laws provide authority for federal and state officials to have access to medical and other records for purposes of public health investigations. These same laws also protect the individual's interest in privacy by placing strict limits on access to medical, hospital, and public health records. Although public health investigations usually rely on the voluntary cooperation of individuals and institutions, federal and state laws do provide authority for the use of compulsory measures when necessary to protect the public health and safety.

Epidemiologists are not expected to know every facet of public health law. However, the use of legal resources that support field work requires an appreciation of the legal issues that pertain to surveillance, privacy of medical records, and the legal responsibilities in the involved jurisdiction(s).

NOTES

a. Because this chapter does not address all possible legal policies and procedures that might exist in a particular jurisdiction or around a specific public health problem, epidemiologists must keep in mind that legal counsel for their respective participating agencies can help determine applicable laws and regulations. Legal counsel for each of these agencies should be identified at the beginning of an investigation and should be enlisted to provide support.

b. Article 1, section 8, clause 1: "The Congress shall have Power to lay and collect Taxes, Duties, Imposts and Excises, to pay the Debts and provide for the common Defence and general Welfare of the United States; but all Duties, Imposts and Excises shall be uniform throughout the United States. . . ."

c. Article 1, section 8, clause 3: "To regulate Commerce with foreign Nations, and among the several States, and with the Indian Tribes."

d. The first 10 Amendments to the US Constitution make up the Bill of Rights.

e. See, for example, 28 Pa. Code § 27.152. Investigation of cases and outbreaks. "(a) The Department or a local health authority may investigate any case or outbreak of disease judged by the Department or local health authority to be a potential threat to the public health. (b) A person may not interfere with or obstruct a representative of the Department or a local health authority who seeks to enter a house, health care facility, building or other premises to carry out an investigation of a case or outbreak, if the representative presents documentation to establish that he is an authorized representative of the Department or the local health authority. (c) In the course of conducting an investigation of a case or outbreak, the authorized representative of the Department or local health authority may conduct a confidential review of medical records. A person may not interfere with or obstruct this review."

f. Ibid.

g. See 45 CFR §§ 164.512(a), (b).

h. IHS is an agency of HHS. IHS provides federal health services to Native Americans and Alaska Natives. The provision of health services to members of federally recognized tribes grew out of the special government-to-government relationship between the federal government and Indian tribes. This relationship, established in 1787, is based on Article I, Section 8, of the Constitution and has been given form and substance by numerous treaties, laws, Supreme Court decisions, and Executive Orders. IHS is the principal federal healthcare provider and health advocate for First Nations people, and its goal is to raise their health status to the highest possible level. IHS provides a comprehensive health service delivery system for approximately 1.9 million Native Americans and Alaska Natives who belong to 567 federally recognized tribes in 35 states. See https://www.ihs.gov/.

i. CDC was involved in investigating an outbreak of Valley Fever in two California Central Valley prisons. They partnered with the California Department of Public Health, the California Correctional Healthcare Services, and the California Department of Corrections and Rehabilitation to investigate the outbreak.

REFERENCES

1. *Bond v. United States*, 134 S. Ct. 2077, 189 L. Ed. 2d 1 (US 2014).
2. Gostin LO, Wiley LF. Public health law in the constitutional design. In: *Public health law: power, duty, restraint*. 3rd ed. Oakland: University of California Press; 2016:73–112.
3. *Holden v. Hardy*, 169 US 366, 392 (1898).
4. *Nebbia v. New York*, 291 US 502, 525, 54 S. Ct. 505, 510 (1934) (footnotes omitted).
5. *Jacobson v. Massachusetts*, 197 US 11; 25 S. Ct. 358 (1905).
6. Gregg MB. *Field epidemiology*. 3rd ed. New York: Oxford University Press; 2008.
7. Chorba TL, Berkelman RL, Safford SK, et al. The reportable diseases: I. Mandatory reporting of infectious diseases by clinicians. *JAMA*. 1989;262:3018–26.
8. Gen Stat of Conn (revised to January 1, 2005), § 19a-2a, Powers and duties, Vol 6, 787.

9. Public Health Code (revised through Sept. 1, 2009). Reportable diseases, § 19a–36, p. 633. http://www.ct.gov/dph/lib/dph/agency_regulations/dph_regulations-9.1.2009.pdf
10. Rousch S, Birkhead GS, Koo D. Mandatory reporting of diseases and conditions by healthcare professionals and laboratorians. *JAMA*. 1999;282:164–70.
11. Thacker SB. Surveillance. In: Gregg MB, Dicker RC, Goodman RA, editors. *Field epidemiology*. New York: Oxford University Press; 1996:16–32.
12. Thacker SB, Berkelman RL. (1988). Public health surveillance in the United States. *Epidemiol Rev*. 1988;10:164–90.
13. Konowitz PM, Petrossian GA, Rose DN. The underreporting of disease and physicians' knowledge of reporting requirements. *Public Health Rep*. 1984;99:31–5.
14. Public Health Service Act, as amended through Pub. L. 114–255 (December 13, 2016).
15. Protection of Human Subjects, 45 CFR Part 46 (2017).
16. Federal Information Policy, 44 USC Sect. 3501 et seq.
17. Controlling Paperwork Burdens on the Public, 5 CFR Part 1320 (2017).
18. Records Maintained on Individuals, 5 USC Sect. 552a.
19. Public Information; Agency Rules, Opinions, Orders, Records, and Proceedings 5 USC Sect. 552.
20. US Department of Justice. Guide to the Freedom of Information Act. https://www.justice.gov/oip/doj-guide-freedom-information-act
21. *NLRB v. Sears, Roebuck & Co.*, 421 US 132, 149 (1975).
22. National Archives and Records Administration, 44 USC Chapter 21.
23. Records Management by the Archivist of the United States, 44 USC Chapter 29.
24. Records Management by Federal Agencies, 44 USC Chapter 31.
25. Disposal of Records, 44 USC Chapter 33.
26. Health Insurance Portability and Accountability Act of 1996, Pub. L No 104-191, 110 Stat. 1936 (1996).
27. General Administrative Requirements, 45 CFR Part 160 (2017).
28. Security and Privacy, 45 CFR Part 164 (2017).
29. HIPAA Privacy Rule. http://www.hhs.gov/hipaa/for-professionals/privacy/
30. CDC. HIPAA Privacy Rule and public health. Guidance from CDC and the U.S. Department of Health and Human Services. *MMWR*. 2003;52:1–12.
31. General Administrative Requirements, 45 CFR Part 160 (2017).
32. Security and Privacy, 45 CFR Part 164, Subparts A and C (2017).
33. General Provisions Respecting Effectiveness, Efficiency, and Quality of Health Services, 42 USC Sect. 242m.
34. Patient Safety Organization Certification and Listing, 42 USC Sect. 299b-24.
35. General Provisions Respecting Effectiveness, Efficiency, and Quality of Health Services, 42 USC Sect. 242m (d).
36. Patient Safety Organization Certification and Listing, 42 USC 299c-3.
37. E-Government Act of 2002, Pub. L. No. 107-347, 116 Stat. 2899 (Dec. 17, 2002).
38. Office of Management and Budget, Memorandum for the Heads of Executive Departments and Agencies, M-07-16, Subject: Safeguarding Against and Responding to the Breach of Personally Identifiable Information (May 22, 2007). https://www.whitehouse.gov/sites/whitehouse.gov/files/omb/memoranda/2007/m07-16.pdf
39. Confidentiality of Alcohol and Drug Abuse Patient Records, 42 CFR Part 2.
40. Public Health Service Act, as amended through Pub. L. 114–255 (December 13, 2016).
41. The Genetic Information Nondiscrimination Act of 2008, Pub. L. 110–233, 122 Stat. 881 (May 21, 2008).
42. Rules and Regulations for Group Health Plans, 29 CFR Part 2590.
43. Pension Excise Taxes, 26 CFR Part 54.
44. Requirements Relating to Health Insurance Coverage, 45 CFR Part 144.
45. Requirements for the Group Health Insurance Market, 45 CFR Part 146.
46. Requirements for the Individual Health Insurance Market, 45 CFR Part 148.

47. General Administrative Requirements, 45 CFR Part 160.
48. Security and Privacy, 45 CFR Part 164.
49. Genetic Information Nondiscrimination Act of 2008, 29 CFR Part 1635.
50. Northwest Center for Public Health Practice, University of Washington. Outbreak investigation. http://www.nwcphp.org/training/tools-resources/uw-epidemiology-competencies/outbreak-investigation
51. Wadl M, Scherer K, Nielsen S, et al. Food-borne norovirus-outbreak at a military base, Germany, 2009. *BMC Infect Dis.* 2010;10:30.
52. Department of Defense Instruction, Number 6200.03, October 2, 2013, SUBJECT: Public Health Emergency Management within the Department of Defense, http://www.dtic.mil/whs/directives/corres/pdf/620003p.pdf
53. CDC. Outbreaks and investigations. http://www.cdc.gov/fungal/outbreaks/
54. Federal Bureau of Prisons. Health Services Division. https://www.bop.gov/about/agency/org_hsd.jsp
55. Goodman RA, Munson JW, Dammers K, Lazzarini Z, Barkley JP. Forensic epidemiology law at the intersection of public health and criminal investigations. *J Law Med Ethics.* 2003;31:684–700.
56. Federal Bureau of Investigation and CDC. Joint criminal and epidemiological investigation handbook. https://www.fbi.gov/file-repository/criminal-and-epidemiological-investigation-handbook.pdf/view
57. CDC. Model memoranda of understanding. https://www.cdc.gov/phlp/publications/type/mmou.html
58. Select Agents and Toxins, 42 CFR Part 73 (2017).
59. Select Agents and Toxins, 42 CFR Sec. 73.5 (Exemptions for HHS select agents and toxins), 73.6 (Exemptions for overlap select agents and toxins) (2017).
60. Regulation of Certain Biological Agents and Toxins, 42 USC Sec. 262a (i) (June 2, 2002).
61. Possession by Restricted Persons, 18 USC Sec. 175b (October 26, 2001).
62. Select Agents and Toxins, 42 CFR Sections 73.3 (HHS select agents and toxins), 73.4 (Overlap select agents and toxins).

COORDINATION OF MULTIPLE STATES AND FEDERAL AGENCIES

TIMOTHY JONES AND CRAIG HEDBERG

INTRODUCTION

Multijurisdictional outbreaks are being increasingly identified. As laboratory technologies for disease surveillance advance and data-sharing tools for interagency communication improve, potential links among widely dispersed cases are more effectively identified. Among foodborne disease outbreaks alone, during 2010–2015, a total of 157 multistate outbreaks were reported, accounting for approximately 10,000 illnesses and 77 deaths (1). However, multistate outbreaks are not limited to foodborne diseases and have been associated with an array of etiologies and sources. Examples include fungal infections associated with contaminated methylprednisolone injections, initially recognized in Tennessee and later reported in 20 states (2); a measles outbreak associated with exposure at an amusement park in California which spread to 17 states (3); a widely dispersed outbreak of tuberculosis among travelers to major metropolitan areas (4); and a combined legionellosis/Pontiac fever outbreak among returning guests living in 26 states and exposed at a hotel in Atlanta (5). Such investigations require cooperation among epidemiologists, laboratory personnel, environmentalists, and regulatory agencies at local, state, and federal levels. Preparing for efficient and effective multijurisdictional coordination is critical for successfully responding to such outbreaks. The success of these efforts should be measured by their ability to identify the etiologic agent, mount a prompt public health intervention, and effectively control the outbreak (6).

In addition to steps involved in all outbreak investigations to identify the source of the outbreak and monitor its progression, particular considerations during multijurisdictional outbreaks include the following (7):

- Rapidly determining when an outbreak is multijurisdictional;
- Identifying potentially involved jurisdictions and agencies;
- Establishing effective and efficient coordination among jurisdictions;
- Clearly identifying a lead outbreak investigation coordinator;
- Monitoring roles and activities in different jurisdictions;
- Managing transitions of the investigation leader or involved parties as the outbreak evolves;
- Coordinating public communications across jurisdictions; and
- Coordinating evaluation of the outbreak investigation and production of a final report, which includes input and data from all involved jurisdictions and agencies.

RAPIDLY DETERMINING WHEN AN OUTBREAK IS MULTIJURISDICTIONAL

A large majority of outbreaks are identified and investigated at the local and state levels and do not involve multiple jurisdictions or outside agencies. Local or state health departments detect approximately 75% of foodborne disease outbreaks through complaints of illness directly by consumers or by healthcare providers aware of clusters of illnesses associated with events or establishments (8). This is the primary detection system for outbreaks caused by norovirus, *Clostridium perfringens*, and other agents for which no pathogen-specific surveillance exists. Relatively few of these outbreaks result in large, complex investigations. For example, an outbreak of norovirus at a restaurant caused by an ill food worker might be an isolated event that can be effectively investigated and controlled by a local health department. However, an outbreak of salmonellosis at a restaurant might herald the interstate distribution of a contaminated fresh produce item

TABLE 14.1 Multijurisdictional[a] foodborne disease outbreaks, United States, 2010–2014

Etiology (pathogen)	Total outbreaks	Multistate, no. (%)		Multicounty, no. (%)	
		Exposure	Residence	Exposure	Residence
Confirmed	2,150	124 (6)	281 (13)	145 (7)	540 (25)
Salmonella	632	65 (10)	86 (14)	77 (12)	184 (29)
Norovirus	834	3 (0)	120 (14)	11 (1)	229 (27)
Staphylococcus aureus enterotoxin	26	2 (8)	0	8 (31)	8 (31)
Suspected	803	3 (0)	70 (9)	9 (1)	146 (18)
Unknown	1,170	0	108 (9)	27 (2)	204 (17)
Multiple	55	0	7 (13)	2 (4)	15 (27)
Total	4,178	127 (3)	466 (11)	183 (4)	905 (22)

[a]Based on the ill person's area of residence or location where the contaminated food was eaten ("exposure").

that will require the efforts of multiple public health and food regulatory agencies to trace to its source. The exposure to a source of infection and/or the location of ill persons can span jurisdictions (Table 14.1). The variety of food- and water-related vehicles and the complexity of their distribution mean that even apparently simple outbreaks can result in complex investigations. Thus, multijurisdictional outbreaks are frequently detected at the local level or by one agency, and subsequent investigation leads to involvement of other parties.

At the other end of the surveillance spectrum, most multistate outbreaks of *Salmonella*, Shiga toxin–producing *Escherichia coli*, and *Listeria monocytogenes* infections are detected through pathogen-specific surveillance, increasingly coordinated through PulseNet (https://www.cdc.gov/pulsenet), created by the Centers for Disease Control and Prevention (CDC). The multistate distribution of cases implies the widespread distribution of contaminated food products or ingredients. Investigation of these clusters is multijurisdictional from the onset.

IDENTIFYING POTENTIALLY INVOLVED JURISDICTIONS AND AGENCIES

"Jurisdictions" can be defined by a variety of criteria. These include geography (e.g., different states), regulatory responsibilities (e.g., the Food and Drug Administration [FDA] and US Department of Agriculture [USDA] have nationwide authorities but over different foods), administrative authority (e.g., FDA Office of Regulatory Affairs Regional Field Offices), and outbreak characteristics (e.g., Federal Bureau of Investigation involvement if a crime is suspected).

Many agencies have overlapping jurisdictions, and even within one agency multiple offices or groups can have different responsibilities or authorities, making coordination of communication among multiple parties exceedingly complex. Likewise, different agencies might have "jurisdiction" over different aspects of an outbreak (Table 14.2). For example, at a wedding party, persons from multiple states might have become ill from eating a food in one state from food produced in yet a different state. In such an instance, each individual state (or county) with ill persons is responsible for conducting the epidemiologic interview of affected persons in its jurisdiction. The local health department could have jurisdiction over the caterer that prepared and served the food. The local department of agriculture might regulate the retail store from which the implicated ingredient was purchased. The FDA might have jurisdiction over the facility that produced the product (as well as the farm at which it was grown, unless it came from another country, in which case the FDA would be responsible for coordinating international communications with the foreign agency regulating that facility).

ESTABLISHING EFFECTIVE AND EFFICIENT COORDINATION AMONG JURISDICTIONS

Rapidly determining which jurisdictions and agencies need to be involved in any outbreak investigation is critical for prompt notification and coordination of investigations (Table 14.3). The agency that detected the outbreak might assume initial responsibility for coordination among jurisdictions. Investigations should be coordinated at the level where relevant investigation steps can be most effectively implemented (6), which requires that the agency have sufficient resources, expertise, and legal authority to collect, organize, analyze, and disseminate data from the investigation.

Coordinating outbreak investigations across jurisdictions requires effective interagency communication. Important tasks include making the initial notifications, establishing roles and responsibilities for each jurisdiction, providing updates on the progress of the investigations, revising priorities for the investigation, and establishing the next steps. Conference calls among collaborating agencies have become a common feature of multistate outbreak investigations. Although these can be an effective way to share information among all parties, the purpose of the call is to facilitate the rapid investigation of the outbreak and focus on issues of import to multiple agencies. In large and prolonged outbreak responses, the number and length of conference calls can impede the investigation's efficiency, and the outbreak Incident Commander (who usually

TABLE 14.2 Roles of selected government agencies that respond to outbreaks[a]

Jurisdiction, agency	Responsibilities
Local/State	
Health departments	
Epidemiology	Conduct surveillance for notifiable diseases and investigation of foodborne, waterborne, and other outbreaks in their county/state; The relative autonomy/authority of local vs. state agencies vary per state.
Regulatory	Conduct licensing, inspection, and environmental investigation of outbreaks in pools, food-service, and other regulated institutions in their county/state.
Departments of agriculture	Conduct licensing, inspection, and environmental investigation of farms, food-production facilities and warehouses, milk-production facilities, water-bottling facilities, grocery stores, and many retail food establishments.
Water regulatory agencies	Regulate drinking water supplies, often including surface water, wells, source water protection, and public water systems.
Federal	
CDC	Assists state and local authorities in surveillance and outbreak investigations; by invitation, provides laboratory and epidemiology support; participates in multistate and international outbreaks.
FDA	Regulates manufacturers, processors, and distributors of human and animal foods, bottled water, pharmaceuticals and medical devices, dietary supplements, tobacco, blood transfusion products. Assists local and state authorities in investigations associated with products they regulate, performs product trace-backs, provides laboratory and regulatory support
USDA-FSIS	Regulates domestic and imported meat, poultry and egg products
FBI	Leads investigations of outbreaks involving criminal acts including terrorism.
International: WHO	Provides technical assistance through the Global Outbreak Alert and Response Network, Disease Control in Humanitarian Emergencies, and diseases reported under International Health Regulations.

[a]Examples of general responsibilities for government agencies frequently involved in investigating outbreaks. All states have unique laws, policies, and organizational structures that will affect investigations, and many other agencies and organizations might play important roles in certain situations.

CDC, Centers for Disease Control and Prevention; FBI, Federal Bureau of Investigation; FDA, Food and Drug Administration; USDA-FSIS, US Department of Agriculture, Food Safety and Inspection Service; WHO, World Health Organization.

TABLE 14.3 Examples of major indicators of foodborne disease outbreaks outbreak and required notification steps

Outbreak detection	Major indicator	Notification steps
Local level	Commercially distributed, processed, or ready-to-eat food contaminated before point of service suspected or implicated as outbreak vehicle.	Immediately notify state health department, relevant state food regulatory agency, CDC, and FDA or USDA-FSIS (depending on product and on local and state reporting requirements).
	Fresh produce item contaminated before point of service is suspected or implicated as outbreak vehicle.	Immediately notify state health department, relevant state food regulatory agency, CDC, and FDA, depending on state and local reporting requirements.
	Ground beef is implicated in an outbreak of *Escherichia coli* O157:H7 infections.	Immediately notify state health department, relevant state food-regulatory agency, CDC, and USDA-FSIS, depending on state and local reporting requirements.
	Molecular subtype characteristics of etiologic agent matches the pattern of an agent independently associated with other foodborne disease outbreaks.	Immediately notify state health department, relevant state food regulatory agency, CDC, and FDA or USDA-FSIS, depending on product and state and local reporting requirements.
	Intentional contamination of food item is suspected or implicated.	Immediately notify state health department, relevant state food regulatory agency, CDC, and FDA or USDA-FSIS (depending on product), local law enforcement, and FBI.
	Illnesses are associated with multiple restaurants or food-service establishments, especially when those establishments are part of the same chain.	Immediately notify state health department, relevant state food-regulatory agency, and CDC, depending on local and state reporting requirements.
State level	Increase of sporadic infections with common subtype characteristics identified across multiple jurisdictions.	Immediately notify affected local agencies, CDC, and state and federal food regulatory agencies.
	Multiple common-source outbreaks linked by common agent, food, or water.	Immediately notify affected local agencies, CDC, and relevant state and federal food regulatory agencies.
	Microbiological food testing by state food regulatory agency prompts recall.	Immediately notify affected state and local public health agencies, CDC, relevant federal food regulatory agencies.

Table 14.3 (Continued)

Outbreak detection	Major indicator	Notification steps
	Illnesses are associated with multiple restaurants or food service establishments, especially when those establishments are part of the same chain.	Immediately notify relevant state food regulatory agency and CDC, depending on product and local and state reporting requirements.
	Intentional contamination of food item is suspected or implicated.	Immediately notify state food regulatory agency, CDC, and FDA or USDA-FSIS (depending on product), local law enforcement, and FBI.
Federal level	Increase of sporadic infections with common subtype characteristics identified across multiple states.	Immediately notify affected state and local public health agencies, federal food regulatory agencies.
	Multiple common-source outbreaks linked by common agent, food, or water.	Immediately notify affected state and local public health agencies, CDC, relevant state and federal food regulatory agencies.
	Microbiological food testing by, or reported to, FDA or USDA-FSIS prompts recall.	Immediately notify affected state and local public health agencies, CDC, relevant state and federal food regulatory agencies.

Source: Adapted from Reference 6.
CDC, Centers for Disease Control and Prevention; FBI, Federal Bureau of Investigation; FDA, Food and Drug Administration; USDA-FSIS, US Department of Agriculture, Food Safety and Inspection Service.

is a formally designated official in the lead coordinating agency) should appropriately manage the frequency and agenda of multijurisdictional discussions.

Important considerations in multistate outbreak investigations include legal barriers to sharing data, which can limit what can be communicated between agencies. Personally identifiable health information is protected under state disease reporting laws and often cannot be shared across jurisdictions (9,10). However, most demographic data, important clinical details, and exposure information can be extracted from case-patient interviews and shared in aggregate form or as a de-identified dataset. In many outbreak investigations, epidemiologists share exposure information with environmental health specialists and regulatory agencies for the purpose of conducting investigational trace-backs to improve the specificity of exposure assessments. In some instances, regulatory agencies are precluded from sharing the results of their investigations with the epidemiologists because of specific restraints within state laws or federal protections for industry trade secrets. FDA has a provision for sharing information (e.g., proprietary or personally identifiable data) with officially designated persons at the state level, but those persons are prevented from sharing specific information with other colleagues. Barriers to sharing results of investigation activities among jurisdictions are a primary challenge to an effective and efficient response. In addition, commercial entities are also protected, and their identity often cannot be disclosed to protect confidentiality of commercial interests. Some of these barriers may be addressed by involving agency attorneys early in an investigation to identify perceived versus actual legal barriers and help develop waivers or de-identification methods to achieve the desired purposes without violating confidentiality laws.

CLEARLY IDENTIFYING A LEAD OUTBREAK INVESTIGATION COORDINATOR

Establishing what agency (and what representative of that agency) is ultimately responsible for coordinating communication and activities of all involved parties is critical. This frequently involves clearly identifying an overall Incident Commander in the Incident Command System (ICS) or an equivalent management structure (see Chapter 16). The Incident Commander is a formally designated position, usually within the agency leading the overall investigation, who is responsible for coordinating overall response activities. Even in multistate outbreaks, the Incident Commander or central outbreak coordinator does not necessarily have to be from a federal agency. For example, in some cases, even in relatively small outbreaks, a local or state agency might invite CDC to lead an investigation. In other situations, for example when one state has a substantial proportion of cases and a robust capacity to investigate, that state might lead the coordination of activities, even across multiple other states and federal agencies. Frequently, the central outbreak coordinator changes as an outbreak response evolves, but any such transitions must be formal and clearly communicated to all participating agencies.

In establishing effective coordination among agencies during a multijurisdictional outbreak response, it is also important to identify a single (or limited number of) point of contact for communication with each agency. Although large numbers of persons might participate in conference calls, meetings, and email communications, it is impossible for a central Incident Commander or outbreak coordinator to ensure that all necessary information reaches the appropriate people in multiple agencies. One point of contact within each agency should be responsible for the "communication tree" within that agency. In all but the simplest outbreaks, the ICS structure should be implemented rapidly. Under such a system, communication can be further coordinated by function (e.g., the Public Information Officer within each agency communicates through the ICS Public Information Officer).

MONITORING ROLES AND ACTIVITIES IN DIFFERENT JURISDICTIONS

Compiling descriptive epidemiology and preliminary exposure assessments are important to generating hypotheses about the source and transmission routes of the outbreak. Early coordination of epidemiologic studies among affected states is important for efficiently gathering data. Most state health departments have developed their own standard questionnaires for routine interviews of persons identified as having reportable diseases, but clearly defining a consistent case-definition across jurisdictions is a critical step. When an outbreak is suspected, more complex hypothesis-generating questionnaires or analytic study questionnaires are needed. If the outbreak involves multiple states, early coordination to use the same questions in all jurisdictions can ensure that data can be combined for overall analyses and minimize the need for repeated interviews of case-patients as additional details are required. Typically, most states prefer (or are required) to investigate case-patients who reside in their jurisdictions. As noted earlier, legal privacy requirements might prevent sharing of personally identifiable data with other jurisdictions, which precludes cross-jurisdictional interviews and requires sharing of only de-identified data for overall analyses. This requires rapid development of a uniform data-collection instrument and a (preferably electronic) mechanism for capturing data quickly from all jurisdictions into one database that the coordinating agency can analyze centrally. Because conducting case-patient interviews is frequently a rate-limiting step in outbreak investigations, the progress of completing interviews should be routinely monitored by the Incident Commander. If agencies or individuals are unable to complete interviews in a timely manner, alternative arrangements should be made.

In addition to compiling the results of interviews, feedback from the interviews might be useful to (1) identify specific exposures that need to be assessed but were not included on questionnaires, (2) guide environmental health specialists investigating establishments, and (3) identify contamination sources and mechanisms of transmission that need to be traced to identify common distribution pathways that can be incorporated into subsequent analyses. As the outbreak investigation evolves from descriptive epidemiology and hypothesis generation to analytical studies and interventions, the leadership of the investigation might change to reflect its focus. As noted earlier, any such transitions must be formal and clearly defined to all participating parties. In general, investigation of reported cases should be coordinated within the appropriate public health agencies (e.g., state and local health departments, CDC). Similarly, investigation of suspected food items or sources of contamination should be coordinated within the relevant regulatory agencies (e.g., FDA, USDA, local food safety regulators), which will help ensure administrative support for determining the root cause of the outbreak and implementing effective control measures. However, because frequently epidemiologic and regulatory activities considerably overlap, sharing of information between public health and regulatory agencies is critical to the effectiveness of these multijurisdictional investigations.

COORDINATING PUBLIC COMMUNICATIONS ACROSS MULTIPLE JURISDICTIONS

Public messaging can be challenging during multijurisdictional outbreaks. It is imperative that media messages or other public communication be consistent and coordinated to prevent widespread confusion. Varying local and agency-specific policies and legal restrictions can complicate such messaging. For example, some states do not routinely release the names of restaurants or implicated establishments in an outbreak unless there is a compelling public safety reason to do so; in other states, such information is not legally confidential. The legal environment and focus of specific agencies also can affect messaging. Public health epidemiologists, for example, often consider early public notification about an outbreak, even if scientific analyses are preliminary, in the hope of preventing ongoing exposure. Regulatory agencies, in contrast, frequently have policy and legal constraints that require additional investigation and evidence before the release of specific information. In such situations, rapid coordinated negotiations among agencies and jurisdictions are necessary to determine the timing and detail of public messages and the audiences to which they are released.

COORDINATING EVALUATION AND REPORTING OF THE OUTBREAK INVESTIGATION

All outbreak investigations should be documented with a written report that summarizes the principal findings. These documents can be used for training and as source material for more extensive evaluations of outbreak response procedures. In addition, multijurisdictional investigations should be reported to CDC, indicating that the investigation was multijurisdictional. Individual state reports should be consolidated as part of a multistate outbreak report and linked to summary reports written by regulatory agencies. In cases in which the investigation leads to new information that is generalizable and of potential interest to a wider audience, consideration should be given to publishing results in a peer-reviewed professional journal.

As a wrap up for the investigation, collaborating agencies should meet or hold a conference call to review findings and actions taken. In particular, lessons learned about the outbreak investigation methods should be discussed and disseminated. After the meeting or conference call, the lead agency should summarize findings in an after-action report (AAR). All collaborators should review the AAR to ensure consensus and common understanding of the findings. AARs, like other outbreak investigation reports, should be available for evaluation to identify common problems that arise during multijurisdictional investigations.

The following case studies of past events highlight many issues that need to be addressed during coordination of investigative activities by multiple states, local health agencies within those states, and the federal public health and food regulatory agencies.

Case Study 1

Large, multistate outbreaks associated with contaminated ingredients incorporated into many different products have emerged as a substantial challenge to investigations of foodborne disease outbreaks. Such outbreaks are increasingly detected through rapidly evolving molecular subtyping laboratory techniques. A well-documented example of this type of outbreak was the 2008–2009 outbreak of *Salmonella enteriditis* serotype Typhimurium infections associated with peanut butter and peanut butter–containing products (11,12).

On November 10, 2008, CDC PulseNet (a food laboratory network for molecular subtyping of foodborne pathogens) identified a cluster of indistinguishable *Salmonella* Typhimurium isolates in 12 states. Two weeks later, a cluster of 27 *Salmonella* Typhimurium cases from 14 states that had a second DNA fingerprint was identified. Epidemiologic assessment of the clusters began on November 25 for the first cluster and on December 2 for the second cluster. Involved states were notified and asked by CDC to identify potentially common sources from routine interviews conducted by state and local health departments. On December 4, the descriptive epidemiology of both clusters was recognized to be similar, and the clusters were effectively joined for investigation purposes.

Hypothesis-generating interviews using a standardized questionnaire were initiated on November 25. During the next 6 weeks, state and local health department personnel interviewed 86 case-patients in 26 states. Local environmental health specialists, state departments of agriculture, the FDA, and the USDA's Food Safety and Inspection Service all participated in trace-back and trace-forward activities to explore hypotheses for suspected food products.

A turning point in the investigation occurred on December 28, when the Minnesota Department of Health recognized several clusters of cases associated with institutional settings, including nursing homes and schools. By January 4, 2009, Minnesota Department of Agriculture investigators identified a common supplier of peanut butter to the institutions. On January 9, the Minnesota Department of Agriculture microbiology laboratory isolated *Salmonella* from the peanut butter, and FDA began an investigation of the facility at which it was produced. On January 10, the distribution company recalled the product.

Concurrently, staff in CDC's Emergency Operations Center conducted a multistate case–control study implicating peanut butter–containing products in the outbreak. FDA investigators at the peanut butter production facility learned that the company also produced peanut paste that was an ingredient used in crackers. On January 18, the Canadian Food Inspection Agency reported isolating *Salmonella* from intact packages of peanut butter crackers.

Multiple recalls and follow-up investigations were conducted during the ensuing few weeks. Ultimately, almost 4,000 products containing peanut butter produced at a single facility were recalled. A total of 714 cases and nine deaths from 46 states and two countries were associated with the outbreak. An AAR was issued May 18, 2009 (13). At least 190 persons within CDC (the lead agency) participated in the response over the course of 127 days, along with innumerable staff from other federal and state agencies. The outbreak substantially affected the political process that led to passage of the national Food Safety Modernization Act in 2011 (14).

Case Study 2

In 2008, a local health department in Florida identified a cluster of patients with symptoms of acute selenium poisoning (including hair loss and nail changes) (15). As the health department began a local investigation, FDA simultaneously initiated an independent investigation as a result of complaints received through its Safety Information and Adverse Events Reporting System (MedWatch). The local health department investigation rapidly identified a specific vitamin supplement marketed by company A as the source of the outbreak. Case finding identified Internet and phone order sales to customers nationwide, with retail distribution primarily in southeastern states. State health departments, CDC, FDA, and poison control centers were notified. CDC coordinated daily conference calls with all involved agencies.

Ultimately, epidemiologic questionnaires were administered to 227 affected persons in nine states, using a questionnaire developed jointly by the state health departments in Florida and Tennessee. Contact information collected from company A, public calls to health departments, and persons calling regional poison control centers was provided to state health departments, and case-patients were interviewed directly. Because identifying information from persons calling MedWatch could not be released to states, the FDA had to contact patients and ask them to call their health departments directly. The FDA conducted trace-back investigation of the implicated product. The product was distributed by company A in Georgia, which received finished product from a manufacturer in Arkansas, which in turn received ingredients from suppliers in Louisiana. No ill persons were identified in either of the latter states. A nationwide recall of the product was issued. At the conclusion of the investigation, 201 poisoning cases resulting from exposure to selenium were identified in 10 states.

These outbreak investigations involved epidemiology, laboratory, environmental, and regulatory investigators from multiple local, state, and federal agencies. They highlight the importance of multijurisdictional coordination of complex and often overlapping activities to ensure rapid and effective response.

CONCLUSION

Multistate outbreaks are becoming increasingly recognized because of improvements to public health surveillance. Whether detected through pathogen-specific surveillance or through consumer complaint systems, the need for ongoing multijurisdictional communication and coordination should be anticipated at the start of every outbreak investigation. Plans for efficient and effective multijurisdictional coordination need to be developed and exercised to successfully respond to these outbreaks.

REFERENCES

1. CDC. Foodborne Outbreak Online Database (FOOD). http://wwwn.cdc.gov/foodborneoutbreaks/
2. Kainer MA, Reagan DR, Nguyen DB, et al. Fungal infections associated with contaminated methylprednisolone in Tennessee. *N Engl J Med.* 2012;367:2194–203.
3. Zipprich J, Winter K, Hacker J, Xia D, Watt J, Harriman K. Measles outbreak—California, December 2014–February 2015. *MMWR.* 2015; 64:153–4.
4. Sterling TM, Thompson D, Stanley RL, et al. A multistate outbreak of tuberculosis among members of a highly mobile social network: implications for tuberculosis elimination. *Int J Tuberc Lung Dis.* 2000;4:1066–73.
5. Benin AL, Benson RF, Arnold KE, et al. An outbreak of travel-associated Legionnaires disease and Pontiac fever: the need for enhanced surveillance of travel-associated legionellosis in the United States. *J Infect Dis.* 2002;185:237–43.
6. Council to Improve Foodborne Outbreak Response. Investigation of clusters and outbreaks. In: *CIFOR guidelines for foodborne disease outbreak response.* 2nd ed. Atlanta: Council of State and Territorial Epidemiologists; 2014:139–65.

7. Council to Improve Foodborne Outbreak Response. Special considerations for multijurisdictional outbreaks. In: *CIFOR guidelines for foodborne disease outbreak response*. 2nd ed. Atlanta: Council of State and Territorial Epidemiologists; 2014:191–204.

8. Li J, Shah GH, Hedberg C. Complaint-based surveillance for foodborne illness in the United States: a survey of local health departments. *J Food Prot*. 2011;74:432–7.

9. Association of State and Territorial Health Officials. Improving your access to electronic health records during outbreaks of healthcare-associated infections. A toolkit for health departments. http://www.astho.org/Toolkit/Improving-Access-to-EHRs-During-Outbreaks/

10. Association of State and Territorial Health Officials. Address patient privacy, authority and security concerns. http://astho.org/Toolkit/Improving-Access-to-EHRs-During-Outbreaks/Address-Patient-Privacy-Concerns/

11. Cavallaro E, Date K, Medus C, et al. *Salmonella* Typhimurium infections associated with peanut products. *N Engl J Med*. 2011; 65:601–10.

12. CDC. Multistate outbreak of *Salmonella* infections associated with peanut butter and peanut butter–containing products—United States, 2008–2009. *MMWR*. 2009;58:85–90.

13. CDC. 2008–2009 *Salmonella* Typhimurium outbreak response, Nov 2008–March 2009: After action report. May 18, 2009. https://www.cdc.gov/salmonella/typhimurium/SalmonellaTyphimuriumAAR.pdf

14. US Food & Drug Administration. US Department of Health and Human Services. https://www.fda.gov/food/guidanceregulation/fsma/ucm247546.htm

15. MacFarquhar JK, Melstrom P, Hutchison R, et al. Acute selenium toxicity associated with a dietary supplement. *Arch Int Med*. 2010;170:256–261.

/// 15 /// MULTINATIONAL OUTBREAK INVESTIGATIONS

FRANK MAHONEY AND JAMES W. LE DUC

INTRODUCTION

Sharing information about infectious disease outbreaks among affected countries dates back to the earliest recorded history and spans the centuries up to the modern era (Table 15.1). More formal coordination of international outbreak response originated in the nineteenth century, when printed materials were widely distributed and publications about analyses of outbreak data and international prevention strategies became widespread. This chapter provides perspective regarding coordination of international outbreak responses, which have evolved substantially since the efforts of the nineteenth and twentieth centuries.

TABLE 15.1 Historical background of sharing information about infectious disease outbreaks among affected countries

Date	Event
430 BCE	Thucydides describes an outbreak with high mortality that ravages Athens, Greece, causing widescale panic and fear among the city's 315,000 residents (1). Symptoms include abrupt onset of fever, headache, fatigue, and pain in the stomach and extremities, accompanied by severe vomiting, diarrhea, and bleeding from the mouth (1–3). Dehydration becomes so profound that men plunge themselves into wells. Illness frequently ends in death in 7–9 days. Healthcare workers are often affected, but those who survive are able to treat others without becoming reinfected. Modern physicians speculate that this rapidly fatal hemorrhagic fever was caused by Ebola virus disease (2,3).
460–370 BCE	Hippocrates describes clinical and epidemiologic features of epidemic-prone diseases and outbreaks (4).
1st century BCE–1st century AD	In a book on agriculture, Marcus Terentius Varro recommends building houses far away from swamps because of creatures too small to be seen with the eye but that enter the body and cause disease (5). Another agriculturist, Lucius Junius Moderatus Columella (4–c. 70 AD), also warns that swamps release pestilential vapors and produce swarms of insects that cause harm (5). During the same era, the Greeks and Romans develop systems for isolation and treatment of patients with epidemic diseases (6), a practice that continues throughout the Middle Ages and into modern times (5,6).
1829–1849	A cholera pandemic furthers development of the principles of modern epidemiologic investigations, including characterization of disease by person, place, and time (7). During the outbreak, in 1832, Amariah Brigham publishes a dot map and trade routes that detail cholera's spread on a global scale (8,9). Commissions are established and information shared within days and sent on ships, trains, and coaches to other affected countries.
1851	The first International Sanitary Conference is convened in Paris to harmonize conflicting and costly maritime quarantine requirements of different European nations (10).
1892	The first international agreement addressing cholera is signed at the seventh International Sanitary Conference in Venice.
1893 and 1894	Conferences in Dresden and Paris result in two additional agreements relating to cholera.
1897	Countries adopt an agreement regarding ways to prevent the spread of plague.
1903	The four previous agreements are consolidated into one international sanitary agreement.

TABLE 15.1 Continued

Date	Event
1907	Government representatives in Rome agree to establish an Office International d'Hygiène Publique (OIHP) in Paris, with a permanent secretariat and a permanent committee of senior public health officials to oversee international rules regarding quarantining of ships and ports to prevent spread of plague and cholera and to administer other public health agreements.
1924	After World War I, the League of Nations Health Organization is established with an initial focus on detection and response to epidemics in Europe; it later becomes an organization in Geneva, Switzerland, laying the foundation for the core functions of the World Health Organization (WHO).
1946	OIHP is dissolved and its epidemiologic service is incorporated into the Interim Commission of WHO.
1948	WHO is formally established and revises and consolidates the International Sanitary Regulations.
1969	The International Sanitary Regulations are renamed the International Health Regulations (IHR); this first version includes a passive reporting system for cholera, yellow fever, and plague. WHO publishes key features of the diseases in the *Weekly Epidemiologic Record* and describes maximally acceptable measures for preventing the diseases from spreading internationally by setting standards for seaports and airports to prevent disease transmission.
2005	With the growth in international travel and trade and the emergence of international disease threats, the World Health Assembly calls for a substantial revision to the IHR; the third edition is established by the 58th World Health Assembly (11).

INTERNATIONAL HEALTH REGULATIONS

The International Health Regulations (IHR) agreement forms the basis for international collaboration and coordination on detection and response to outbreaks (Box 15.1). As an international agreement, IHR is binding for all 196 World Health Organization (WHO) Member States. IHR focuses on preventing, protecting against, controlling, and responding to the international spread of disease without unnecessary interruptions to traffic and economic trade. The 2005 edition contains key changes from the previous two versions, including

---

BOX 15.1

INTERNATIONAL RESPONSE TO SEVERE ACUTE RESPIRATORY SYNDROME

While the International Health Regulations (IHR) were being developed, the global community was responding to an outbreak of unknown origin that was named severe acute respiratory syndrome (SARS) (12). The rapid spread of SARS highlighted the importance of coordination and collaboration on international outbreak response as the virus spread across the globe in 2003. During the outbreak, information was shared electronically, thus providing detailed knowledge about the outbreak's causative agent, mode of transmission, and other epidemiologic features. The real-time sharing of information was essential for providing guidance about clinical management and protective measures to prevent further spread. The World Health Organization issued a series of recommendations to stop international spread, and airports screened passengers for a history of contacts who were ill with SARS or clinical illness compatible with SARS. Despite remarkable spread, the outbreak was successfully contained within 4 months and represents a good example of how the IHR mechanisms can be successfully applied during coordination of outbreak responses (12).

- Not limiting the scope to specific diseases or manners of transmission, but covering "illnesses or medical conditions, irrespective of origin or source,"
- Member States' obligations for developing core public health capacities to detect and respond to outbreaks,
- Member States' responsibility for notifying WHO of events that might constitute a public health emergency of international concern.
- WHO authorization for considering unofficial reports of public health events and obtaining verification from Member States' Parties concerning such events,
- Procedures for WHO's Director-General to declare a "public health emergency of international concern" and issuance of corresponding temporary recommendations (11).

A *public health emergency of international concern* is defined as an extraordinary event that might constitute a public health risk to other countries through international spread of disease and require an internationally coordinated response (11). Although the current IHR includes considerable responsibilities for Member States and WHO, no provisions are included for ensuring Member States comply with the legally binding agreement.

Mechanisms of Cooperation in International Outbreak Investigations

As outlined in IHR, the responsibility for detecting, investigating, and responding to outbreaks resides within the nation's health authority where the outbreak is occurring. At times, a nation's capacity for responding might be overwhelmed, necessitating outside technical assistance. National health authorities might be hesitant to request assistance because of economic and political concerns, including the impact outbreaks can have on different sectors. The roles and responsibilities of different partners for international support during outbreak responses are outlined in the following sections.

Ministries of Health

Management of outbreaks by national health authorities has evolved, and most countries use some type of structured management system to respond. During the recent Ebola virus disease outbreaks, Nigeria, Liberia, Sierra Leone, and Guinea established emergency operations centers (EOCs) and an incident management system (IMS) to coordinate outbreak response and international support. Within the IMS, EOC managers established technical working groups, co-chaired by technical partners, for managing different aspects of the response (e.g., clinical management, surveillance, laboratory support, communication, and contact tracing) (13). During complex outbreaks such as Ebola, most countries coordinate requests for assistance through WHO; however, authorities might directly request assistance from partners or Member States. In addition, Member States can offer unsolicited support through diverse channels, including WHO.

WHO

The Emergency Response Directorate at WHO provides technical assistance to Member States for early detection and response to infectious disease outbreaks of international concern. In the aftermath of the Ebola epidemic, WHO experienced criticism about weak initial response and underwent a reform process for responding to outbreaks of international concern (14). This reform culminated in a World Health Assembly resolution in 2016 to adopt the Health Emergencies Programme "to deliver rapid, predictable, and comprehensive support to countries and communities as they prepare for, face or recover from emergencies caused by any type of hazard . . ." The reorganization in Geneva convened infectious disease subject-matter and emergency response experts under a centralized management system that is organized into five areas of work:

- Infectious hazard management.
- Country health emergency preparedness.
- Health emergency information and risk assessment.
- Emergency operations.
- Core services.

This organizational structure is generally mirrored within WHO's regional offices. WHO also maintains a roster of technical experts through the Global Outbreak Alert and Response Network (GOARN) who can support all aspects of international outbreak responses (15).

GOARN

In April 2000, WHO established a formal network of partners to respond to infectious disease outbreaks, natural disasters, and other humanitarian emergencies. GOARN is a collaboration of institutions and networks, constantly alert and ready to respond rapidly to outbreaks. Key partners include academic and scientific institutions, medical and surveillance initiatives, laboratory networks, United Nations (UN) organizations, the Red Cross (the International Committee of the Red Cross, the International Federation of Red Cross, the Red Crescent Societies, and other national assistance societies), and international humanitarian nongovernmental organizations (e.g., Médecins sans Frontières, the International Rescue Committee, Medical Emergency Relief International [also known as MERLIN], and Epicentre). The network combines human and technical resources for rapid identification, confirmation, and response to outbreaks to prevent international spread and to develop capacity regarding long-term epidemic preparedness in selected Member States. All activities are aligned with the six work streams, including

- Strengthening GOARN policies, operational procedures, and secretariat functions.
- Expanding participation in the network.
- Engaging partners in alert and risk assessment activities.
- Engaging stakeholders through communications and advocacy.
- Developing operational research and tools.
- Preparing training programs in outbreak response.

Each of the WHO regional offices participates in GOARN, with many having a dedicated GOARN coordinator. In WHO's Western Pacific Region, GOARN is a component of the Asia Pacific Strategy for Emerging Diseases work plan. GOARN receives multiple requests annually to support capacity-building in emergency preparedness.

Since GOARN was created, its partners have provided support during many public health emergencies, including the West Africa Ebola epidemic (Box 15.2). In partnership with WHO, GOARN deployed more than 1,100 experts in response to Ebola, including experts in surveillance, epidemiology, case finding, contact tracing, and information management and analysis. The GOARN Emerging and Dangerous Pathogens Laboratory

---

BOX 15.2

INTERNATIONAL RESPONSE TO THE EBOLA VIRUS DISEASE OUTBREAK (2014–2016)

Whereas the response to severe acute respiratory syndrome (SARS) highlighted the effectiveness of the International Health Regulations (IHR) mechanisms, the outbreak of Ebola virus disease across West Africa highlighted remarkable shortcomings of global response capacity. Few countries had capacity to detect and respond to the outbreak as obligated in the legally binding regulations.

Key challenges included response coordination, early detection and isolation of patients, clinical management of patients, and development of a skilled workforce to support clinical care and surveillance. All countries had logistical challenges regarding building and equipping treatment centers. Early in the response, national health authorities and partners were challenged by trying to reach a consensus regarding specific strategies for the overall response.

In addition to the limited capacity of affected countries, shortcomings existed in the World Health Organization's response, including inadequate funding, limited staffing for operational support, and limited scale of the initial response (14). Bilateral support from several countries and the Global Outbreak Alert and Response Network (GOARN) helped address operational gaps.

During the response, more than 60 Ebola treatment centers were established in Sierra Leone, Liberia, and Guinea, and more than 40 organizations and 58 foreign medical teams were deployed, including 2,500 personnel to operate these centers. In response to outbreaks in settings without treatment units, community care centers were established (16).

Despite support from GOARN and partners, the outbreak highlighted the need for stronger international surge capacity for times when countries are overwhelmed by an outbreak and the importance of improving infection control capacity in developing countries.

Network deployed more than 25 mobile laboratories with more than 200 experts for providing diagnostic assistance for rapid case confirmation (16).

UN Cluster System

Outbreaks of international concern often occur in countries experiencing a humanitarian emergency. In 2005, the UN General Assembly adopted a cluster system to improve capacity for responding to humanitarian emergencies (17). The system includes groups of humanitarian organizations (UN and non-UN) working in the main sectors of humanitarian response. On occasion, the cluster system has been involved in managing outbreak response, particularly when outbreaks occur during a humanitarian emergency (e.g., the 2017 outbreak of cholera in Somalia). Historically, outbreaks often lead to such humanitarian crises as the Ebola outbreaks in West Africa. The cluster system was not activated during the Ebola outbreaks; however, the UN established its Mission for Ebola Emergency Response, which helped coordinate the response.

GLOBAL OR REGIONAL DISEASE SURVEILLANCE AND LABORATORY NETWORKS FOR DISEASES OF INTERNATIONAL CONCERN

Multiple global laboratory networks support early detection and response to infectious disease outbreaks. WHO organizes and supports many of these networks, including laboratory networks for polio, measles, influenza, invasive bacterial disease, and yellow fever (18). The European Center for Disease Prevention and Control also maintains multinational surveillance networks for Legionnaires' disease, tuberculosis, antimicrobial resistance, Creutzfeldt-Jakob disease, diphtheria, and invasive bacterial vaccine-preventable diseases (19). In 1999, the US Department of Defense established the Global Emerging Infections Surveillance and Response (GEIS) system in its overseas laboratories and medical institutions. GEIS has made key contributions during multiple outbreaks, including the first report of a new strain of pandemic influenza in 2009 (20).

Development of capacity for molecular characterization of bacterial pathogens has led to formation of surveillance networks for foodborne disease (21,22). PulseNet International is a network of seven national and regional laboratory networks dedicated to tracking reported foodborne illness cases worldwide. Participating laboratories are supported by the Centers for Disease Control and Prevention ([CDC] US Department of Health and Human Services) and use standardized genotyping methods. Subtyping and epidemiologic information are shared in real-time among participating laboratories. PulseNet provides early warning of international foodborne and waterborne disease outbreaks through detection of case clusters associated with specific subtypes. This network of networks is an efficient means of defining the international scope of such outbreaks and is a crucial component of international outbreak investigations.

FIELD WORK DURING INTERNATIONAL INVESTIGATIONS

Field work during international outbreak investigations can be challenging and thus requires unique skills for effectively contributing to the response. Deployed personnel should learn as much as possible before deployment, not only about the disease they will be investigating but also about the country and culture in which they will be working. Challenges experienced in the field often are related to the cultural context of the outbreak and involve working in settings with limited laboratory, data management, informatics, and human resource capacity. Field staff need to be flexible and learn how to be effective despite these constraints. Key challenges related to preparedness and field work include the following:

- *Clarifying roles and responsibilities.* Outbreaks frequently stress national response capacity, and, at times, who is responsible for performing which tasks is unclear. International teams might receive instructions with conflicting strategies coming from different parts of the government and experience a lack of cohesion regarding the overall response. Nigeria experienced such a crisis in 2014, with the arrival of a Liberian diplomat who had Ebola virus disease. The country lacked a disease importation plan and did not have capacity for safely isolating patients. Roles and responsibilities between federal and state officials lacked clarity. The initial response included different plans for establishing treatment centers, none of which was realistic in addressing the urgent need to isolate febrile contacts of the Liberian traveler. At one point, eight febrile contacts of the Liberian traveler were living in the community without a suitable place to receive care. After considerable debate about treatment options, the health ministry established an incident command team structure by using staff from the polio EOC to manage the outbreak (23). The team quickly identified an approach for isolating patients and containing the outbreak by converting an abandoned hospital ward into a treatment center as a stop-gap measure until a more suitable location was identified (Figure 15.1). During such crisis situations, consultants should establish and maintain strong relationships with different counterparts within the response, even when contentious problems arise and disagreements occur among partners.

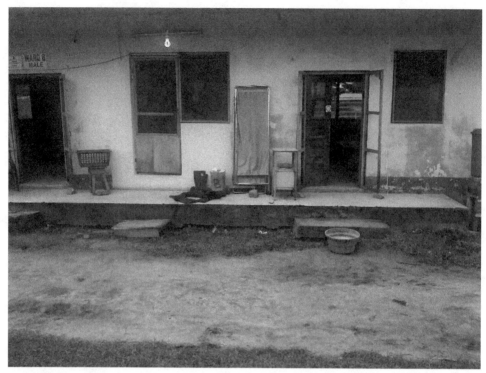

FIGURE 15.1 Emergency Ebola treatment center using an old hospital ward with impro-
vised water, sanitation, and hygiene (WaSH) stations until a more suitable center could be
set-up: Nigeria, 2014.

- *Ensuring adequate technical capacity.* Field epidemiologists deployed to outbreak
  settings might realize they are ill-equipped to address unique challenges they face
  in the field. When asked to accept an international assignment, candidates should
  receive clear tasks or terms of reference (TORs) and only accept assignments with
  TORs they are able to address. This was a problem during the Ebola response
  where specific technical skills were needed to support safe burials, water and sanitation procedures, clinical management of patients, and infection control. To address this concern, response partners developed training programs for personnel
  before their deployment. Despite this training, staff sometimes needed mentoring
  and guidance from experienced staff during their deployment.
- *Cross-cultural sensitivity.* When conducting a field investigation, field staff must be sensitive to the cultural norms of the community where they are deployed and suitably
  adapt their approaches to field investigations and response. For example, unique burial
  practices had to be considered when designing safe burial interventions during the
  Ebola outbreak. When designing interventions, recognizing that local counterparts
  might have different and equally valid approaches to problem-solving is vital.

- *Working in fragile settings.* Outbreaks frequently occur in fragile states or settings within a country where government systems and service delivery might be limited. Field staff need to navigate complicated security and political concerns carefully because of mistrust and tension between the government and the communities it serves. In such settings, engaging civil society organizations or community leaders as interlocutors to support field work and the response is often helpful. Neutral access negotiators (e.g., the Red Cross) can communicate with community leaders in affected areas and help recruit local teams from the affected communities to assist with the response.

- *Data and sample sharing.* Nothing will get a field investigator a premature airplane ride home quicker than inappropriate sharing of data or clinical samples. Data or clinical sample sharing is often a contentious concern, and recognizing the sovereignty of national data and seeking permission of health authorities are crucial. Data sharing between institutions can also be contentious. Best practices include submitting all requests in writing and have a data sharing agreement with national health authorities; these actions will help ensure that everyone has a firm understanding of what data and clinical samples can be shared.

CONCLUSION

Although considerable progress has been made on coordinating international outbreak response, the publication and revision of the IHR did not prevent the spread of Ebola in West Africa and highlights the need for continued refinement of global response to international outbreaks. Since 2009, there have been four declarations of public health emergencies of international concern. With each declaration, WHO and the global community have gained experience and learned lessons on coordinating response. Key efforts to support WHO include the work of GOARN, the global laboratory networks, and support from key organizations and Member States.

REFERENCES

1. Thucydides. *History of the Peloponnesian War.* Book 2. Oxford: Clarendon Press; 1900:137–40.
2. Kazanjian P. Ebola in antiquity? *Clin Infect Dis.* 2015;61:963–8.
3. Olson PE, Hames CS, Benenson AS, Genovese EN. Thucydides syndrome: Ebola déjà vu? (or Ebola reemergent?). *Emerg Infect Dis.* 1996;2:155–6.
4. Pappas G, Kiriaze IJ, Falagas ME. Insights into infectious disease in the era of Hippocrates. *Int J Infect Dis.* 2008;12:347–50.
5. Dehnhardt WL. ¿Hubo infectólogos en la Antigua Roma? [in Spanish]. *Rev Chil Infect.* 2010;27:165–9.
6. Sabbatani S. Excursus sull'organizzazione dell'assistenza in tempi di pestilenza [Italian]. *Le Infezioni in Medicina.* 2003;3:161–7.

7. McLeod KS. Our sense of Snow: the myth of John Snow in medical geography. *Soc Sci Med.* 2000;50:923–35.

8. Koch T. 1831: The map that launched the idea of global health. *Int J Epidemiol.* 2014;43:1014–20.

9. Brigham A. *A treatise on epidemic cholera. including an historical account of its origin and progress, to the present period: compiled from the most authentic sources.* Hartford, CT: H and F J Huntington; 1832.

10. WHO. Origin and development of health cooperation. http://www.who.int/global_health_histories/background/en/

11. WHO. International Health Regulations (2005). 3rd ed. Geneva, Switzerland: WHO; 2016. p. 84. http://www.who.int/ihr/publications/9789241580496/en/

12. Heymann DL. The international response to the outbreak of SARS in 2003. *Philos Trans R Soc Lond B Biol Sci.* 2004;359:1127–9.

13. Centers for Disease Control and Prevention. CDC's response to the 2014–2016 Ebola epidemic—West Africa and United States. *MMWR Suppl.* 2016;65(Suppl 3):1–112.

14. Woodall J. WHO reform: bring back GOARN and Task Force "Scorpio." *Infect Ecol Epidemiol.* 2016;6:30237.

15. WHO. Global Outbreak Alert and Response Network (GOARN). http://www.who.int/ihr/alert_and_response/outbreak-network/en/

16. WHO. 2015 WHO Strategic Response Plan, West Africa Ebola outbreak. http://www.who.int/csr/resources/publications/ebola/ebola-strategic-plan/en/

17. United Nations. Strengthening the coordination of humanitarian emergency assistance of the United Nations. Resolution 46/182. http://www.un.org/Docs/journal/asp/ws.asp?m=A/RES/46/182

18. WHO. Laboratory networks. http://www.who.int/immunization/monitoring_surveillance/burden/laboratory/en/

19. European Centre for Disease Prevention and Control. EUVAC.Net. http://ecdc.europa.eu/en/healthtopics/vaccine-preventable-diseases/euvac/Pages/index.aspx

20. Fry AM, Hancock K, Patel M, et al. The first cases of 2009 pandemic influenza A (H1N1) virus infection in the United States: a serologic investigation demonstrating early transmission. *Influenza Other Respi Viruses.* 2012;6:e48–53.

21. Swaminathan B, Barrett TJ, Hunter SB, Tauxe R V. PulseNet: the molecular subtyping network for foodborne bacterial disease surveillance, United States. *Emerg Infect Dis.* 2001;7:382–9.

22. Kirk MD, Little CL, Lem M, et al. An outbreak due to peanuts in their shell caused by Salmonella enterica serotypes Stanley and Newport—sharing molecular information to solve international outbreaks. *Epidemiol Infect.* 2004;132:571–7.

23. Shuaib F, Gunnala R, Musa EO, et al. Ebola virus disease outbreak—Nigeria, July–September 2014. *MMWR.* 2014;63:849–54.

/// 16 /// EMERGENCY OPERATIONS CENTERS AND INCIDENT MANAGEMENT STRUCTURE

JEFFREY L. BRYANT, DANIEL M. SOSIN,
TIM W. WIEDRICH, AND STEPHEN C. REDD

INTRODUCTION

Public health emergencies are often complex, protracted, and can overwhelm public health systems typically staffed and equipped for routine operations. Recent US and international responses to polio eradication (2011–present), the Ebola virus disease outbreak in West Africa (2014–2016), and Zika virus disease in the Americas (2016–2017) required extended field operations and response structures to bring partners together in a coordinated effort. Applying the concepts of emergency management, including the use of Emergency Operation Centers (EOCs) and Incident Management Systems (IMS) can help national and subnational public health systems protect populations impacted by a public health threat (1). For the United States, the National Response Framework (NRF) outlines the common structures national, state, and local governments use to respond to natural disasters, public health, medical, and other emergency situations (2). The NRF includes roles, responsibilities, and legal authorities used by different agencies within the US government during a response and applies to national, state, and local governments.

National-level organizations in the United States, such as the Centers for Disease Control and Prevention (CDC) consider an "All Hazards" approach to preparedness and response because epidemiology expertise is needed in diverse response activities ranging from traditional infectious disease outbreak investigations to chemical spill and natural disaster responses. Although every public health response has unique considerations, a functional knowledge of emergency management principles can help field epidemiologists integrate effectively into national and subnational emergency response structures.

EMERGENCY MANAGEMENT PROGRAMS

An organization's Emergency Management Program (EMP) comprises both preparedness and response activities. Preparedness activities, such as exercises and training, can help prepare field epidemiologists for response operations. The EMP facilitates efficient, coordinated public health activities for the duration of a response. Most EMPs use a tiered level of activations; in the United States, these generally range from Level 3 (lowest activation level) to Level 1 (highest activation level). This flexibility enables an organization to right-size response operations to meet changing response requirements. Most national-level agencies in the United States use the following activation levels:

- *Level 3 (lowest level)*: This level implies that, with modest augmentation, the lead agency or program can address the primary needs of the response. In the United States, many small natural disasters or environmental responses fall into this activation level. An example is the CDC response to the 2016 water contamination crisis in Michigan.
- *Level 2 (intermediate level)*: This level implies substantial augmentation is required for the lead agency or program to meet response requirements. For CDC, the response to the 2011 Japan earthquake, tsunami, and nuclear disaster was a Level 2 activation.
- *Level 1 (highest level)*: This level requires an agencywide response and often includes domestic and international partners. As an example, CDC has recorded four Level 1 activations: Hurricane Katrina (2005), influenza A (H1N1) pandemic (2009–10), Ebola virus disease outbreak (2014–2016), and Zika virus outbreak (2016–2017).

> **BOX 16.1**
>
> **NATIONAL EMERGENCY MANAGEMENT COMPONENTS AND PRINCIPLES**
>
> - Defined modular management structures that are scalable and flexible
> - Standardized national response doctrine, including common terminologies
> - Focus on communication, information management, and resource management
> - Importance of operating from one set of objectives and priorities
> - Understanding of joint limitations in a multipartner environment
> - Protection of agency's legal authorities to conduct response operations
> - Optimization of unity of effort among partners under a single plan

The demands and complexity of a response influence the transition between levels. It is common for a response to transition between levels as operations escalate and deescalate. For example, the 2016 Zika virus response evolved from activation of the EOC at Level 3 in late January 2016 to Level 2 by the first week in February, and to Level 1 a week later because the size, scope, and complexity of activities warranted an agencywide response for CDC (CDC, unpublished data). For the 2014 Ebola outbreaks, the EOC was activated at Level 3 in July 2014 and in August of the year moved directly to a Level 1 response (CDC, unpublished data).

In the United States, government entities respond to public health emergencies using the structures and guidance in the NRF, which by design are scalable and flexible to fit the full spectrum of emergency responses (2). Familiarity with the basic emergency management components and principles outlined in the NRF (Box 16.1) can help field epidemiologists integrate into response structures at national, state, and local levels.

EMPs organize response structures in different ways. In the United States, most national and state systems use the common organizational designations in the NRF, which characterize necessary response functions according to major systems. For example, the national transportation, communication, or public health and medical systems all have a place in the overall structure. For public health organizations, common elements of a response may include epidemiologic investigations, laboratory services, medical care, medical countermeasure (such as vaccines, antiviral, and antimicrobial drugs) distribution, public messaging and risk communications, and partner communication—all organized in a series of task forces or similar structures within an IMS. For example, CDC organizes these response elements under a Scientific Response Section (Box 16.2), and understanding the relationships between the task forces or structures can benefit field epidemiologists. Within the

---

BOX 16.2

SCIENTIFIC RESPONSE SECTION TASK FORCES[a]

- Epidemiology and surveillance
- State coordination
- Vaccine
- Modeling
- Environmental health
- Laboratory
- Medical care and countermeasures
- International operations
- Global migration and quarantine
- Infectious diseases

---

[a]*Individual task forces might not be part of every Incident Management System structure.*

CDC response structure, the task forces include subject matter experts, operational coordinators, and evaluators; whether an epidemiologist is forward deployed to conduct field investigations or works in the Atlanta-based EOC, he or she will be assigned to a given task force for guidance, assistance, and direction.

In addition to subject matter expert–led task forces, other key positions, and teams fall under the Incident Manager and the CDC IMS structure (Box 16.3).

BOX 16.3

CDC IMS RESPONSE POSITIONS AND TEAMS

- Joint Information Center
- Deployment Risk Mitigation Unit
- Safety
- Liaison Officers
- Ethics
- Chief Science/Health Officer
- Policy
- Medical Investigations Team
- Security
- Office of General Counsel
- Associate Director for Science
- Deputy Incident Manager(s)

National and subnational EMPs also typically have a professional cadre of emergency managers who conduct preparedness activities (e.g., training and exercises) and serve in response leadership roles including senior positions in planning, logistics, operations, situational awareness, resource management, and communications. In the US emergency management system, these cadres are referred to collectively as the General Staff.

EMERGENCY OPERATION CENTER ACTIVATIONS

EOCs around the world are activated for public health responses when routine systems and structures become overwhelmed (Box 16.4). As an example, during the Ebola outbreak during 2014–2016, Liberia developed an incident management structure operating from its EOC to manage response activities (3). Activation of the EOC facilitates overall response operations by providing the working platform and resources to support response staff through established structures, capabilities, and procedures. The EOC also provides the opportunity to bring relevant response partners together to establish common objectives and strategies, thus creating unity of effort. Each year in the United States, many public health emergency responses are handled efficiently using state and local resources without the need for national assistance. When national assistance is required, it is scalable and flexible and can be provided in many forms ranging from remote epidemiologic consultations to on-the-ground field epidemiology work in addition to other response capabilities.

Field epidemiologists can accelerate integration into national, state, and local response operations by understanding how working in an EOC environment differs from

---

BOX 16.4

COMMON ACTIVATION TRIGGERS FOR EMERGENCY OPERATIONS CENTERS

- Requests for assistance from overwhelmed cities, states, or countries
- Need for significant external partner coordination
- High political or media interest expected
- Need to coordinate risk communication messages with diverse response partners
- Need for significant internal coordination (multiple agency programs involved)
- New agents or known agents exhibiting different characteristics
- Activation of other Emergency Operations Centers by external response partners

routine program conditions. For most public health organizations, day-to-day routines and activities are insufficient to successfully manage an emergency response. In the emergency response environment:

- Response staff work in a rapid-pace setting for extended periods of time.
- Decisions are needed quickly within a context of ambiguous and incomplete information.
- Hiring, acquisition, contract, and other business processes must be expedited.
- Working relationships expand to include new and external response partners.
- Tensions can arise between response requirements and normal, daily obligations.

MEETING STATE EXPECTATIONS

In the US response system, there is a very strong relationship between the national response systems and the subnational (state and local) response systems. Although most state and local public health agencies use the standard NRF organizational structure, the state and local systems vary greatly in relation to activation triggers, authority, and autonomy. Successful response depends on a strong understanding of the incident management approach used in an individual state system, the field epidemiologist's relationship with these state and local systems, and agreement on the role of the field epidemiologists in these jurisdictions.

State and Local Incident Management Environments

In the United States, most (76%) state health officials are appointed by the state governor. The remainder are appointed by other state agency heads, state legislatures, or commissions (4). These governance relationships influence the day-to-day and emergency operations of state health departments. State public health incident managers receive authority from their respective governing and policy bodies, and this authority affects the specific system functions within each state. States vary in relation to the autonomy and delegated authority of local public health: in about 30% of states, local public health departments are highly subordinated centrally to the state health department, and the remainder are decentralized (4). These organizational differences between centralized and decentralized structures influence coordination between state and local public health jurisdictions and, consequently, how IMS structures are established to manage public health emergency responses. When field epidemiologists deploy, operational performance can be optimized through attentiveness to key considerations in advance of arrival in the affected field area and during work in the field. Using the US model between national and state governments, the following two sections describe issues national field epidemiologists should consider when deploying to subnational jurisdictions.

Before Arriving in the Field

- Determine whether the IMS in a state or local jurisdiction was triggered and is activated.
  - If triggered, identify the incident management and liaison officer and agree on the reporting requirements and operating authorities (chain of command) that exist within the national and state response structures.
  - If not triggered, identify who has leadership responsibility for the state response and review the reporting requirements and operating authorities (chain of command) that are in place within the national and state response structures.
- Clearly define the goals that the state and national public health systems hope to achieve in the field.
- Establish the frequency, communications channels, location, and format for progress reports and updates.
- Establish who has decision authority for and custody of collected data. Determine whether the response will use national or state information technology systems and files.
- Review the supplies, equipment, work space, information technology, and transportation assets needed and identify who (national or state) will meet those needs.
- Define a process for developing and approving public information messages.
- Determine who has the authority to release information and data and agree on the methods used for data release.
- Review arrival dates, location, and work hours.
- Determine how the field epidemiology position fits into the state or local response operations. These positions can be embedded within a state team or can operate independently. If embedded, understand the role, team member roles, reporting systems, and the chain of command.
- Identify environmental and safety conditions that might affect the responder and the response (i.e., weather, clothing, and transportation).

During the Field Operations

- As soon as possible after arrival, secure a briefing with the state incident manager or, if the IMS was not triggered, with other state leadership.
  - Request an incident briefing, summary of findings, and recommendations for a work plan. Remain open and unbiased to this information.
  - Review and revise the issues covered in the prearrival discussions to ensure they are current and appropriate to evolving situations.
  - Confirm the frequency, communications channels, location, and format for progress reports and updates.
- Participate in the situational awareness and progress update meetings. If unable to attend, notify and provide leadership with a written summary of activities or information to update the group, if possible.
- Consider state operational suggestions if they do not conflict with national policies or procedures. State officials will have a foundational understanding of the limitations and challenges for response within their jurisdiction, which will help optimize the response work.
- Respect the authority of the state and its leadership. The state may choose a course of action that does not have unanimous approval for reasons specific to the state.
- Conduct an exit briefing shortly before departure.
  - Review what was accomplished and what remains to be done.
  - Establish frequency and channels for future communication.
  - Establish a procedure for approval and publication of any postevent media releases, academic publications, and poster presentations.

NATIONAL AND INTERNATIONAL COMPLEXITIES OF PUBLIC HEALTH EMERGENCY RESPONSE

The United States has legislation that establishes the legal authorities and responsibilities of the national government to conduct emergency response operations. The Robert T. Stafford Disaster Relief and Emergency Assistance Act, enacted in 1988 and last amended in 2013 (5), is the authority the Federal Emergency Management Agency uses to deliver national-level assistance to state governments. Such authorities might not exist in every country, and field epidemiologists should work with the Ministry of Health or international partners, such as the World Health Organization, to understand how response operations fit into national government or international structures. This includes considerations involving data collection, data analysis, information sharing, and potential publications. It also could include issues involving custody of laboratory samples, specimen transport, and customs and border implications for shipping or receiving medical countermeasures. Taking time to understand the field epidemiologist's role in the context of a specific response operation involving multiple levels of government could help sort through complex issues such as these. In addition, field epidemiologists should understand reach-back mechanisms to their national governments as another resource to help work through complex national or international situations.

Another aspect of field epidemiology is knowing what resources might already be in place at a deployed location. Domestically in the United States, national public health personnel are embedded within state and local public health agencies. Knowledge of and outreach to these other field staff can accelerate integration into local response operations. Similarly, when field epidemiologists deploy to another country, there might be response partners permanently assigned to specific locations that can equally accelerate integration into the response.

UNIQUE ASPECTS OF EPIDEMIOLOGIC FIELD INVESTIGATIONS DURING AN EMERGENCY RESPONSE

Although IMS was not designed specifically for outbreak responses or public health emergencies, it does provide a clarifying framework for reporting and organizing the investigative work of an outbreak response. The basic purpose and methods are the same for epidemiologic field investigations undertaken during large-scale public health emergencies and in smaller programmatic response events. When an epidemiologic field investigation is conducted as part of a larger public health emergency response, the context and situation differ from those in routine investigations, particularly in the urgency, speed, and scale of the investigation (Box 16.5).

Because field investigations during emergency responses must be designed to answer questions in a timeframe sufficient to inform near real-time decision-making and interventions, they can constrain the adequacy of standard data collection and information analysis procedures. The team lead or senior field epidemiologist must decide which initial operational questions are most important and prioritize investigative efforts to answer those questions first. Most responses also carry Director's Critical Information Requirements, or the equivalent, which are determined early in response operations and can change as the response develops. The Director's Critical Information Requirements immediately and automatically trigger notification of senior agency leadership (Box 16.6).

Large and complex emergency responses can involve many national and subnational agencies. Under such circumstances, the epidemiologic investigation must be integrated

BOX 16.5

UNIQUE ASPECTS OF EPIDEMIOLOGIC FIELD INVESTIGATIONS DURING AN EMERGENCY RESPONSE

- Rapid information gathering enables near real-time decisions and interventions.
- Scale and speed of response activities are paramount.
- Parallel and simultaneous investigations must be coordinated within the larger response effort and within the existing Incident Management System structure to avoid duplication of effort.
- Wide media coverage and political pressures should be managed effectively by an experienced spokesperson/team for the response.
- Increased leadership attention may result in greater access to resources, potentially augmenting demands on reporting and coordination requirements.
- Investigation results or interim results may be used immediately to influence decisions by senior leaders.

into the larger response structure. For emergencies and investigations occurring simultaneously in multiple locations, activities sometimes require additional coordination and communication in the field and with the epidemiologist's parent agency headquarters. In addition, complex responses will also require additional time to prepare and present progress reports to responsible authorities and time to speak with and receive guidance from the parent agency headquarters.

An epidemiologic field investigation during an emergency response also might attract intense media interest. Preparation is critical and should entail planning for the following:

BOX 16.6

EXAMPLES OF CDC DIRECTOR'S CRITICAL INFORMATION REQUIREMENTS

- Serious illness or injury in deployed CDC staff member
- Identification of new routes of transmission for infectious disease agents
- Unexpected infectious disease cases or clusters
- Infectious disease cases or clusters in new geographic areas
- Major genetic sequencing changes for infectious disease agents
- Initial requests for deployment of CDC assets
- New security threats to areas where CDC staff are deployed
- Communicable disease outbreaks in temporary shelter populations

- A predetermined, experienced media spokesperson.
- Coordination with other agencies and state and local officials.
- Help from health communicators to plan what information and public messaging strategies should be presented.
- Assurance that all personally identifiable information is protected according to applicable laws.

Greater interest by the media, local officials, and others can add additional coordination and information burdens but also can create opportunities to marshal greater resources than in a lower profile event. Response leadership might be able to deploy more epidemiologists, have access to more data management specialists, add communications specialists to the investigative team, and provide logistics experts to support the investigation.

Finally, epidemiologic field investigations conducted during emergencies often result in actionable findings that have immediate implications for the public health response. Examples include the influenza A(H1N1) pandemic response in 2009–2010 that generated recommendations such as school closures and cancellations of large social gatherings, and the Ebola response in 2014–2016 that resulted in acceptable interventions for contact tracing, active case finding, and safe burial practices.

CONCLUSION

In the United States, national emergency management programs, including EOCs and incident management structures, have been refined during the past 40 years and today provide an efficient and effective system for responding to public health emergencies. Standardization of emergency management components and principles across national, state, and local jurisdictions creates a common foundation for both public health and emergency management professionals. Field epidemiologists can accelerate their preparation for and integration into public health response operations by understanding the basic fundamentals:

- National governments can have unique response systems, and field epidemiologists should remain flexible and strive to quickly integrate into national or subnational operations.
- Functional knowledge of emergency management principles can help field epidemiologists integrate effectively into national, state, local, and international emergency response structures.

- In an emergency response environment, routine daily systems and processes are often inadequate because:
  - Response staff work in a rapid-pace setting for extended periods.
  - Decisions are needed quickly within a context of ambiguous and incomplete information.
  - Hiring, acquisition, contract, and other business processes must be expedited.
  - Working relationships expand to include new and external response partners.
  - Tensions can arise between response requirements and normal, daily obligations
- State, local, and international response environments can vary greatly and preparation for deployments should include an understanding of specific jurisdictions' structures and authorities.
- Public health emergency responses can be complex, and national systems designed to respond to natural disasters might require modification to be used successfully in a public health emergency.
- Because national-level staff might live and work in jurisdictions to which an epidemiologist deploys, these staff understand the unique considerations of those communities and can help with response operations.
- The IMS was not designed specifically for outbreak responses or public health emergencies, but it does provide clarity and a framework for reporting and organizing the investigative work of an outbreak response.
- When an epidemiologic field investigation is undertaken as part of larger public health emergency response, the context and situation differ from routine operations, particularly in the urgency, speed, and scale of the investigation.
- Epidemiologic field investigations undertaken during emergencies often offer the opportunity for the results to affect a public health response immediately.

REFERENCES

1. CDC. CDC's Emergency Management Program activities—worldwide, 2003–2012. *MMWR*. 2013;62:709–13.
2. Federal Emergency Management Agency. National Response Framework, third edition. http://www.fema.gov/media-library/assets/documents/117791
3. Pillai SK, Nyenswah T, Rouse E, et al. Developing an incident management system to support Ebola response—Liberia, July–August 2014. *MMWR*. 2014;63:930–33.
4. Association of State and Territorial Health Officials. State health agency structure, governance, and priorities. In: ASTHO profile of state public health, volume 3. Washington, DC: Association of State and Territorial Health Officials; 2014:17–28.
5. Robert T. Stafford Disaster Relief and Emergency Assistance Act, Pub. L. 93–288 (November 23, 1988), as amended.

GEOGRAPHIC INFORMATION SYSTEM DATA

STEPHANIE FOSTER, ERICA ADAMS, IAN DUNN, AND ANDREW DENT

INTRODUCTION

Place is one of the basic tenets of a field investigation. Both the *who* and the *when* of disease are relative to and often dependent on the *where*. Geographic information science, systems, software (collectively known as GIS) and methods are one of the tools epidemiologists use in defining and evaluating the *where*. This chapter reviews GIS applications as they pertain to the 10 steps of a field investigation.

STEP 1. PREPARE FOR FIELD WORK

Generating Maps for Situational Awareness

Standard mapping techniques will produce informative visualizations and provide orientation for studying the location, the physical attributes of the investigation area, and descriptive characteristics of the population(s) of interest. Field staff should begin by creating general reference maps (1,2). Google Maps (Google, Inc., Mountain View, CA), OpenStreetMap (an open-source wiki software by the OpenStreetMap Foundation), or county geographic files serve as reasonable starting points. These maps can include information about road networks, hotels, airports, and other points of interest to familiarize the field team with the area in which it will be investigating the disease or injury occurrence. Reference maps can be useful in both domestic and international settings, especially in unfamiliar areas.

Additionally, such maps are useful for establishing the boundaries of the investigation area (2–4). Using geographic information science, systems, or software (collectively known as GIS), boundaries can be drawn for the area of interest and from which specific GIS data files, known as *shapefiles*, can be created (2,4,5). These boundary files can then be used to evaluate variables of interest (e.g., estimating the number of persons residing within a particular area or examining the extent of contamination from a harmful exposure) (Figure 17.1).

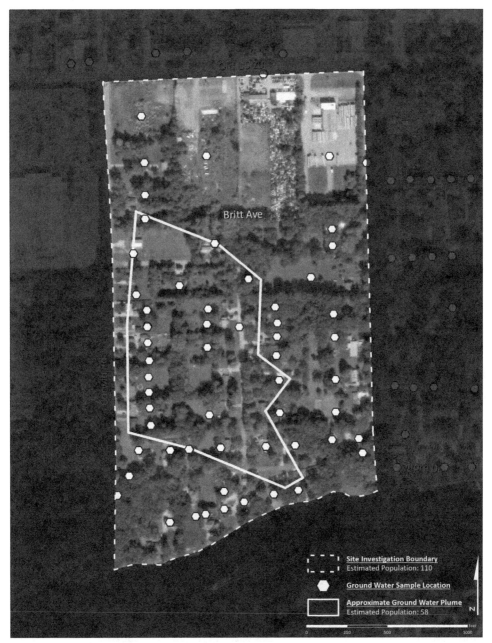

FIGURE 17.1 General site profile maps not only provide an overview of the location and spatial association of the study area to other general points of reference, but also present estimates of general characteristics of an affected population.

Identifying and Acquiring Pertinent Supplemental Data

Time permitting, the field team might consider gathering pertinent data sets useful beyond general reference data. For example, incorporating such sociodemographic characteristic data as population counts, age, sex, race/ethnicity, sensitive populations, language/translation needs, and measures of poverty by specific state, county, or other census boundaries is possible by using US Census data (Figure 17.2). The US Census Bureau makes these data available with a unique geographic identifier, thereby enabling easy association between the population data and the location data in GIS (6).

Understanding the influence of the natural and built environment is possible with GIS (1–3). For example, exploring the distribution of persons in communities and neighborhoods, school locations, childcare facilities, or senior living facilities relative to the locations of industry might prove key to the investigation. During a natural disaster or a chemical release, imagery can be useful for understanding the extent of damage, to track population movements, and to guide the planning and logistics of travel for fieldwork. Furthermore, identifying transportation routes and locations of public utilities might be pertinent to understanding potential transmission modes (Figure 17.3).

GIS can be a principal resource for generating a sampling plan. By using GIS, investigators can select homes or areas within communities for sampling activities (Figure 17.4).

Similarly, investigators can use road network data to develop optimized routes for data collection. Before fieldwork in Panama, for example, researchers used GIS to characterize varying levels of forestation adjacent to villages for study site selection (7). Additionally, the researchers used maps to determine each village's accessibility.

Depending on the study area's location (i.e., domestic vs. international), different levels of data might be available. In domestic situations, current and historic data from the US Census Bureau and satellite imagery may be readily available. This might also be true in certain international settings; however, obtaining this information before deployment might be difficult. In those instances, investigators might need to rely on dated or minimally detailed information before beginning fieldwork. Under these circumstances, the team should consider collecting pertinent data after arriving at the location.

Selecting GIS Software and Equipment

Both commercial and open-source GIS packages offer useful software options (4,8). Additionally, statistical software packages with spatial analysis capabilities exist. When selecting a GIS package, the user should consider data collection, analysis, and visualization needs, as well as available technical and financial resources, in determining which package is most feasible.

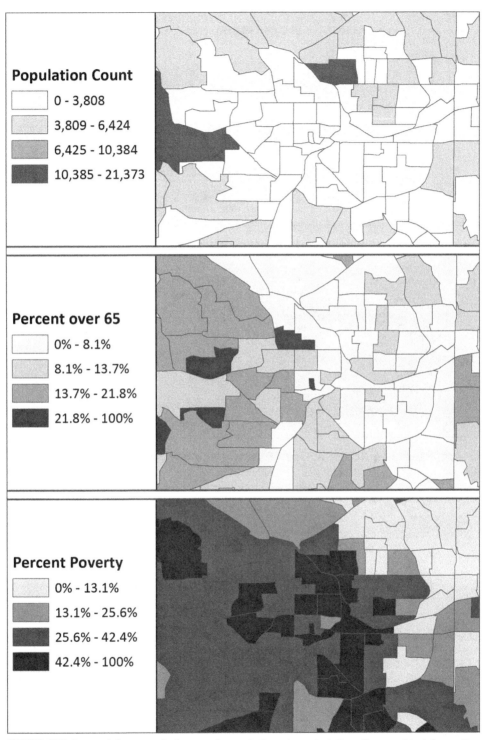

Population Count

- 0 - 3,808
- 3,809 - 6,424
- 6,425 - 10,384
- 10,385 - 21,373

Percent over 65

- 0% - 8.1%
- 8.1% - 13.7%
- 13.7% - 21.8%
- 21.8% - 100%

Percent Poverty

- 0% - 13.1%
- 13.1% - 25.6%
- 25.6% - 42.4%
- 42.4% - 100%

FIGURE 17.2 Determining populations and population characteristics. Geographic information system methods provide the means for determining population estimates within specific geographic areas for populations of particular interest. In these maps, population count, percentage of people 65 years old, and percentage of people in poverty based on 2014 American Community Survey Estimates are shown by census tract.

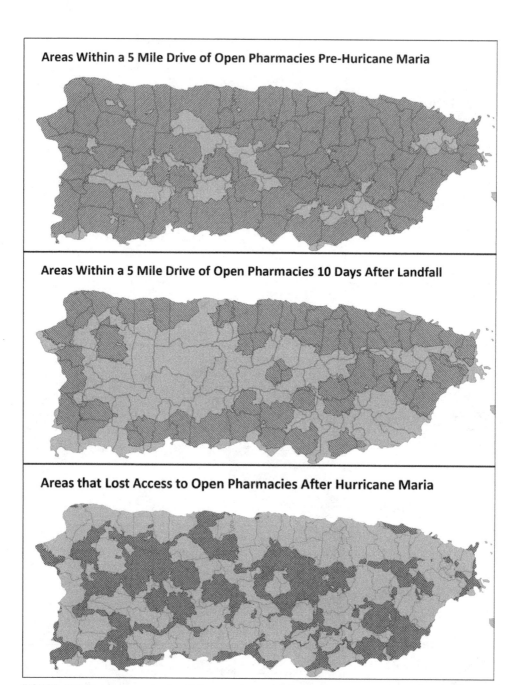

FIGURE 17.3 Network analysis. Using road or public transportation networks provides a more accurate analysis of travel times, distances, and connectivity over more traditional buffer methods. Through network analysis, this series of maps demonstrate the change in access to pharmacies as a result of Hurricane Maria's impact on the island of Puerto Rico.

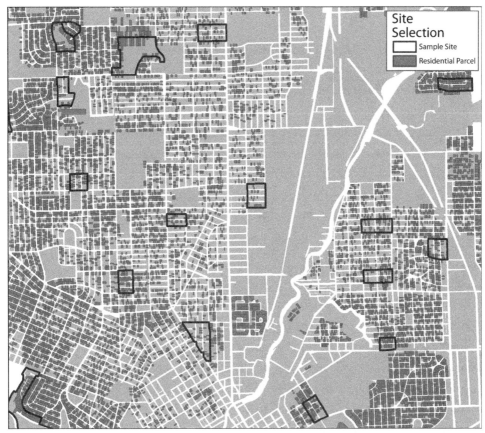

FIGURE 17.4 Using geographic information systems for sampling. As shown here, housing data, roads, and neighborhood information can be used to develop a sampling plan when conducting fieldwork.

Developing GIS Capacity

The beginning of the investigation is often the best time to collaborate with a GIS subject matter expert (SME) because that person can provide advice regarding pertinent maps, data, and analysis plans. Engaging GIS SMEs from the beginning can also build GIS capacity among the field team. During 2017, for example, a team from the Center for Global Health of the Centers for Disease Control and Prevention (CDC) collaborated with GIS SMEs in the Geospatial Research, Analysis, and Services Program to determine the best methods for collecting, storing, and analyzing locations where sex workers were active in Papua, New Guinea (9). That collaboration resulted in a plan to determine locations to conduct the surveys, to implement methods for collecting location data, and to enable spatial data analysis, which led to development of an interactive mapping tool. After completion, not only were relevant data collected, but the team began to develop internal GIS capacity.

Summary

- General reference maps can provide situational awareness.
- Maps can be useful for setting the boundaries of the investigation area.
- Maps can be instrumental in developing a sampling plan.
- Publicly available data (e.g., US Census Bureau and health outcome data) can be mapped and evaluated for the particular area of interest.
- Imagery data also might be informative, especially when attempting to assess damage from natural disasters.
- Inviting GIS SMEs to participate in the planning process can build field team capacity.

STEP 2. CONFIRM THE DIAGNOSIS

The field investigator might begin extracting location information provided directly from laboratory reports. The patient's residential street address at the time of diagnosis is often collected along with specimens for laboratory testing. Therefore, these data should be readily available when a laboratory or hospital reports its results. If this information is unavailable through laboratory reports or other electronic records, the field team should consider whether location information will be important to the analysis and determine methods for collecting those data.

STEP 3. DETERMINE THE EXISTENCE OF AN EPIDEMIC

GIS for Determining Populations at Risk

When determining whether a particular health outcome is occurring at a greater than expected rate, the correct population at risk must be determined. This often involves estimating a population within a specified geographic area. Census data are readily available at varying geographic units (e.g., block, census tract, county, and state) in files easily processed in GIS (6). Similarly, evaluating census data with GIS can assist in identifying a relevant comparison population. Often, these preexisting geopolitical boundaries are sufficient for estimating population characteristics. However, this is not always the case. For example, wind patterns may carry a contaminant to only a portion of a county or across multiple census tracts, creating nonstandard shapes. GIS can calculate the area of interest and be used to estimate the proportion of area of interest relative to known

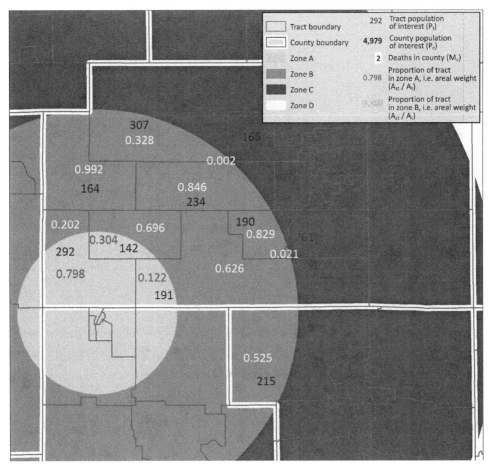

FIGURE 17.5 Applying geographic information systems (GIS) to estimate populations of interest within specified areas. Through GIS, it is possible to estimate sociodemographic characteristics when boundaries of interest do not conform to standard political boundaries. These estimates can be calculated by allocating the same proportion of geographic area included in the boundary of interest to sociodemographic characteristics. *Source*: Reference 10.

geopolitical boundaries. This proportion can then be applied to population data to estimate the population of interest (Figure 17.5).

Exploring Rates Across Space and Time

Preliminary spatial and temporal analyses of baseline rates can be useful at this early investigation stage for establishing an outbreak's existence. Through spatial and temporal methods, estimates of changing rates of diseases or injury across time might become apparent. A series of static maps can present temporal trends of disease distributions (Figure 17.6).

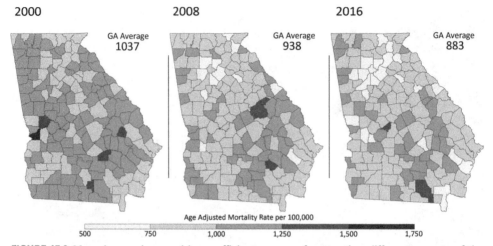

FIGURE 17.6 Maps in a series provide an efficient means of presenting different aspects of the same data simultaneously. The series can represent rates among populations with different sociodemographic characteristics, or it might be used to explore changes over time. The decrease in age-adjusted mortality rates in Georgia can be seen in data from 2000, 2008, and 2016.

Linked micromaps, another type of map series, can display rates of disease in the same area across time or different population groups (3,8,11). Additionally, interactive software is available for animating disease distributions across time.

Uncovering Risk Factors

Analysis of environmental risk factors (e.g., wind direction, wind speed, or drinking water sources) can assist in uncovering a common exposure route. GIS can also be used for exploring and defining social networks crucial in understanding disease spread. As the transmission source is determined, a common location might also be revealed. At the least, the field investigator can begin thinking of methods for obtaining location information of patients and suspected locations where infection might be occurring to begin generating hypotheses regarding exposure and transmission factors.

Summary

- Geographic boundaries can be customized to the particular study area and can be used to estimate underlying population counts and characteristics.
- Preliminary spatial and temporal analyses can provide evidence of unusual disease rates across time.
- Visualization can inform the team of potential transmission factors and changing disease patterns across different places and times.

STEP 4. IDENTIFY AND COUNT CASES

Collecting and Geocoding Location Data

The street address at the time of disease diagnosis, whether a residence or common establishment, is usually part of routine data collection efforts; however, remembering that location information should be collected in a standardized format is crucial (3). After collection, these data can be converted into points or shapes for mapping, a process known as *geocoding* (3,12,13). Providing specific instructions for collecting complete and accurate address information can influence correct point placement (3,12).

The field team can determine early on the preferred method for collecting geographic coordinates during data collection in the field (2). Given inconsistencies in complete and accurate address data availability, variability in geocoding software accuracy, and the wide availability of handheld global positioning system (GPS) devices, collecting GPS coordinates might prove better than address data. Additionally, obtaining address-level data for analysis in international settings can be challenging, especially in remote locations where standardized addresses may not be available for data collection or for the geocoding process. For example, throughout the Ebola virus disease epidemic during 2014–2016, infection spread rapidly. In one particularly remote village, the rapid identification of infected persons and their isolation was essential for limiting transmission. During that fieldwork, the investigator was able to use a GPS device to collect the latitude and longitude of each household location while collecting interview data (14). Having these household locations enabled spatiotemporal analysis of transmission risk factors. Without the point locations, examining risk factors at the household level may not have been possible.

In addition to GPS data, network location information from a cellular device might be used to identify location. Today, almost any standard cellular device can generate geographic data. In one instance of fieldwork in Africa, the field investigators used the geotagging function on their cellular phones to take pictures inside their pockets to document their locations.

Beyond Points on a Map

A common misconception is that location can represent only a single position. Collecting spatial data in formats other than points (e.g., lines or polygons) is additionally informative (2–4). Moreover, certain spatial data can represent abstract ideas (e.g., activity space) (15,16). Activity space can include places of employment, houses of worship, residences, restaurants, points of food purchase, recreational areas, friends' residences, and anywhere else the persons of interest might have frequented. Therefore, when in the field, an investigator should not be limited to recording a street address or assigning a single georeference point.

Visualizing distribution points of contaminated products through road network data can be informative during the case identification process. Other spatial data that might be of interest reflect the movement of materials between facilities and the points of interaction with affected populations. Food products can undergo a lengthy trip from production or harvesting to the consumer and every location along the route. Even the route itself can be a source of risk. Processing locations (e.g., water treatment plants or heating, ventilation, and air conditioning handlers) also can be sources of risk. Collecting data about the locations of and connections between these networks can aid the team's understanding of the risk factors.

In addition, GIS and location information can be useful in understanding the impact of specific interventions or changes in the natural or built environment. For example, in Atlanta, Georgia, GIS and location information was used to study possible health impacts to residents resulting from the development of a city "Beltline" to improve urban walkability and enhance active commuting (17,18). Field data collection efforts included location and measurement of sidewalk characteristics, walkability, and aesthetics (Figure 17.7). Data were collected for specific road segments, mapped, and spatially analyzed to examine the possible impact of the "BeltLine" on local residents' health.

Summary

- GIS can be used to specify the place associated with the case definition.
- GIS can be informative for planning field data collection methods.
- The type of analysis will influence spatial data needs and spatial data collection tools.
- Geographic-level data collected during fieldwork will affect the specificity of visualization and the spatial statistical methods during analysis.
- Field investigators should think beyond collection of latitude and longitude, point-level data.

STEP 5. TABULATE AND ORIENT THE DATA IN TERMS OF TIME, PLACE, AND PERSON (DESCRIPTIVE EPIDEMIOLOGY)

Characterizing the Geographic and Sociodemographic Distribution of Disease

Often, the first look at the data involves creating a map visualizing the disease distribution. Maps can comprise points representing the location of each case or display the geographic

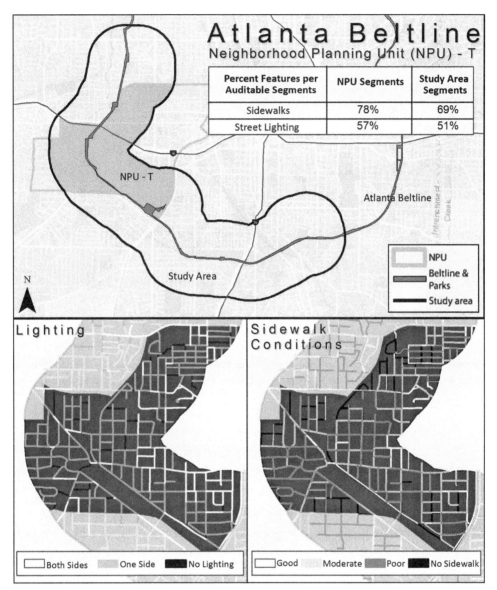

FIGURE 17.7 Collecting data regarding the natural or built environment. Geographic information system data about the natural or built environment can be collected in the field, mapped, and spatially analyzed. This map characterizes data about walkability in a study area around the Atlanta BeltLine.

distribution of rates or changes in the distribution of counts or rates across time (1–3,8). Both count and rate data can be aggregated to different geographic units (e.g., census tracts, counties, or zip codes). The technique known as *choropleth mapping* visualizes the intensity of the counts or rates by using boundary aggregations (Figure 17.8) (1–3,8). Selecting classification breakpoints and color schemes are chief considerations (8,19).

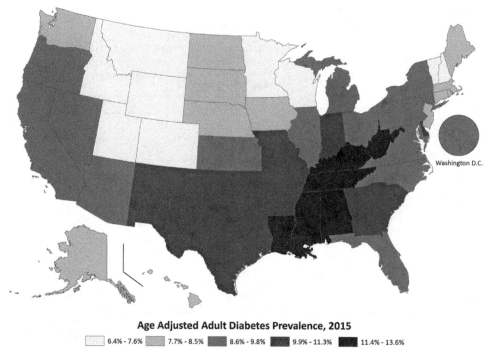

Age Adjusted Adult Diabetes Prevalence, 2015

| 6.4% - 7.6% | 7.7% - 8.5% | 8.6% - 9.8% | 9.9% - 11.3% | 11.4% - 13.6% |

FIGURE 17.8 Choropleth maps offer an overview of the variation in disease distribution through the use of color to denote value differences. Darker colors are often associated with greater values.

Analyses do not have to be restricted to commonly used geopolitical boundaries. For example, mapping the accumulation of cases among homes within a village might be useful. With this information, choropleth maps of the number of cases, or rates, within each home can be compared with the quantity in other homes within the study area. Another possibility is for the map to represent the location of cases in rooms in a building (e.g., in a hospital or nursing home).

GIS Operations and Their Utility

Point-level analyses of cases can provide an overview of the extent of disease distribution. Point-level data also are needed for evaluating spatial clustering of disease. Alternatively, service area or activity space analyses can help characterize the extent of disease distribution on a more relative and temporal scale. As previously mentioned, another advantage of GIS is incorporating other spatially related information into the analysis, thus providing context for disease patterns and insights regarding place-based risk factors. For example, during the 2016 Flint, Michigan, shigellosis outbreak, cases were aggregated by census area for reporting and visualization. In doing so, the team was able to examine the case rates in relation to reported water-quality events, thus leading to more in-depth spatial analysis (20).

Providing Context with Supplemental Data

Analyzing supplemental data (e.g., environmental or infrastructure data) enables further contextualization of the public health problem. For example, during the investigation of elevated lead levels in Flint, Michigan, water supply system data were important for understanding the common source of contamination and identifying particularly vulnerable populations (i.e., child residents). Similarly, waterline information was used to model chlorine residuals to understand a later outbreak of shigellosis in the same area (20).

Another resource is *remotely sensed data*. Remotely sensed data can include aerial and satellite images, or they can be data collected by sensors on satellites orbiting in space (2). Remote sensing techniques can aid in locating key geographic features or monitoring change across time. Imagery can be particularly useful in preparing for responses to natural disasters by providing an aerial view of environmental and infrastructural damage and stranded populations. For example, after Hurricane Harvey's landfall in Texas in 2017, field investigators analyzed satellite imagery to predict and prevent mold exposure. After the 2010 earthquake in Haiti, satellite imagery was used to locate stranded populations and to identify the locations to which affected residents were moving to find shelter. During the 2016–2017 Zika virus infection response in Puerto Rico, spectral signature remote sensing techniques were used to locate standing water, which served as a breeding ground for *Aedies egypti* mosquitos potentially carrying the Zika virus (Figure 17.9).

Visualizing Disease Across Time

GIS can be used to visualize disease progression, changing concentrations, or distribution of risk factors across time. Static map series, linked interactive micromaps, and animations are methods for such visualization. An animation of the spread of Ebola virus infection among households and the institution of household-wide and village-wide isolation and quarantine efforts in Sierra Leone was particularly informative in understanding the outbreak's epidemiologic curve (14). New tools are also being developed to visualize the slope of an epidemiologic curve for every geographic unit within a study area. As the direction and magnitude of this slope is mapped, a visualization of the stage, magnitude, and geographic distribution of an outbreak can be realized.

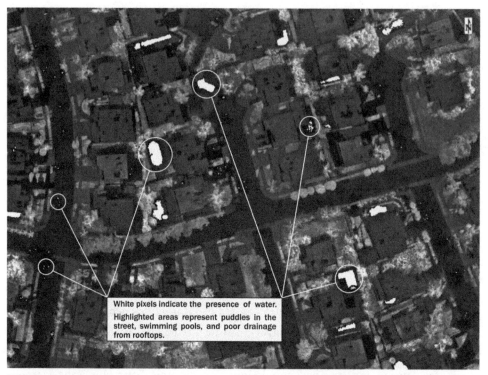

White pixels indicate the presence of water.

Highlighted areas represent puddles in the street, swimming pools, and poor drainage from rooftops.

FIGURE 17.9 Imagery analysis. Aerial photography and satellite imagery can provide data to extract key features in the environment. In this example, image classification of aerial imagery was used to identify potential mosquito habitats given the presence of water.

Summary

- Mapping count and rate data describe disease distribution and potential risk factors whether at the county, household, or room level.
- Supplemental data add another dimension to the analysis, enabling further contextualization of the public health problem.
- Environmental, infrastructure, transportation networks, water systems, and satellite imagery are common supplemental resources.
- Linked micromaps and animations are helpful for describing disease distributions across time.

STEP 6. CONSIDER CONTROL MEASURES

Selecting Control and Prevention Locations

Maps and geostatistical results can guide decisions about when and where to implement control, prevention, and surveillance measures. During outbreaks related to environmental exposures or vectorborne diseases, results can delineate areas of highest need or uncover potentially new reservoirs of disease spread. During the 2016–2017 Zika virus infection outbreak, the vector-control unit in Puerto Rico used GIS techniques to delineate population-based regions for placing mosquito traps. Data collected from these traps were visualized, and the resulting maps were used to estimate Zika virus in a heavily affected area of Puerto Rico. During that same response, the epidemiology unit used GIS to intersect data characterizing women of childbearing age and weekly changes in Zika virus infection incidence by county to determine where to focus educational interventions and to distribute Zika virus infection prevention kits.

Summary

- Visualization of rates through mapping enables identification of probable locales for implementing control and prevention measures.
- Results from geospatial analyses are useful for determining areas of highest need, predicting future locations of concern, and identifying particular populations at risk.

STEPS 7 AND 8. DEVELOP AND TEST HYPOTHESIS(ES) AND PLAN STUDIES

Using Geospatial Descriptive Results to Generate Hypotheses

Maps generated from descriptive results can assist in generating theories about possible routes of exposure and interactions between risk factors and susceptible populations. Using maps and the results of the descriptive analysis can guide hypothesis development regarding disease-causing agents, the transmission mode, and exposure locations. With this information, the field team might determine the need for additional analyses, perhaps applying other advanced geospatial statistics to further understand the spatial and temporal associations between suspected risks and disease.

Geospatial Analytical Methods for Study Design

Creating risk maps by using spatial overlays and using interpolation methods to estimate values in an unsampled location or spatial regression techniques can be used to further understand the geographic distribution of potential risk factors or disease processes (3,21). *Cluster analysis* provides the researcher with quantifiable, statistical estimates to evaluate whether similar values occur near one another and whether these occurrences are nonrandom (3,21). Cluster analysis can be highly useful in hypothesis generation and risk factor evaluation regarding place and time. An overview of selected advanced and inferential spatial techniques that can be useful in hypothesis redefinition and development of additional studies is provided (Table 17.1).

Summary

- Results of mapping and spatial analyses provide information pertinent to generating study hypotheses.
- Geospatial methods can generate estimates for areas where only limited data might be available, thus assisting in generation of additional investigations.
- Cluster analysis is useful in providing statistical evidence of nonrandom disease processes.

STEP 9. IMPLEMENT AND EVALUATE CONTROL AND PREVENTION MEASURES

Short- and Long-Term Geospatial Approaches for Evaluation

Geospatial methods described thus far are also useful for understanding the impact of control and prevention efforts. In particular, visualization of rates by location can highlight locales where control measures might be more or less effective. Identifying these places and then uncovering factors influencing the efficacy of such measures can be useful in determining whether changes to control measures are required, and, if so, where changes might be necessary. For example, researchers can track changes in opioid-related death rates in different locales to identify where efforts are working or not (22).

Spatiotemporal analysis provides researchers tools for exploring and quantifying complex associations between disease risk factors and prevention activities. Using the opioid overdose epidemic example, geospatial methods revealed the impact of the placement of prevention measures (e.g., treatment locations, recovery resources, or prescription drop boxes) (22). Researchers can use time-series animations, map series, linked micromaps, and spatiotemporal modeling to evaluate these types of trends. Transit times and healthcare service area analyses can reveal missed opportunities for prevention or highlight areas where specific interventions are successful. Such information can be useful in determining where additional resources and control measures are necessary.

TABLE 17.1 Geospatial operations for field epidemiology

Research question	Geospatial operation	Description
What is the geographic distribution of the data in the study area?	Mean/median center	Identify a geographic center
	Directional distribution; standard deviational ellipse; linear directional mean	Summarize directional trends
Does any clustering or uniformity exist anywhere in the study area? That is, does spatial autocorrelation exist?	Global Moran's I (polygon); Ripley's K Function (point); Weighted K (count, incidence)	Detect whether clustering or uniformity exists across an area
Where are hot spots (or cold spots) specifically located in the study area?	Local Indicators of Spatial Association (LISA Statistic); Getis Gi-Ord	Reveals areas of clustered high values and clustered low values within a defined region
Do nearby data tend to occur at about the same time? That is, are the data clustered in space and time?	Space-time statistics: k nearest neighbor; Kulldorf's spatial scan; Knox test	Reveals whether data are clustered in space and time (even if not clustered in space or time individually)
What is the most likely value of a variable at an unsampled location?	Mean or median statistics or Voronoi diagram	Uses input data points to divide the study area in to polygons such that the area within each polygon is closer to the control point than any other point
	Kernel density estimation; inverse distance weighting	Estimate density of events or their values, per unit area
	Kriging	Empirically calculates and fits a model to create a surface of predictions and error
How is an observed value at a specific location explained by various other factors, considering that they have different values at different locations?	Spatial regression models: ordinary least squares; generalized linear mixed models; geographically weighted regression	Regression models can be applied to spatial data to determine what independent variables might explain a spatially dependent outcome
	Bayesian statistics; conditional and simultaneously autoregressive models	Spatially aware models that account for space in the model by using weighted distance matrices

Summary

- Locales where control measures prove effective can be identified through mapping.
- Mapping and spatial analyses can uncover factors influencing the efficacy of control measures, thus enabling researchers to modify programs accordingly.
- Network analysis, time-series animations, map series, linked micromaps, and spatiotemporal modeling are methods for evaluating long-term trends.

STEP 10. COMMUNICATE FINDINGS

Efficient and Effective Communication Through Mapping

Maps are one of the most efficient ways to quickly guide situational awareness and communicate place-related information about incidence, prevalence, environmental or infrastructural exposures, and other related spatial information. During major disease outbreaks (e.g., Zika and Ebola virus infection outbreaks), weekly maps helped visualize incidence and geographic shifts in disease presence. After Hurricane Maria devastated Puerto Rico in 2017, CDC's Medical Care and Counter Measures Task Force used interactive Internet-based maps to access open-source data regarding the location and status of pharmacies, hospitals, and other health infrastructure. The information these maps provided was essential in determining where best to direct medical resources.

Maps provide essential situational awareness and communicate findings to response agencies and local authorities. Moreover, they can be used to readily share information with affected populations. For example, during the 2016–2017 Zika virus infection outbreak in Puerto Rico, the island's health department published weekly Internet-based maps of case counts and incidence, providing the public with updated information about how the outbreak was changing (23).

Summary

- Maps quickly reveal and communicate place-related information about disease distributions and disease processes.
- Maps provide essential information for directing healthcare resources and focusing prevention and control measures.
- Maps are useful in communicating with multiple stakeholders.

CONCLUSION

This chapter has highlighted GIS techniques, resources, and methods integral to the 10 steps of the field investigation process. GIS can provide the tools to further identify and define the where of a field investigation. Striking the balance between the need for situational awareness with rapid, yet complete and accurate spatial data is an art. It requires consideration of the strengths and limitations of data collection instruments, facility of locational data collection, accuracy of locational data, and pertinent attributes for understanding disease risk.

Ultimately, collecting relevant location data is only one part of a field investigation, but location data are nonetheless a principal part and should be considered from the very beginning of an investigation. One solution does not fit all field investigations. No one single spatial data collection method or analysis is best suited for every field investigation scenario. Therefore, GIS is one tool in the field investigator's toolkit not to be overlooked.

REFERENCES

1. Dent BD, Torguson JS, Hodler TW. *Cartography: Thematic Map Design*. 6th ed. New York: McGraw-Hill Higher Education; 2008.
2. Campbell J, Shin M. Essentials of geographic information systems. https://open.umn.edu/opentextbooks/BookDetail.aspx?bookId=67
3. Cromley EK, McLafferty SL. *GIS and Public Health*. 2nd ed. New York: The Guilford Press; 2012.
4. de Smith MJ, Goodchild MF, Longley PA. Geospatial analysis: a comprehensive guide to principles, techniques and software tools. 5th ed. http://www.spatialanalysisonline.com/HTML/index.html
5. Mitchell A. *The ESRI guide to GIS analysis. Volume 1: geographic patterns & relationships*. Redlands, CA: ESRI Press; 1999.
6. US Census Bureau. TIGER products. https://www.census.gov/geo/maps-data/data/tiger.html
7. Dyer J, Tanner S, Runk J, Mertzlufft C, Gottdenker N. Deforestation, dogs, and zoonotic disease. *Anthropology News*. 2016;57:344–7.
8. Geography and Geospatial Science Working Group. Cartographic guidelines for public health. https://www.cdc.gov/dhdsp/maps/gisx/resources/cartographic_guidelines.pdf
9. White RG, Hakim AJ, Salganik MJ, et al. Strengthening the reporting of observational studies in epidemiology for respondent-driven sampling studies: "STROBE-RDS" statement. *J Clin Epidemiol*. 2015;68:1463–71.
10. Hallisey E, Tai E, Berens A, et. al. Transforming geographic scale: a comparison of combined population and areal weighting to other interpolation methods. *Int J Health Geogr*. 2017;16:29.
11. Pickle L, Carr D. Visualizing health data with micromaps. *Spat Spatiotemporal Epidemiol*. 2010;1:143–50.
12. Goldberg D. A geocoding best practice guide. https://20tqtx36s1la18rvn82wcmpn-wpengine.netdna-ssl.com/wp-content/uploads/2016/11/Geocoding_Best_Practices.pdf
13. Rushton G, Armstrong MP, Gittler J, et al. *Geocoding Health Data: The Use of Geographic Codes in Cancer Prevention and Control, Research and Practice*. Boca Raton, FL: CRC Press; 2008.
14. Gleason BL, Foster S, Wilt GE, et al. Geospatial analysis of household spread of Ebola virus in a quarantined village—Sierra Leone, 2014. *Epidemiol Infect*. 2017:145:2921–9.

15. Lewin K. *Field Theory in Social Science*. Cartwright D, ed. New York: Harper and Row; 1951.

16. Schönfelder S, Axhausen KW. *Urban Rhythms and Travel Behaviour: Spatial and Temporal Phenomena of Daily Travel*. Burlington, VT: Ashgate; 2010.

17. Wilkin HA, Gallashaw C, Gayman M, Mingo C, Steward J, Kolling J. Community engagement and inclusion in research about the potential impact of changes in the built environment on the community. Presented at the American Public Health Association Annual Meeting and Exposition, November 7, 2017, Atlanta, Georgia. https://apha.confex.com/apha/2017/meetingapp.cgi/Paper/385571

18. Kanchik M. A Secondary Analysis of walkability data for the Atlanta BeltLine communities. https://scholarworks.gsu.edu/iph_capstone/79/

19. Brewer CA. Designing better maps: a guide for GIS users. Redlands, CA: ESRI Press; 2005.

20. McClung RP, Castillo C, Miller A, et al. *Shigella sonnei* outbreak investigation in the setting of a municipal water crisis—Genesee and Saginaw Counties, Michigan, 2016. Presented at the 66th Annual EIS Conference, April 24–27, 2017, Atlanta, Georgia. https://www.cdc.gov/eis/downloads/eis-conference-2017.pdf

21. Waller LA, Gotway CA. *Applied Spatial Statistics for Public Health Data*. Hoboken, NJ: John Wiley and Sons; 2004.

22. Lindemann J. Oakland County, Michigan using data and maps to help understand and combat the opioid epidemic. New America Public Interest Technology blog. https://www.newamerica.org/public-interest-technology/blog/oakland-county-michigan-using-data-and-maps-help-understand-and-combat-opioid-epidemic

23. Gobierno de Puerto Rico, Departamento de Salud. Informe semanal de enfermedades arbovirales [in Spanish]. http://www.salud.gov.pr/Estadisticas-Registros-y-Publicaciones/Pages/VigilanciadeZika.aspx

/// 18 /// HEALTHCARE SETTINGS

BRYAN E. CHRISTENSEN AND RYAN P. FAGAN

INTRODUCTION

The term *healthcare setting* represents a broad array of services and places where health-care occurs, including acute care hospitals, urgent care centers, rehabilitation centers, nursing homes and other long-term care facilities, specialized outpatient services (e.g., hemodialysis, dentistry, podiatry, chemotherapy, endoscopy, and pain management clinics), and outpatient surgery centers. In addition, some healthcare services are provided in private offices or homes.

Within each type of setting, specific locations or services might be the focal point of an epidemiologic investigation. Acute care hospitals are complex organizations that can have multiple specialized areas for triage and emergency care, inpatient and outpatient surgical procedures, management of immunosuppressed populations (e.g., oncology or transplant recipients), rehabilitation services, and intensive care units. An understanding of the types of patients and clinical services provided in a given setting is crucial for recognizing infectious disease transmission risks. Problems identified within a healthcare setting also can be related to use of medications or devices that became contaminated at the point of manufacture or other locations outside the setting of interest.

This chapter is an overview of outbreak investigations in healthcare settings. Although most reported outbreaks in healthcare settings are caused by infections, outbreaks also can be associated with exposures to noninfectious chemical and other toxic agents. This chapter mainly addresses epidemiologic investigations of infections but includes some noninfectious disease examples as well.

CONTEXT FOR INFECTIONS ASSOCIATED WITH HEALTHCARE SETTINGS

Defining Healthcare-Associated Infections (HAIs)

Healthcare-associated infections (HAIs) are one of the leading causes of unnecessary death and avoidable harm for patients receiving medical care. They are a serious threat to public health, and each year millions of patients are affected by HAIs worldwide.

An HAI is an infection associated with healthcare delivery in any setting. This term reflects the inability to always determine with certainty where the pathogen is acquired because patients might be colonized (i.e., microorganisms on or in a person without causing a disease) or exposed outside the healthcare setting, and patients frequently move among different settings within a healthcare system (1). HAIs might appear after discharge, and HAIs transmission can involve visitors and healthcare personnel (HCP) in addition to patients.

HAIs Causes

During the course of receiving medical care, patients are exposed to different microorganisms, and infectious agents can be acquired from

- Infected or colonized HCP or another patient (cross-infection);
- The patient's own microbiome (endogenous infection);
- Environmental surfaces or objects contaminated from another human (e.g., bed rails, intravenous poles, countertops, or bathroom surfaces);
- Contaminated medical devices (e.g., central venous catheters, urinary catheters, endoscopes, surgical instruments, or ventilators);
- Contaminated medications;
- Contaminated water sources; or
- Air from heating, ventilation, or air-conditioning systems.

A vast number of agents have been implicated in HAIs transmission scenarios; these include a constantly evolving list of bacteria, fungi, viruses, parasites, and prions. HAIs outbreaks can be caused by pathogens that are common in the community or by pathogens that are rarely observed outside of healthcare environments and specific patient populations. The likelihood of infection after exposure is related to (1) the characteristics of the microorganisms, including resistance to antimicrobial agents, intrinsic virulence, and amount of infective material; (2) patient factors, including immune status, wounds, other underlying comorbidities, duration of care, prior antimicrobial exposures, and whether their care involves surgical or other invasive procedures or devices; and (3) facility-level factors, including inattention to individual or environmental hygiene, crowding, lack of an effective infection control program, and shortage of trained infection control practitioners.

HAIs Prevalence

Despite progress during the past decade in preventing certain types of HAIs through improved surveillance and infection prevention and control practices, HAIs remain common. The Centers for Disease Control and Prevention's (CDC) HAI Prevalence Survey of 2014 regarding the burden of HAIs in US hospitals reported that, during 2011, an estimated 722,000 HAIs occurred in US acute care hospitals (Table 18.1) (2). Additionally, approximately 75,000 patients with HAIs died during their hospitalizations. More than half of all HAIs occurred outside of intensive care units (2).

TABLE 18.1 Healthcare–associated infection estimates in US acute care hospitals, 2011

Major infection site	Estimated no.
Pulmonary	157,500
Gastrointestinal	123,100
Urinary tract	93,300
Primary bloodstream	71,900
Surgical from any inpatient surgery	157,500
Other	118,500
Estimated total no. infections in hospitals	721,800

Source: Adapted from Reference 2.

OVERVIEW OF SEQUENCE OF STEPS INVOLVED IN AN HAI INVESTIGATION

Typically, the state, territorial, local or tribal public health authority is notified of a potential HAI outbreak by a healthcare provider or facility on the basis of laboratory or other HAIs surveillance data or as a result of recognizing an unusual infection cluster. Health departments might also detect potential outbreaks through surveillance or after being directly contacted by affected patients. The public health department can contact CDC for additional technical assistance. In certain instances, however, the healthcare facility's administrator contacts CDC directly; in that instance, CDC subject matter experts can provide technical advice, but they must coordinate with the state or local public health department before becoming involved in a field investigation. Depending on the scenario, initial steps taken by a public health authority might include the following:

1. Public health department epidemiologists gather information and provide consultation to the healthcare facility reporting the potential outbreak.
2. The public health department official begins an on-site investigation and considers inviting CDC to assist.
3. The public health personnel and healthcare facility staff gather and analyze information through interviews, chart reviews, observations, and environmental sampling to identify a point source or practice that might have caused the outbreak.
4. The public health personnel recommend new or revised measures to stop the outbreak and prevent additional HAIs.

FIELD INVESTIGATION

The basic steps of epidemiologic field investigations that are described in Chapter 3 are adapted here for investigations in healthcare settings.

- Step 1. Verify the diagnosis.
- Step 2. Confirm presence of an HAI outbreak.
- Step 3. Alert key partners about the investigation.
- Step 4. Establish case definition(s).
- Step 5. Identify and count cases.
- Step 6. Organize data according to person, place, time, and size.
- Step 7. Conduct targeted observations, review key concerns with setting healthcare providers, and develop abstraction forms.
- Step 8. Formulate and test hypotheses.
- Step 9. Infection control assessment and implementation of control measures.
- Step 10. Follow-up, communicate findings, and notify patients.

Step 1. Verify the Diagnosis

Early in the investigation, identify as accurately as possible the specific nature of the disease by

- Ensuring that the diagnosis is correct;
- Evaluating for possible laboratory error as the basis for increased diagnoses;
- Evaluating possible changes in surveillance and case definitions; and
- Reviewing clinical findings and microbiological testing results.

Step 2. Confirm Presence of an HAI Outbreak

- An early major step in the investigation is verifying that a suspected outbreak is real. Cases in excess of historical or predicted levels might not necessarily indicate an outbreak.
  - Some cases might be part of an actual outbreak with a common cause, whereas others might be unrelated.
  - Reporting might be increased because of changes in local reporting procedures, changes in the case definition, increased interest reflecting local or national awareness, or improvements or other changes in diagnostic procedures.

- Possible community-associated or other explanations for illness not associated with healthcare should be investigated. Public health surveillance data sometimes can inform investigators about an increase in infections that is initially recognized in healthcare settings but actually is part of a broader community outbreak.
- Pseudo-outbreaks (e.g., those caused by laboratory processing errors or contamination of clinical diagnostic equipment, such as bronchoscopes, without clinical illness) are important to investigate and control because they can lead to unnecessary antibiotic prescriptions, diagnostic procedures, and other potentially harmful interventions to patients. Pseudo-outbreaks also represent opportunities to recognize and correct inadequate infection control processes (e.g., device reprocessing).

Step 3. Alert Key Partners About the Investigation

After confirming an HAI outbreak, investigators should inform key partners.

- Include relevant facility staff (e.g., hospital epidemiologist, infection control practitioner, environmental services department staff, medical staff, administrative leaders, media relations director, and department leads for the affected facility area).
- Ask the clinical laboratory director to save all isolates that might be related to the outbreak.
- Notify local, state, national, and international public health officials, as required.
- Notify regulatory partners (e.g., Food and Drug Administration, Environmental Protection Agency) if the investigation involves regulated medical devices or products.
- Notify professional oversight organizations, as required (e.g., pharmacy boards, clinician licensing boards).

Step 4. Establish Case Definitions

A case definition is used to identify persons who are, or might be, infected and to characterize them in relation to the disease, time and location of exposure or illness onset, and other persons affected. A case definition usually includes

- Clinical information about the disease (e.g., laboratory test results, symptoms, and signs);
- Demographic characteristics of affected patients (e.g., age, race/ethnicity, sex, and occupation);

- Information about the location of possible exposure or time of onset (e.g., what part of an intensive care unit, radiology suite, operating room, ward, or other unit); and
- A defined time during which exposure or onset occurred.

Ideally, the case definition initially should be broad enough to include most if not all cases; it can then be refined as the investigation progresses and more relevant information is accumulated.

The case definition also should be based on the etiologic agent, if known, and can include clinically infected and colonized patients. The specificity of the definition can vary.

- A stratified case definition (e.g., confirmed vs. probable vs. possible [i.e., suspected], or confirmed vs. probable) can be applied to account for the uncertainty of certain diagnoses.
  - *Confirmed*: Usually must have laboratory verification.
  - *Probable*: Usually has typical clinical features and an epidemiologic link to confirmed cases but lacks laboratory confirmation.
  - *Possible*: Usually has fewer of the typical clinical features or weaker epidemiologic links to confirmed cases.

The following are example case definitions:

- A methicillin-resistant *Staphylococcus aureus* bloodstream infection in a patient in Hospital A's neonatal intensive care unit during January 1–December 31.
- Isolation of *Burkholderia cepacia* complex matching the outbreak strain in a hospitalized patient who received Medication A any time during January 1–June 30.
- Fever (temperature ≥ 38.5ºC) and compatible symptoms in a patient who had been in an Ebola virus infection–affected country 21 days or less before symptom onset.

Step 5. Identify and Count Cases

Outbreaks often are first recognized and reported by perceptive HCP or identified during surveillance activities. Additional cases related to the outbreak can be identified through multiple types of data and records, for example,

- Central service or supply records,
- Occupational health records,
- Hospital billing records,
- Operative notes,

- Infection control assessment,
- Pathology reports,
- Interviews with physicians,
- Pharmacy reports,
- Log books,
- Purchasing records,
- Medical records,
- Radiology reports,
- Microbiology data, and
- Surveillance records.

Step 6. Organize Data According to Person, Place, Time, and Size

Step 6.1. Create a Line Listing

The *line listing*, which typically involves using a spreadsheet program so that data can be sorted easily during data analysis, helps guide the outbreak investigation and permits rapid examination of exposures. For each case, collect and array the following types of information encompassed by the case definition:

- *Location information.* Location within the facility (e.g., room number, bed number, and adjacent rooms).
- *Demographic information.* Typically, age, sex, race/ethnicity, and occupation, plus other relevant characteristics of the affected population or others at risk.
- *Clinical information.* Symptoms, signs, and laboratory tests (e.g., culture, serology, or polymerase chain reaction results).
- *Risk factor information.* Adjust the investigation to the specific disease in question.

Develop a standard questionnaire if patients are to be contacted and interviewed. Box 18.1 summarizes data that should be obtained for a line listing in an HAI investigation.

Collect the information described previously on a standard case-report form, questionnaire, or data abstraction form (Table 18.2).

- *Abstract selected key items to build a table.* Each column represents a variable, and each row represents a case.
- *Add new cases as they are identified.* This simple format allows the investigator to scan key information on every case and to update it easily.

BOX 18.1

EXAMPLE DATA TO OBTAIN FOR A LINE LISTING

- Patient characteristics (e.g., age, sex, race/ethnicity, comorbidities, birthweight)
- Date of admission
- Date of illness onset
- Date of discharge
- Facility locations/units (i.e., room number, bed, and adjoining room numbers)
- Medications
- Procedures
- Consults (e.g., laboratory or nursing)
- Attending healthcare personnel (e.g., specific nursing staff, respiratory therapists, and physicians)

An example HAI outbreak abstraction form and user guide are available with the Healthcare-Associated Infection Outbreak Investigation Toolkit (3).

Step 6.2. Construct an Epidemic Curve

Create an *epidemic curve* (*epi curve*) to visually demonstrate the outbreak's magnitude and time course. The epidemic curve

- Illustrates the course of the epidemic by day, week, or month and can help project its forward trajectory;
- Might help estimate a probable exposure period and, therefore, focus a questionnaire on that period, especially when an approximate incubation period is known or suspected.

TABLE 18.2 Example line listing for healthcare-associated infection investigations

			Illness onset			
				Patient		
Patient	Age, yrs	Sex	Date	location	Comorbidities	Current status
1	26	M	June 9, 2016	ICU Bed 2	Diabetes, renal disease	Hospitalized
2	35	F	June 11, 2016	ICU Bed 3	Cardiovascular disease	Discharged
3	42	M	June 12, 2016	ICU Bed 3	HIV infection	Hospitalized

ICU, intensive care unit; HIV, human immunodeficiency virus.

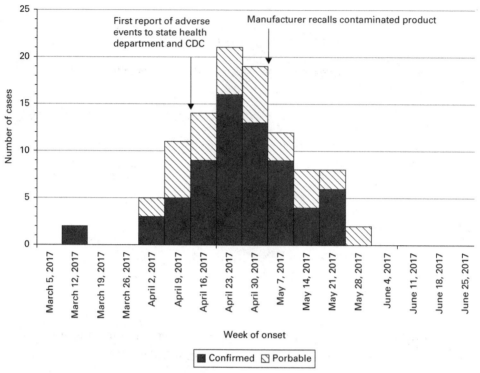

FIGURE 18.1 Example epidemic curve of patient adverse events associated with a contaminated medical product. *Source*: Adapted from Reference 4.

- Might enable inferences about the epidemic pattern (e.g., whether common source or person-to-person).

In the example (Figure 18.1), confirmed and probable cases are plotted over time to show the onset of adverse events associated with a contaminated medical product, including markers for key events during the investigation. This example was adapted after a published field investigation (4).

Step 7. Conduct Targeted Observations, Review Key Concerns with Setting Healthcare Providers, and Develop Abstraction Forms

- Healthcare setting investigations often are complex and hypotheses elusive. Most outbreaks are solved through rigorous observation and discussion of procedural concerns with facilities' HCP.
  - Focus on whether actual practices deviate from recommended infection control practices and the facility's policies. Such discrepancies are best identified

through a combination of direct observations and review of HCP self-reported practices.

- Examine whether practices differ among HCP.
- Review recent scientific literature related to the key concerns involved with the outbreak.
- Observe key activities (e.g., medication preparation, care of vascular access, hand hygiene, adherence to isolation precautions, device and equipment reprocessing, environmental services, and respiratory therapy) related to suspicions about likely transmission pathways that might be involved in the outbreak.
- In addition to available local and setting-specific tools, use general infection control assessment tools available through CDC to assist with both prevention programs and response scenarios (5).
- Review key concerns with facility HCP to help generate hypotheses about the source and mode(s) of transmission.
  - Are protocols accurate and up-to-date?
  - How does actual practice compare with written or verbal protocols?
  - Are procedures consistently adherent to protocols?
  - Do instances exist where procedures must be performed differently?
  - Have other HCP been observed to perform procedures differently from protocol?
  - What are the challenges with maintaining accurate and consistent techniques?
  - What do you think is the root cause of the outbreak?
  - What procedures or medications might not be documented in the medical record?
  - Is all information in patients' medical records accurate and current?
- Develop, modify if necessary, and complete abstraction forms. Abstraction forms can include additional details about patients' illnesses that provide information for analytic studies. Abstraction forms can be adapted from information collected on the line listing to help determine which fields or sections of the abstraction form to include.

Step 8. Formulate and Test Hypotheses

Step 8.1. Conduct Analytic Studies

A case–control study is the approach most commonly used for hypothesis testing for field investigations in healthcare settings. The frequency of exposure to a risk factor among a group of case-patients (i.e., persons with the HAIs) is compared with the frequency of exposure to that risk factor among a group of controls (i.e., persons without the HAIs). Controls must be selected carefully to limit bias; for example, two or more controls for each case-patient might be needed to provide sufficient statistical power. Cohort studies might also be useful in HAIs investigations.

However, analytic studies are labor-intensive and in healthcare settings not always necessary to identify the likely source of an outbreak and to institute control measures. For example, a combination of laboratory evidence and observations of serious lapses in infection control practices that are known to be associated with transmission are frequently sufficient to recommend and implement control measures. The following considerations can influence the decision to conduct an analytic study:

- Will an analytic study add to what is already known about the cause of the outbreak or contribute to the control recommendations?
- Is the necessary technical and statistical support available?
- Is the number of cases large enough to support statistical inferences?
- Can enough controls be selected to minimize bias?
- Is information available for testing possible risk factors?

Step 8.2. Conduct Environmental Sampling and Testing

A major tool available for HAIs investigations is environmental sampling and laboratory analysis. An environmental sampling strategy (i.e., where and what should be cultured) should always be influenced by epidemiologic findings. Molecular methods (e.g., polymerase chain reaction or pulsed-field gel electrophoresis) can be deployed in certain investigations to link environmental samples to clinical specimens. Optimal methods should be discussed with laboratory personnel experienced in environmental sampling to determine how specimens should be obtained and where the cultures can be processed. Often, public health laboratories are needed to support specialized sampling of surfaces, devices, water, or air or when substantial numbers of samples should be obtained. A plan for correctly processing and interpreting results should be established before sample collection. When developing a sampling plan, specify the following:

- Ensure protocols are in place for safe and correct collection and processing of environmental samples. Many environmental pathogens need special procedures for collection, handling, storage, and media for culture growth. Contamination of samples is possible if procedures are inadequate, and overgrowth of organisms in the samples can obscure results for the pathogen of interest. Safety precautions for personnel collecting the samples also need to be followed.

- Use epidemiologic findings to guide testing so that laboratory resources are used appropriately and results can be meaningfully interpreted. Interpretation of results should consider the following:
  - Positive environmental samples are not necessarily evidence of transmission from a particular source; thus, understanding how patients are most likely being exposed to the organism from the environment is crucial. Organisms can be polyclonal even from the same source; for example, biofilms in plumbing systems frequently have many different species and strains of coexisting microorganisms.
  - Conversely, negative environmental samples do not rule out that the pathogen of interest is present or was present at the time of transmission.
  - Samples that test negative must be confirmed to be true-negatives and not inactivated by environmental disinfectants or media preservatives.
  - Laboratory analyses (e.g., pulsed-field gel electrophoresis for DNA finger-printing) can be used to determine whether environmental isolates match those from patients; however, organisms can be polyclonal.
- Even with correct methods and materials, sensitivity can be low, and negative results do not necessarily rule out environmental reservoirs.

Analytic studies can support a hypothesis even if a source cannot be confirmed by environmental testing.

Step 8.3. Considerations for Testing of HCP

Testing HCP can further support or confirm possible associations between HCP colonization and infection transmission to patients. These scenarios are most readily recognized in point-source outbreaks involving colonized HCP and absence of other clear links among infected patients. Possible transmission from HCP to patients should be considered in the context of the type of organism and investigation into other possible transmission routes.

- HCP testing should only be undertaken after careful consideration of (1) how the results will help control the outbreak, (2) what duty or work restrictions might need to be applied, and (3) a known decolonization or other specific control strategy to undertake for personnel who test positive.

- Testing of HCP provokes anxiety, and positive results can be highly stigmatizing. The rationale for testing should be clearly explained to HCP, and strict discretion should be emphasized when obtaining samples and communicating results.
- Positive results should not necessarily be regarded as evidence of causality because HCP frequently acquire microorganisms from infected patients.
- Because of limitations in the sensitivity of cultures and the potential for transient contamination, negative results can be reassuring in certain scenarios but should not be regarded as excluding the possibility that HCP were involved in transmission.

Step 9. Infection Control Assessment and Implementation of Control Measures

Step 9.1. Infection Control Assessment

When investigating an HAI outbreak, an understanding of infection prevention and control is crucial to determine which control measures need to be implemented. A setting-specific infection control assessment tool can help accomplish this task (5,6). Such tools provide a framework for assessing major areas of infection control and help guide a facility infection control assessment. Box 18.2 summarizes major infection control domains to consider when performing an assessment. A physical walkthrough of the specific health-care setting should be targeted for specific domains, depending on the hypothesized

---

'BOX 18.2

INFECTION CONTROL DOMAINS FOR ASSESSMENT

- Infection control program review
- Infection control training
- Hand hygiene
- Personal protective equipment use, availability, quality, and training
- Prevention of catheter-associated urinary tract infection
- Prevention of central line–associated bloodstream infection
- Prevention of ventilator-associated event
- Injection safety
- Prevention of surgical site infection
- Prevention of *Clostridium difficile* infection
- Environmental cleaning
- Waste management
- Device reprocessing
- Multidrug-resistant organism surveillance

source of transmission (i.e., care locations or others areas hypothesized to be involved in the outbreak), including

- Triage and emergency care departments,
- Inpatient areas,
- Device reprocessing and storage areas,
- On-site or off-site compounding pharmacies,
- Operating or other procedure rooms, or
- Management areas for specific equipment (e.g., hemodialysis machines or ventilators).

Step 9.2. Defining Infection Control Measures

Control measures should be implemented as soon as deficiencies or gaps are identified; these should be aimed at specific links in the infection chain, the agent, the source, or the reservoir. Multiple control measures might be required.

Ultimately, the primary goal is to stop transmission, even when the specific source remains unidentified. Therefore, implementing multiple control measures targeting different possibilities based on the initial observations might be necessary. Table 18.3 provides key examples of immediate control measures that can be used to manage an outbreak.

Certain new or targeted multidrug-resistant organisms warrant consultation with public health departments, and control measures can extend into the community or across healthcare systems. Control measures might include contact tracing, lower thresholds for screening patients and HCP, specialized environmental testing, and implementing systems to adhere to contact precautions or enhanced environmental cleaning and disinfection. A tiered approach for investigating and controlling transmission of such pathogens also might be needed (7).

Step 10. Follow-Up, Communicate Findings, and Notify Patients

Step 10.1. Stages of the Follow-Up Investigation

1. *Refining the case definition*. Refine the case definition on the basis of data gathered from initial case-patients, controls, and HCP. Capturing all cases and optimizing the power of analytic studies might require narrowing or expansion of the definition.
2. *Continuing case finding and surveillance*. Continue case finding and surveillance efforts on the basis of the refined case definition. Surveillance should continue, for

TABLE 18.3 Immediate control measures for outbreak management

Type of transmission suspected	Suggested action
Cross-transmission (transmission between persons)	Patient isolation and transmission-based precautions determined by infectious agent(s)
	Certain scenarios might require closure of locations to new admissions
Hand transmission	Improvements in handwashing and nonsterile glove use where needed
Airborne infections (e.g., tuberculosis or emerging viral pathogens)	Triage, detection, and patient isolation with recommended ventilation type (positive or negative air pressure)
Agent present in water, waterborne agent	Assessment of premise water system, liquid products, or medications
	Use of disposable devices where reusable equipment is suspected
Foodborne agent	Elimination of the suspected food
Environmental reservoirs	Review and enhancement, as needed, of cleaning and disinfection processes
	Interruption of suspected mode of delivery from environment to patient
Colonized or infected healthcare personnel	Review of facility policies and discussion of work restrictions, duty exclusions, treatment, personal hygiene, or other steps
High-risk infection control breaches for risk of bloodborne or other pathogen transmission	Immediate cessation of risky practice until corrective action can be instituted
	Patient notification
	Assurance that occupational health staff are aware

example, for 1 month, 3 months, or even 1 year (e.g., in a long-term care facility) after the outbreak to ensure it has ended.

3. *Reviewing control measures.* Assess adherence and determine whether control measures need to be further enhanced or relaxed.

Step 10.2. Communication of Findings

Findings should be communicated to all partners involved in the investigation. This communication typically takes two forms: (1) an oral briefing for local health authorities and (2) a written report (e.g., for CDC or the state or local health department). The final report, which might await laboratory confirmation, should describe (1) the outbreak characteristics, (2) infection control problems that most likely contributed to the outbreak, and (3) any interventions that were instituted and their effects. Additionally, the report should make recommendations for preventing future occurrences (8).

Step 10.3. Patient Notification

Notification of patients potentially exposed to infectious organisms and their healthcare providers should be considered during investigation of HAIs outbreaks, cases involving pathogens of public health concern, or unsafe infection prevention and control practices. Although the circumstances of each outbreak and infection control breach vary, communication needs during notifications are more predictable. CDC has published considerations for when to notify patients and a patient notification toolkit to support HCP and public health personnel throughout the notification process (9).

Depending on the scenario, typical reasons for conducting notifications can include one or more of the following:

- Identify potentially exposed or infected patients who will derive a health benefit through follow-up testing or other clinical evaluation.
- Establish transparency between healthcare providers and patients and other stakeholders.
- Limit the spread of multidrug-resistant organisms or other pathogens of public health concern by identifying exposed patients and their contacts who should be managed under recommended precautions.
- Improve case finding by informing patients and providers about the outbreak and associated exposures and clinical signs and symptoms that might signify the infection of interest.
- Use the notification scenario as an educational and prevention opportunity by reminding healthcare providers about the importance of infection prevention and control.

Examples of recently conducted patient notification scenarios include lapses in injection safety, drug diversion, contact with other patients with drug-resistant organisms, and exposure to contaminated or incorrectly processed devices (e.g., cardiopulmonary bypass heater-cooler units, endoscopes or surgical instruments, and exposure to contaminated medications).

The objectives of patient notifications are to deliver a consistent message quickly to all affected patients and to inform patients about testing or other follow-up actions that should be taken. Major steps include

- Verifying that exposures have occurred and confirming the type of procedure or substances involved;
- Determining the timeframe of the breach and the number of patients potentially exposed;
- Determining the severity of potential risks to patients;
- Determining whether testing or other further evaluation is available or warranted;
- Identifying any options for prophylactic treatment of exposed persons; and
- Determining how and what entity will provide the initial and follow-up care if testing, evaluation, or postexposure prophylaxis are to be offered.

Guidance for assessing unsafe injection practices and other serious infection control breaches includes how to assess whether a breach warrants patient notification and a sample notification letters and other materials (10,11).

Step 10.4. Legal Concerns

HAIs outbreaks can result in litigation and have broad financial and public relations implications for affected facilities. This concern often increases the scrutiny and number of interested stakeholders in the investigation. Pressure might be applied not only to investigate rapidly, but also to implement necessary control strategies quickly. Additionally, public health records of HAIs outbreak responses frequently are the subject of Freedom of Information Act requests. Investigators should keep records of all steps taken, exercise care and discretion in how emails and other communications are used, and assume that any investigation records might become publicly available or used as part of litigation proceedings.

COMMON OUTBREAK SETTINGS AND RESPONSE

Wide variability exists across types of healthcare settings with regard to patient susceptibility to infection, infectious exposures, types of healthcare services provided, and pathogenic organisms likely to be present. Additionally, care locations can differ within the same facility. For example, acute care hospitals often have operating rooms, neonatal intensive care units, oncology wards, and burn units. Understanding these different settings when investigating HAIs outbreaks is crucial. Tables 18.4 and 18.5 summarize some of the common outbreak and exposure scenarios that result during epidemiologic consultations with health facility managers.

TABLE 18.4 Examples of cross-cutting outbreaks across multiple types of healthcare settings

Healthcare setting type	Exposure or risk factor	Examples of related outbreak and response scenarios
Any	Infected or colonized persons (healthcare personnel, patients, or visitors) Contaminated environmental surfaces	Contact-spread organisms (e.g., *Staphylococcus aureus*, drug-resistant gram-negative bacteria, *Clostridium difficile*, Group A S*treptococcus* infections, common respiratory viruses, or norovirus
	Airborne infectious agents	Measles or tuberculosis contact investigations; might require large-scale notification and laboratory testing of contacts
	Serious, high-risk infection transmission breaches, with or without known infectious agents	Patient notification, including considerations for bloodborne pathogen testing and prophylaxis
	Contaminated water sources (e.g., sinks, ice machines, whirlpool bathtubs and hydrotherapy locations), aqueous medication preparation areas, or any device that generates mist	Outbreaks of nontuberculosis mycobacterium skin and soft-tissue infections; *Legionella*; *Pseudomonas* species; *Acinetobacter* species; and other gram-negative bacteria
	Movement of patients across different healthcare facilities	Multifacility transmission of multidrug-resistant organisms across acute care, long-term care, dialysis, or outpatient settings
	Emerging pathogens with potential for human-to-human transmission	Initial patient presentation for new influenza viruses, severe acute respiratory syndrome, Middle East respiratory syndrome, or viral hemorrhagic fever
Any setting where injections are administered	Contamination of injectable medications or solutions at point of manufacture, compounding pharmacy, or healthcare facility level	Outbreaks of different environmental organisms (e.g., gram-negative bacteria or fungi); syndromes might reflect mechanism of transmission (e.g., bloodstream infections after administration of contaminated intravenous medications, abscesses, or infections localized at the injection site)
	Reuse of single-patient blood glucose monitoring devices on multiple patients	Outbreaks of bloodborne pathogens, especially hepatitis B or C virus, in long-term care settings
	Diversion of narcotic drugs by healthcare personnel	Outbreaks of bloodborne pathogens, especially hepatitis C virus

(continued)

TABLE 18.4 (Continued)

Healthcare setting type	Exposure or risk factor	Examples of related outbreak and response scenarios
Surgical and other invasive procedure settings (e.g., inpatient and outpatient surgical, podiatry, dental, ophthalmologic, plastic or cosmetic, or orthopedic centers)	Perioperative contamination of surgical wounds by healthcare personnel, the operative environment, or inadequately cleaned and sterilized instruments	Surgical site infections related to colonized healthcare workers (e.g., *S. aureus*, group A *Streptococcus, Pseudomonas aeruginosa*, nontuberculosis mycobacteria); contaminated devices (e.g., environmental bacteria or fungi), or other medical products (e.g., bandages or wound dressings); transmission of drug-resistant bacteria; adenovirus outbreaks in ophthalmology clinics and neonatal intensive care units; or nontuberculosis mycobacteria infections from contaminated heater–cooler units in open-chest surgeries
Endoscopy settings	Endoscope reprocessing errors or device design problems that prevent adequate cleaning and disinfection	Outbreaks of multidrug-resistant organisms associated with duodenoscopes; outbreaks of upper- and lower-respiratory tract infections associated with bronchoscopes; reported reprocessing errors and patient notification; pseudo-outbreaks of nontuberculosis mycobacteria

TABLE 18.5 Additional setting-specific outbreak and exposure scenarios

Healthcare setting type	Exposure or risk	Examples of related outbreak and response scenarios
Transplant units	Dust exposure or air-handling problems for severely immunocompromised patient populations (e.g., during building construction or renovation)	Invasive mold infections in bone-marrow transplant units
Long-term care facilities	Group residential setting and limited infection control infrastructure or patients with high comorbidities	Outbreaks of multidrug-resistant bacteria, transmission across long-term care and acute care settings, respiratory viruses (especially seasonal influenza), or norovirus
Hemodialysis clinics	Lapses in injection safety, maintenance of dialysis machines, or central-line and other vascular access care	Bloodborne pathogens, especially hepatitis C virus and bloodstream infections

TABLE 18.4 (Continued)

Healthcare setting type	Exposure or risk	Examples of related outbreak and response scenarios
Dental clinics	Biofilm formation in inadequately maintained dental unit waterlines Inadequate cleaning and sterilization of dental surgical instruments	Outbreaks of nontuberculosis mycobacteria infections among children after pulpotomy procedures; or bloodborne pathogen exposures
Laboratory	Specimen collection, handling, or culture-related activities Contamination of microbiological specimens during collection, handling, or culture	Unintentional laboratory staff and other healthcare personnel exposures to bloodborne pathogens through needlesticks and splashes to mucous membranes; culture of tularemia or brucellosis; pseudo-outbreaks resulting in inappropriate invasive diagnostic procedures, antibiotic prescriptions, or extended hospitalizations

CONCLUSION

This chapter provided an overview of outbreak investigations of infections across various healthcare settings that may include acute care hospitals, urgent care centers, rehabilitation centers, nursing homes and other long-term care facilities, and specialized outpatient services (e.g., hemodialysis, dentistry, podiatry, chemotherapy, endoscopy, and pain management clinics). Investigations of outbreaks in these settings require special attention in comparison with traditional community outbreaks. In particular, investigations in healthcare settings may include other patients, healthcare personnel, medical devices, environmental surfaces, and environmental reservoirs (e.g., surfaces, air, and water). Additionally, healthcare investigations often require case finding, detailed line lists, infection control assessments, environmental sampling, implementing control measures, and patient notification. The chapter also emphasized coordination with the facility staff and leadership, as well as local and state public health when conducting the investigation. Investigating an outbreak in a healthcare setting requires a step-by-step process from verifying the diagnosis to identifying cases to notifying patients.

REFERENCES

1. Siegel JD, Rhinehart E, Jackson M, Chiarello L; the Healthcare Infection Control Practices Advisory Committee. 2007 Guideline for isolation precautions: preventing transmission of infectious agents in healthcare settings. https://www.cdc.gov/infectioncontrol/pdf/guidelines/isolation-guidelines.pdf

2. Magill SS, Edwards JR, Bamberg W, et al. Multistate point-prevalence survey of healthcare–associated infections. *N Engl J Med.* 2014;370:1198–208.

3. CDC. Healthcare-associated infection (HAI) outbreak investigation toolkit. https://www.cdc.gov/hai/outbreaks/outbreaktoolkit.html

4. Blossom DB, Kallen AJ, Patel PR, Edward A, Robinson L. Outbreak of adverse reactions associated with contaminated heparin. *N Engl J Med.* 2008;359:2674–84.

5. CDC. Infection control assessment tools. https://www.cdc.gov/hai/prevent/infection-control-assessment-tools.html

6. CDC. Setting-specific guidelines. Guidelines library. https://www.cdc.gov/infectioncontrol/guidelines/index.html

7. CDC. *Interim Guidance for A Public Health Response to Contain Novel or Targeted Multidrug-Resistant Organisms (MDROs).* Atlanta: US Department of Health and Human Services, CDC; [undated]. p. 1–9. https://www.cdc.gov/hai/outbreaks/docs/Health-Response-Contain-MDRO.pdf

8. Institute of Medicine Forum on Microbial Threats. Summary and assessment. In: *Global Infectious Disease Surveillance and Detection: Assessing the Challenges—Finding Solutions, Workshop Summary.* Washington, DC: National Academies Press; 2007. http://www.ncbi.nlm.nih.gov/books/NBK52862

9. CDC. Patient notification toolkit. https://www.cdc.gov/injectionsafety/pntoolkit/index.html

10. Patel PR, Srinivasan A, Perz JF. Developing a broader approach to management of infection control breaches in healthcare settings. *Am J Infect Control.* 2008;36:685–90.

11. CDC. Outbreaks and patient notifications: resources for state health departments investigating healthcare-associated infection outbreaks and patient notifications. https://www.cdc.gov/hai/outbreaks/outbreak-resources.html

/// 19 /// COMMUNITY CONGREGATE SETTINGS

AMRA UZICANIN AND JOANNA GAINES

INTRODUCTION

Settings and patterns of human congregation are risk factors and determinants for infectious and other diseases in communities because they can modulate the scope and extent of spread through modes of exposure and transmission (e.g., person-to-person, airborne, foodborne, waterborne, and vectorborne). Except for households, which are the elemental unit of human congregation, among the most notable community settings associated with regular, nonrandom congregation are educational institutions and workplaces. Other community congregate settings include places where people gather occasionally or without a prevailing pattern in terms of time, place, or membership (e.g., entertainment and mass gathering venues, such as movie theaters and concert halls, or commercial venues, such as shopping malls). Some congregate settings accommodate larger groups of people with limited access to the surrounding community (e.g., jails, prisons, and other detention facilities).

Comprehensively enumerating all congregate settings and congregation behaviors that could become relevant in a field investigation is difficult; therefore, this chapter reviews field investigations in four types of congregate settings: (1) educational institutions, (2) workplaces, (3) mass gatherings, and (4) detention facilities. For investigations in each setting, practical and legal implications are discussed, followed by a summary of one or more illustrative investigations.

EDUCATIONAL INSTITUTIONS

Educational institutions are virtually ubiquitous and are the key settings where children and youth regularly congregate in large numbers. For example, 75.2 million students were enrolled in schools and colleges in the United States in 2014; of these, an estimated 55 million were elementary and secondary school students (pre-kindergarten through grade 8, and grades 9–12, respectively) (1). These institutions and facilities also employ many adults; for example, in 2014, almost 10 million teachers and other staff worked in educational institutions (1).

The intense social density that characterizes schools, combined with age-related biological, behavioral, and environmental factors, can facilitate infectious disease transmission within schools and lead to secondary spread into households and the wider community. School-based outbreaks have involved a multitude of infectious pathogens, and correlation between school opening dates and communitywide disease activity has been reported for influenza and other seasonally occurring respiratory infections (2–4). Educational institutions are therefore important venues for epidemiologic field investigations of disease outbreaks in communities and priority settings for encouraging appropriate disease prevention measures, such as vaccination, environmental hygiene, and healthy behaviors. Educational institutions also can be settings for implementing or evaluating some public health interventions (e.g., vaccination).

Implications for Field Investigations

- *Practical*:
  - School-based records can provide information useful for field investigations, and school nurses might be able to assist the public health team.

- Since some case-patients may seek care elsewhere rather than contact a school nurse, investigators may need to work simultaneously with the affected schools and the local healthcare providers to evaluate a school-based outbreak and obtain relevant case-based information.
- The fact that some school nurses serve on a part-time basis in multiple schools can pose a logistical challenge for collaboration with investigators.
- School-based investigations can interfere with routine educational activities and processes; accordingly, public health teams should strive to minimize that interference by coordinating thoroughly with education officials.
- *Legal*:
  - In addition to general legal requirements (see Chapter 13), public health staff preparing to conduct an investigation in schools should be aware of the privacy protection laws that apply in schools. The federal Family Educational Rights and Privacy Act protects the privacy of student education records (5), including school attendance records, which might be relevant in some investigations.
  - School nurses are particularly important for data collection that must adhere to requirements of both the Health Insurance Portability and Accountability Act of 1996 (6) and the Family Educational Rights and Privacy Act.
  - Because educational institutions employ staff, legal considerations pertinent for worksites might apply.

Illustrative Field Investigation

Because school-based outbreaks often herald wider disease spread, school-based investigation may yield critical early insights into wider community outbreaks and even major epidemics. In April 2009, an investigation of a febrile respiratory illness outbreak was initiated in a New York City high school comprising 2,686 students and 228 staff, days after Centers for Disease Control and Prevention (CDC) confirmation of an initial eight cases of human infection with a novel swine-origin influenza A(H1N1) virus, subsequently termed influenza A(H1N1)pdm09, in Texas and California. During April 22–24, a total of 222 students visited the school nursing office because of fever and respiratory symptoms and subsequently left school. Because of suspicion that the new influenza A virus might have caused the outbreak, public health officials visited the school on April 24 and collected nasopharyngeal swab samples from five newly symptomatic students identified by the school nurse and from an additional four students at a nearby physician's office. On April 26, CDC confirmed seven of these nine initial samples as the new influenza A(H1N1) virus. Nasopharyngeal swab collection kits were provided to local physicians' offices and emergency departments. During April 26–28, they collected an additional 42 samples, of which 37 (88%) subsequently tested positive for the new virus, bringing the total number of confirmed cases in this cluster to 44—approximately half of all US cases of this novel influenza A(H1N1) virus detected by April 28. Field investigators conducted telephone interviews with these 44 persons with laboratory-confirmed illness, which helped determine that the clinical presentation in this cluster (in a population known to be at low risk for severe disease from seasonal influenza) appeared to be similar to seasonal influenza (7). An enhanced surveillance for self-reported influenza-like illness (ILI) was subsequently launched, including two online surveys to all students and staff administered on April 26 and May 2, which identified that approximately 800 students and staff (35% of student respondents and 10% of employee respondents) had ILI during that period. A link with travel to Mexico, where the new virus was known to be circulating widely, was established for five students with ILI and symptom onset during April 20–23; one of these students also had laboratory-confirmed infection. The data on laboratory-confirmed cases collected through this school-based investigation helped describe the natural history of the 2009 outbreak of a novel influenza A(H1N1) in New York City (8). The new virus subsequently spread throughout the United States and worldwide, causing the first influenza pandemic of the twenty-first century.

During the response to the 2009 influenza A(H1N1) pandemic in the United States, school-aged children were designated as one of the priority groups for the monovalent pandemic vaccine. An estimated 85% of local health departments held school-located vaccination clinics starting in October 2009. Approximately one-third of all US children aged 5–17 years who received pandemic vaccine were vaccinated at school (9). School-based field evaluations undertaken in 2010 in Maine by public health officials in close collaboration with schools, most notably with school nurses, helped to document that the vaccine was effective in preventing laboratory-confirmed pandemic influenza and in reducing student and teacher absenteeism (10,11).

WORKPLACES

In 2015, of 81.4 million families in the United States, 80% had at least one employed member (12). Places of employment range from small family-owned businesses with few or no employees to large companies with tens of thousands of employees in offices, production plants, or other facilities. Availability of workplace-based employee services also varies and can include employee cafeterias, occupational health clinics, and other on-site health and wellness facilities. Epidemiologic field investigations in workplaces most frequently involve occupational disease and injury issues (see Chapter 21). However, workplaces may be associated with occurrence of nonoccupational diseases, most notably infectious disease outbreaks that prompt field investigations. Initial case-patients in workplace-associated infectious disease outbreaks frequently are identified by the local healthcare facilities where employed adults receive primary care or by emergency departments. Information about the place of employment obtained from adult patients with an infectious disease is the key piece of the puzzle in identifying and investigating workplace-related outbreaks.

Implications for Field Investigations

- *Practical*:
  - Preparatory steps include gathering information about the workplace setting of the investigation and identifying opportunities for collaboration with an on-site occupational health team (if available), as well as with local healthcare providers and facilities where affected employees might have sought care.
  - Because epidemiologic investigations in a workplace can interfere with, or even interrupt, business processes, coordination with the workplace leadership can help avert or minimize disruption and ensure compliance with business-specific rules and regulations.
  - At the onset of workplace-based investigations, field teams should determine which business records might aid the investigation and what additional information should be collected about worksites, employees, and/or clients. In addition, on-site occupational health clinics might be able to assist with conducting field investigations and implementing outbreak responses.
- *Legal*: In addition to legal requirements (see Chapter 13), field investigators should be aware of rules and regulations that apply to investigations in a workplace setting (see Chapter 21).

Illustrative Field Investigations

Although workplaces are not commonly thought of as venues for spread of infectious diseases that are prevented through routine childhood vaccination, under some circumstances clusters of vaccine-preventable disease can occur among adults in work settings and spread into surrounding communities. In 1999, a 29-year-old man sought treatment in three healthcare facilities for what he thought was a sexually transmitted disease. At his third visit, he was noted to have a maculopapular rash, low-grade fever, and lymphadenopathy, and he subsequently tested IgM positive for rubella. He was employed at a meat-packing plant in a county that had no cases of rubella reported for the previous 9 years and had high rubella vaccination rates among children. In the following 2 months, 83 confirmed rubella cases occurred in the county, all among unvaccinated persons. Of those cases, 52 (63%) were in meat-packing plant employees or their household contacts, mainly foreign-born Hispanic men from countries without childhood rubella vaccination at the time they were born. The meat-packing plant had an attack rate of 14.4/1,000 persons, compared with the countywide attack rate of 0.19/1,000 persons. Field investigation documented that vaccine failure was not associated with this outbreak originating in a workplace but rather lack of rubella vaccination among some of the employees. Crowded working and living conditions further facilitated rubella transmission. During outbreak response, vaccination campaigns targeted seven meat-packing plants with 3,000 workers (13). In this example, the workplace was the setting where many unprotected (unvaccinated) adults congregated and acquired rubella infection after the virus was introduced in that setting despite little rubella circulation in the surrounding community. The workplace component of this field investigation helped elucidate the actual risk factors associated with this outbreak.

The built environment of community congregate settings, including workplaces, may be an important determinant for disease exposure. After reports of illness of unknown etiology among several military base employees, Legionnaires' disease (LD) was confirmed in two persons. An epidemiologic field investigation identified 67 cases of *Legionella*-related disease, including LD and Pontiac fever. Cases clustered on the base's eastern office complex. Subsequently, *Legionella* colonies grew from environmental samples collected from two cooling towers serving the eastern office complex; isolates from one of two towers matched the same species and serogroup as clinical isolates. A retrospective cohort indicated that the risk for *Legionella* infection was associated with occupancy in the building closest to that cooling tower (14). This example illustrates how understanding a workplace layout and distribution of cases can help epidemiologists develop and test a hypothesis during a field investigation in workplaces and other settings.

MASS GATHERINGS

Mass gatherings range in size and purpose; no minimum number of people constitutes a "mass gathering." The World Health Organization defines a mass gathering as any event during which people gather at a specific place for a set time in sufficient numbers to strain the resources or infrastructure (including healthcare) of the host community or country

(15). Medical and public health efforts in advance of mass gatherings focus primarily on preparedness and response. Risk assessment is a critical component in planning for mass gatherings and should follow an iterative process in which feedback informs the focus of public health surveillance and response efforts (15).

Implications for Field Investigations

- *Practical*:
  - The multiplicity of factors associated with different mass gatherings (e.g., location, number of venues, number and mobility of participants, length of planning time, indoor or outdoor setting, weather and seasonal considerations, number of government jurisdictions) directly influence public health preparations and potential epidemiologic field investigations.
  - Potential partners for public health surveillance and response include traditional public health systems (e.g., health departments, hospitals) and agencies and event-specific entities (e.g., Olympic organizing committees).
  - The public health risks associated with a mass gathering include environmental health issues, infectious diseases, and other domains (16,17).
  - Because existing public health surveillance systems sometimes are of limited value for timely detection of outbreaks associated with mass gatherings, retrospective surveys often are needed to complete epidemiologic field investigations involving mass gathering attendees. For that reason, enhancement of existing surveillance systems to ensure timeliness and accuracy might be required for some mass gatherings (18,19). These enhanced systems typically increase the speed of reporting of existing surveillance systems (20).
- *Legal*: Multiple government and administrative levels (e.g., local, state, federal, multinational) might have jurisdiction in mass gatherings, and their response roles will depend on such factors as their capacities and legal authorities.

Illustrative Field Investigation

Surveillance systems using preestablished criteria can expedite the speed of outbreak detection and response. A syndromic surveillance system was used in 2005 for a camping event in Virginia attended by approximately 43,000 youths and adults. Public health personnel screened arriving attendees for symptoms such as vomiting, diarrhea, rash, fever, pinkeye or red eyes, and cough. If any group of arriving attendees (e.g., a bus) had three or more persons with symptoms associated with communicable disease during the previous 48 hours, the entire group was referred for additional screening. Public health personnel also established a syndromic surveillance system to quickly identify communicable disease outbreaks. These screening processes rapidly identified four clusters of gastrointestinal illness, and symptomatic persons were restricted from handling food for the remainder of their time in camp. Screening on the hottest day of the event identified a surge in heat-related illnesses, leading to rescheduling of an event and provision of additional shade structures, cooling stations, and water sources. These efforts to mitigate heat-related illnesses resulted in one of the lowest rates of heat-related exhaustion and heatstroke during the entire 10-day event (21). These rapid public health responses demonstrate the value of syndromic surveillance at a mass gathering event. Health risks were quickly and effectively identified through judicious planning and use of resources, and steps were taken to reduce the risk to other attendees.

DETENTION FACILITIES

Disease surveillance and outbreak response in detention facilities require collaboration and coordination between public health agencies and the criminal justice system, sometimes at multiple jurisdictional levels. Prisons, jails, and other detention facilities involve tight regulation of populations, with special protections to ensure the population's vulnerability is not exploited. The US Department of Health and Human Services defines a prisoner as "any individual involuntarily confined or detained in a penal institution"—such persons include those detained pending arraignment, trial, or sentencing (22). Oversight of prisoners depends on jurisdiction of incarceration. For example, at the federal level, the federal Bureau of Prisons operates federal facilities; provides essential medical, dental, and psychiatric services; and monitors for infectious disease outbreaks (23). State and local detention facilities—including prisons and jails—usually are operated at respective levels of jurisdiction.

Implications for Field Investigations

- *Practical*:
  - Health officials have limited access to prisoners. They might be able to speak with prisoners only within sight of guards. Prisoners might be distrustful and unwilling to disclose possible exposures, particularly if an exposure was related to a prohibited activity (e.g., brewing alcohol) (24,25).

- Field investigators may be able to closely track points of contact for prisoners because of their controlled movements; however, many prisons have large populations and therefore many opportunities for contact among prisoners.

- In some detention settings, limitations in access to medical records for prisoners and workers also can complicate outbreak detection and response.

- Workers in detention facilities can share exposures with prisoners (e.g., environmental conditions or person-to-person contact), adding an additional layer of complexity to the response as the two populations are treated differently within detention facility systems.

- Investigations in these settings require collaboration between criminal justice authorities and public health officials, sharing resources and information when appropriate to identify and mitigate public health threats (26).

- *Legal*:
  - Public health practitioners need to be aware of the unique regulations for prison populations and ensure that their efforts comply with applicable rules and laws.

  - Specific regulations provide additional protections to prisoners involved as subjects in Department of Health and Human Services–conducted or – supported research (27). These regulations also apply if a person becomes a prisoner during the course of an investigation (27).

  - Law enforcement officials also should be consulted to ensure prisoners are adequately protected.

Illustrative Field Investigation

Public health investigations in prison populations pose unique challenges and require close collaboration between public health entities and the criminal justice systems. For example, consumption of prison-made alcohol, known as *pruno*, was related to multiple outbreaks of botulism among prison inmates during 2011 and 2012 (24,25). Botulism, a potentially life-threatening illness, is caused by a toxin produced by the bacterium *Clostridium botulinum*. In previous outbreaks, prisoners have been hospitalized and intubated (25). Pruno is made primarily from fruit, sugar, and water; root vegetables sometimes are added. An investigation of a cluster of eight prisoners sickened in Utah found that they had added to their pruno a baked potato saved from a meal, which was the likely source of the *C. botulinum* (24). Partnership with law enforcement officials and prison authorities enabled epidemiologists to understand patient connections and identify possible exposures.

CONCLUSION

The systematic approach to conducting an epidemiologic field investigation (see Chapter 3) applies to epidemiologic investigations of congregate settings. However, investigations involving congregate settings also can face unique challenges, such as the potential for interference with normal business processes, limits on data availability and access, and additional legal and confidentiality requirements. Field investigations of congregate settings can be aided by the following:

- Online information can help investigators learn about community and congregate settings affected by the public health issue under investigation.
- Initial meetings with local public health officials can verify and supplement information found online and facilitate contact with key persons responsible for congregate settings of interest.
- Understanding setting-specific legal and practical implications is important at the onset of investigations of congregate settings.
- Depending on the situation, field investigators might need to research and document the characteristics of the congregate settings, including physical layout, environmental aspects (e.g., air, water, sanitation), on-site ancillary services (e.g., food and healthcare), relevant schedules, and attendance and/or absenteeism.
- A field investigation in a congregate setting must take into consideration behaviors and other potentially relevant factors for disease exposure or transmission within that setting and community.
- Close coordination and collaboration with officials responsible for the congregate setting during all investigation stages—from planning to completion—are critical to ensure the investigation's efficiency and minimizing disruptions of the gathering.

REFERENCES

1. National Center for Education Statistics. Digest of education statistics: 2014. https://nces.ed.gov/programs/digest/d14/index.asp
2. Heymann A, Chodick G, Reichman B, Kokia E, Laufer J. Influence of school closure on the incidence of viral respiratory diseases among children and on healthcare utilization. *Pediatr Infect Dis J.* 2004;23:675–7.
3. Wheeler CC, Erhart LM, Jehn ML. Effect of school closure on the incidence of influenza among school-age children in Arizona. *Public Health Rep.* 2010;125:851–9.

4. Chao DL, Halloran ME, Longini IM Jr. School opening dates predict pandemic influenza A(H1N1) outbreaks in the United States. *J Infect Dis*. 2010;202:877–80.

5. US Department of Education. Laws & guidance/General: Family Educational Rights and Privacy Act (FERPA). 2015. http://www2.ed.gov/policy/gen/guid/fpco/ferpa/index.html

6. Health Insurance Portability and Accountability Act of 1996, Pub. L No 104–91, 110 Stat. 1936 (1996).

7. CDC. Swine-origin influenza A (H1N1) virus infections in a school—New York City, April 2009. *MMWR*. 2009;58:470–2.

8. Lessler J, Reich NG, Cummings DA, et al. Outbreak of 2009 pandemic influenza A (H1N1) at a New York City school. *N Engl J Med*. 2009;361:2628–36.

9. Vogt TM, Wortley PM. Epilogue: school-located influenza vaccination during the 2009–2010 pandemic and beyond. *Pediatrics*. 2012;129 Suppl 2:S107–9.

10. Uzicanin A, Thompson M, Smith P, et al. Effectiveness of 1 dose of influenza A (H1N1) 2009 monovalent vaccines in preventing reverse-transcription polymerase chain reaction–confirmed H1N1 infection among school-aged children in Maine. *J Infect Dis*. 2012;206:1059–68.

11. Graitcer SB, Dube NL, Basurto-Davila R, et al. Effects of immunizing school children with 2009 influenza A (H1N1) monovalent vaccine on absenteeism among students and teachers in Maine. *Vaccine*. 2012;30:4835–41.

12. US Department of Labor. Employment characteristics of families—2015. https://www.bls.gov/news.release/archives/famee_04222016.pdf

13. Danovaro-Holliday MC, LeBaron CW, Allensworth C, et al. A large rubella outbreak with spread from the workplace to the community. *JAMA*. 2000;284:2733–9.

14. Ambrose J, Hampton LM, Fleming-Dutra KE, et al. Large outbreak of Legionnaires' disease and Pontiac fever at a military base. *Epidemiol Infect*. 2014;142:2336–46.

15. World Health Organization. *Public Health for Mass Gatherings: Key Considerations*. Geneva: World Health Organization; 2015.

16. Milsten AM, Maguire BJ, Bissell RA, Seaman KG. Mass-gathering medical care: a review of the literature. *Prehosp Disaster Med*. 2002;17:151–62.

17. Arbon P. Mass-gathering medicine: a review of the evidence and future directions for research. *Prehosp Disaster Med*. 2007;22:131–5.

18. Memish ZA, Zumla A, McCloskey B, et al. Mass gatherings medicine: international cooperation and progress. *Lancet*. 2014;383:2030–2.

19. Fleischauer AT, Gaines J. Enhancing surveillance for mass gatherings: the role of syndromic surveillance. *Public Health Rep*. 2017;132(1_suppl):95S–8S.

20. Schenkel K, Williams C, Eckmanns T, et al. Enhanced surveillance of infectious diseases: the 2006 FIFA World Cup experience, Germany. *Euro Surveill*. 2006;11:234–8.

21. CDC. Surveillance for early detection of disease outbreaks at an outdoor mass gathering—Virginia, 2005. *MMWR*. 2006;55:71–4.

22. US Department of Health and Human Services. Prisoner involvement in research. 2003. https://www.hhs.gov/ohrp/regulations-and-policy/guidance/prisoner-research-ohrp-guidance-2003/

23. Federal Bureau of Prisons. https://www.bop.gov/

24. CDC. Botulism from drinking prison-made illicit alcohol—Utah 2011. *MMWR*. 2012;61:782–4.

25. CDC. Notes from the field: botulism from drinking prison-made illicit alcohol—Arizona, 2012. *MMWR*. 2013;62:88.

26. CDC. Influenza outbreaks at two correctional facilities—Maine, March 2011. *MMWR*. 2012;61:229–32.

27. Protection of Human Subjects, 45 CFR 46 (2009).

/// 20 /// EXPOSURES AND CONDITIONS OF ACUTE ENVIRONMENTAL ORIGIN

SHARON M. WATKINS AND JERRY FAGLIANO

CHARACTERISTICS OF ENVIRONMENTAL HEALTH FIELD INVESTIGATIONS

Field investigators face special challenges when confronted with exposures or disease clusters that might be related to contaminants or environmental factors. Challenges can include accurately assessing human exposure and determining a case definition and linking exposure to adverse health effects. Communication with potentially affected populations about risk and about actions to reduce risk is particularly challenging in environmental field investigations (1).

The scope of this chapter is limited to the investigation of short-term exposures and resultant acute diseases or symptom clusters of environmental origin. Early, important examples of such investigations include the mass methylmercury poisoning of the population around Minamata Bay in Japan (2) and exposure to dioxins after an industrial accident in Seveso, Italy (3). In acute events, exposures are likely to be high and episodic, and the adverse health outcome might be detectable or measurable immediately or within days or weeks. Guidance documents for the public health investigation of clusters of disease of long latency are available for suspected clusters of cancer or birth defects but will not be discussed here (4,5). Similar to these guidance documents, this chapter emphasizes a stepwise approach to investigation and transparent communication with potentially affected communities at all stages.

For this chapter, the "environment" includes contaminants that could cause an adverse health outcome in air, water, soil, food, or consumer products. Exposure factors can be physical (e.g., radiation or extreme weather) biological, or chemical. Chemical factors can be synthetic (e.g., organophosphates) or naturally occurring (e.g., arsenic and biological toxins).

The trigger for an environmental field investigation might be the *unusually increased occurrence of acute symptoms or characteristic set of symptoms (syndromes) in a population*, which is suspected to be causally related to some environmental factor. Community members, alert clinicians, or a disease surveillance system might bring these symptoms to the attention of health investigators. Syndromic surveillance systems can be particularly useful and are commonly used to detect syndrome increases for public health action. The data sources for syndromic surveillance vary by jurisdiction but might include monitoring data from hospital emergency departments, poison control centers, over-the-counter drug sales records, or other sources (6). The field investigator will have the following objectives, which are in common with most epidemiologic investigations:

- Developing a working case definition.
- Identifying who has become ill.
- Defining the disease or symptom cluster in space and time.
- Identifying the likely causal agent of the adverse health outcomes.
- Recommending or taking actions to prevent further exposure and prevent additional cases of disease.
- Considering conducting an environmental assessment, where appropriate.

However, the trigger for an environmental field investigation also might be *exposure* or *suspicion of exposure to an environmental agent*, rather than knowledge that a cluster of symptoms or disease already has occurred. Exposure itself might be sufficient grounds to initiate immediate public health interventions, for example, when a release of a highly toxic chemical has occurred (Box 20.1). Like disease clusters, exposures also might come

BOX 20.1
BIOLOGICAL MONITORING OF CHILDREN EXPOSED
TO MERCURY AT A DAYCARE CENTER

PUBLIC HEALTH PROBLEM

Children and staff of a daycare center in New Jersey were exposed for many months to elevated levels of elemental mercury in indoor air. The building was previously used for thermometer manufacturing and had been vacant before its inappropriate conversion to use as a daycare facility. State environmental officials notified health officials of elevated mercury vapor concentrations in rooms occupied by children and staff.

PUBLIC HEALTH RESPONSE

Daycare operations were halted immediately on the advice of state health officials. Inspectors found liquid mercury in the structure. Within days, state and federal health investigators obtained specimens from 72 children and 9 staff for measurement of mercury in urine by the laboratory at the National Center for Environmental Health, Centers for Disease Control and Prevention. Urine mercury concentrations well above the background range demonstrated exposure to mercury. Health investigators conducted serial urine testing for mercury among exposed children and adults for several months, until all urine mercury levels had decreased to background. Reduction in body burden was consistent with the known half-life of elemental mercury.

TAKE-HOME POINTS

Immediate actions are warranted to stop exposure to a known toxicant. Biological monitoring can be an important tool to assess exposure and to track the reduction in body burden once interventions to stop exposure have been implemented.

_____

Source: Reference 7.

to the attention of health investigators from community members or alert clinicians or through partners (e.g., environmental protection agencies or poison information centers), environmental monitoring systems, or emergency response personnel. In these circumstances, the field investigator might have one or more of the following objectives:

- Identifying the likely environmental causes of the adverse health outcomes.
- Confirming and (if possible) quantifying the magnitude of exposure and route of exposure, taking into account processes that may have changed the intensity of exposure such as dispersion or dilution.
- Defining the potentially exposed population.

- Determining whether exposure is sufficient to result in adverse health effects (includes assessment of inherent toxicity of the exposure, suspected dose, and pathway and duration of exposure).
- Determining whether exposure has in fact resulted in symptoms or disease in the exposed population, if sufficient time has elapsed for occurrence.
- Recommending or taking actions to prevent further exposure and prevent additional cases of disease.

Environmental health investigations usually require assembly of multidisciplinary teams whose makeup will depend on the exposure and health concern. Understanding exposure might require expertise in chemistry and the environmental or biological fate of the contaminant, and likely transport of contaminants in various environmental media (air, water, or soil), or methods of exposure measurement or modeling. Understanding the potential for health impacts requires expertise in toxicology, epidemiology, and environmental or occupational medicine.

Investigation teams also need staff trained in risk communication and community or media relations to gather and disseminate health information during and after acute exposure events. These skills are especially important because environmental health field investigations often are conducted while communities experience fear, uncertainty, mistrust, and anger, and during intense media attention.

Environmental health field investigations should follow a stepwise approach. Some steps should be performed simultaneously because of the acute nature of some situations; some investigations might not entail all steps.

COLLECTING PRELIMINARY EXPOSURE AND DISEASE INFORMATION

Regardless of the initial trigger, capture as much information as possible from the initial alerting source (community member, clinician, the media, emergency responders, or surveillance and monitoring systems). Gather information from several corroborating sources, including reports of responses to previous, similar events, for more reliable situational awareness. The sources will be dictated by the specific circumstances but might include local, state, and federal environmental regulatory authorities, health agency surveillance programs, emergency response on-scene coordinators, hazardous materials units, local hospital emergency departments, and poison control centers. Early in the response, keep an open mind about the possible nature, magnitude, and source of exposure. Exposures can occur from an unexpected source, such as a misapplied pesticide or imported product (Box 20.2).

BOX 20.2
METHYL BROMIDE POISONING FROM PESTICIDE MISAPPLICATION

PUBLIC HEALTH PROBLEM

A family of four vacationing at a resort was hospitalized with severe neurologic symptoms (including muscle weakness, twitching, and sensory alteration), vomiting, and diarrhea. Three required mechanical ventilation.

PUBLIC HEALTH RESPONSE

Food contamination by pesticides or biological toxins was suspected but ruled out. Investigation revealed that the condominium unit below the family's had been fumigated with methyl bromide 2 days before the family became ill. No one other than the family occupied the fumigated building. Symptoms were consistent with exposure to methyl bromide. Methyl bromide was detected in the indoor air of the occupied and fumigated units several days after fumigation and remained high enough to cause acute illness. Based on fumigation records, investigators discovered previous incidents of methyl bromide–related poisoning. The US Environmental Protection Agency did not permit methyl bromide to be used as a residential fumigant.

TAKE-HOME POINT

When looking for possible causative exposures, investigators must be aware of the potential for misapplication or misuse of pesticides or other products. In addition, investigators should be aware that poisonings have occurred from substances banned in the United States that might be in imported products.

Source: Reference 8.

When reports of symptoms or disease are the trigger, gather information about the number and ages (and other relevant demographic factors) of persons reporting disease or symptoms, dates and times of symptom onset or disease diagnosis, the nature and severity of illnesses, whether ill persons have sought medical attention or care, and locations or settings where persons became ill. Gather duration of symptoms and timing of onset for each symptom because this progression could be a key to contaminant identity.

Initial exposure information might include eyewitness reports of visible plumes of gases or particulates, accounts of unusual odors or tastes, and discoloration of soils or water. Emergency responders might have collected data using portable air monitors indicating nonspecific contamination of air or gathered samples from surfaces or other contaminated media. Such information can be useful to reconstruct exposure patterns retrospectively. As early as possible during the investigation, document specific measurements of chemical contaminants in environmental media.

Initial impressions of the magnitude of an event might be based on incomplete information and appear minimal; further investigation, including review of all relevant surveillance and monitoring data, might reveal a wider impact. As early as possible, consider protective interventions and mitigation actions, even when information about exposure and illness is preliminary. Early mitigation to contain exposure can be important given that some environmental exposures have delayed effects, concern might exist about additional exposures, or the population at risk has not yet been fully described (e.g., with potential product tampering or contamination). Examples of mitigation actions include elimination of a point source, evacuation, sheltering in place, and engineering controls. Appropriate interventions also can build or maintain public confidence and trust.

DEVELOPING A RISK COMMUNICATION PLAN

In the age of widespread use of social media, frequent class action litigation, and sensationalized movie portrayals of environmental contaminant impacts, there is renewed emphasis on effective public health risk communication on environmental issues. In any field investigation, developing and implementing a risk communication strategy as early as possible is essential, emphasizing transparency, good listening skills, and assurance that public health investigators are actively looking into an issue (9). The risk communication plan is critical to build trust and support that investigation findings will be credible and accepted by affected communities. Situations that trigger formation of an incident management structure will require coordination of communication with a joint information center. An effective risk communication approach during an environmental investigation will adhere to the following principles (10):

- Accept and involve the public as a legitimate partner. Community members may have critical insights about local environmental exposure issues.
- Listen to the community's specific concerns. Find out what people are thinking and what they want to know.
- Be honest, frank, and open. As soon as possible, disclose what is and is not yet known about environmental risks.
- Coordinate and collaborate with other credible sources. Involve independent communication partners (e.g., community physician) whom the community might already trust.

- Meet the needs of the media. Be accessible to reporters and prepared with concise messages.
- Speak clearly and with compassion. Avoid technical jargon, acknowledge and respond to emotions expressed, and emphasize actions under way to reduce risk.

As part of risk communication planning and preparation, develop specific objectives for particular stakeholder audiences. Whenever possible, be prepared with pretested risk messages that are adaptable to emergent situations.

Fear and outrage are magnified when exposure to contaminants is imposed and outside of individual control and when a community's expectation of safe air, water, food, or consumer products is violated (Box 20.3). Stressful events reduce the ability of community members to process and assimilate information, so state the most important public health messages first and repeat them frequently.

ASSEMBLING A MULTIDISCIPLINARY INVESTIGATION TEAM

To the degree possible, assemble an internal team with skills in epidemiology and environmental exposure assessment that address the specific situation. From the outset, include a risk communication or media relations specialist on the team. Team members also could include representatives of local or state health and environmental agencies and emergency response units. Try to establish partnerships with, and obtain assistance from, federal health and environmental resources.

As early in the investigation as possible, assemble independent or outside subject matter experts whose assistance might be needed. This team could include environmental and laboratory-based scientists, industrial hygienists, physicians or other clinicians trained in occupational or environmental medicine, toxicologists, and poison control directors. Some incidents may require coordination with law enforcement.

DEVELOPING CASE DEFINITIONS AND CONFIRMING DIAGNOSES

Use preliminary information about the nature of symptoms and illnesses to establish a working case definition for further analysis of the situation. The case definition can be tightened, expanded, or otherwise modified as information emerges, but it should include symptoms or sets of symptoms, the period of onset, and geographically relevant information. If an environmental exposure is known or suspected, the case definition should take into account what is known about the toxic effects or biological responses after exposure, taking latency, exposure pathway, and suspected dose into consideration.

BOX 20.3

EXPOSURE TO LEAD IN DRINKING WATER AMONG CHILDREN, FLINT, MICHIGAN

PUBLIC HEALTH PROBLEM

In April 2014, the city of Flint, Michigan, switched its drinking water source as a cost-saving measure. The new source, however, was not treated appropriately to reduce corrosivity. Consequently, residents—including children—were exposed for many months to lead and other corrosion products leaching from plumbing and service lines.

PUBLIC HEALTH RESPONSE

Government officials were slow to recognize the developing problem and to respond to concerns expressed by residents about the quality of drinking water, triggering anger and fear for children's well-being. Independent researchers working with community members demonstrated that lead concentrations at drinking water taps were elevated throughout the city and that the proportion of elevated blood lead measurements among Flint children increased after the water source switch. Community outrage forced the city to switch back to the original water source in October 2015, though corrosion-related damage to the water infrastructure may be long-lasting. Officials began providing residents with bottled water and point-of-use filters and agreed to replace lead service lines and other damaged water system infrastructure. Subsequent analyses of Flint children's blood lead levels have confirmed that the proportion of children with elevated blood lead returned to pre-switch levels once the original water source was restored and other exposure reduction actions had been implemented.

TAKE-HOME POINTS

It is essential to listen and respond appropriately and early to community concerns. Public trust may be irretrievable once lost. Environmental and biological monitoring information can be useful to understand exposure and spur timely preventive or corrective actions.

Source: References 11–13.

Interview each person whose illness meets a working case definition. In an investigation driven by exposure information, consider interviewing persons with suspected exposure to gather information about symptoms or illnesses, including those possibly related to the exposure of concern (Box 20.4). To facilitate data collection, develop or refine a case interview and abstraction form that addresses demographics, symptoms,

BOX 20.4

VINYL CHLORIDE EXPOSURE AND ACUTE SYMPTOMS AFTER A TRAIN DERAILMENT

PUBLIC HEALTH PROBLEM

A freight train carrying dozens of chemical tank cars derailed on a railroad bridge at dawn. One car ruptured, releasing 24,000 gallons of vinyl chloride into the air. Within minutes, a cloud of vinyl chloride vapors moved through the adjacent diverse community in New Jersey. Although air measurements of vinyl chloride were not taken until several hours after the vinyl chloride gas plume was released, dispersion models indicated that air concentrations probably were high enough to produce acute illness nearly a mile from the derailment site.

PUBLIC HEALTH RESPONSE

Emergency responders issued recommendations to shelter in place. Late in the day, nearby residents were evacuated. After the scene was stabilized days later and residents were able to return to their homes, state and federal health officials conducted surveys of residents and emergency responders to determine the frequency of symptoms. More than half of the town's residents experienced symptoms; those living closer to the derailment site were more likely than those living farther away to report symptoms. The most commonly reported symptoms were headache; irritation of the eyes, nose, and throat; cough and difficulty breathing; dizziness; and nausea. Although nonspecific, these symptoms were consistent with the acute effects of exposure to vinyl chloride. Medical records review found that more than 250 residents and emergency responders sought medical care at hospital emergency departments.

TAKE-HOME POINT

Even nonspecific symptoms can be used in a case definition when other discrete details can define time and place for exposure. Combining symptoms, time, and place in a case definition enables estimation of the number exposed and symptomatic persons after a discrete exposure event.

Source: References 14–16.

symptom onset, risk factors, possible exposures, and medical system encounters in relation to time and place. When useful as part of a case definition, consider collecting and analyzing biological specimens for appropriate measures.

When considering the collection and use of health records, know the jurisdictional authority for collecting and inspecting these records and any limits placed on this authority by law or regulation. This understanding is particularly important in regard to conditions not specifically reportable in the state. Many states require reporting of specific noninfectious diseases to public health authorities. Additionally, most states have laws and regulations that require reporting of unusual clustering of disease or unusual health events to public health authorities.

CHARACTERIZING EXPOSURE: WHO HAS BEEN EXPOSED AND TO HOW MUCH

Regardless of whether an apparent increase in disease or an exposure event triggers an investigation, accurate assessment and quantification of the population's exposure to an environmental agent is critical. However, exposure assessment can be difficult or impossible in many circumstances. For example, chemical releases during disaster incidents can occur quickly and disperse before sampling or monitoring equipment can be brought to the scene. In some situations, no scientifically reliable or validated environmental or biological monitoring measure (for example, of a chemical in air, water, blood, or urine) may be available, making characterization of the exposure even more difficult.

When applicable, case definitions should include clinical measurements of human exposure, particularly for situations involving exposure to chemicals with relatively clear relationships between exposure level and clinical outcome, such as for certain pesticides, metals (lead, mercury), or carbon monoxide (17,18). For example:

- Exposure to organophosphate pesticides can be defined on the basis of changes in cholinesterase values.
- Evidence of unusual mercury exposure might include a clinical measurement of urine mercury.
- Carbon monoxide poisoning definition might include assessment of the carboxyhemoglobin value.

Biomonitoring or chemical measurements in people can also help determine that exposure has not resulted in widespread contamination (19,20). Biological measurements of chemicals or metabolites must be understood in the context of the chemical's pharmacokinetics, which dictates the timing of specimen collection and the biological medium to be sampled (for example, blood, urine, exhaled breath, or hair). For chemicals with short half-lives, specimens might need to be collected and measurements made within hours of exposure to be interpretable as an exposure metric. For some chemicals, clinical laboratory measurements might not be relevant because an analytical method is unavailable or testing could not be done in a time period relevant to the assessment of exposure.

The National Center for Environmental Health of the Centers for Disease Control and Prevention has established national reference values for many environmental chemicals (21). These values can be used as cutoff concentrations in a case definition or as comparison for population exposure results in community surveys that use biological monitoring.

COMPLETING CASE ASCERTAINMENT

Once a case definition is established, attempt to ascertain all possible cases by using all relevant sources of data. These data sources might include syndromic surveillance systems (Box 20.5), other potentially relevant surveillance data systems that collect laboratory findings, emergency department medical records and poison control center information

---

BOX 20.5
EYE INJURIES SUSTAINED AT A FOAM PARTY

PUBLIC HEALTH PROBLEM

Attendees of a nightclub foam party were exposed to sprayed foam (concentrated sodium lauryl sulfate). Partygoers sustained serious eye injuries that required emergency medical treatment.

PUBLIC HEALTH RESPONSE

Calls from local officials and law enforcement alerted public health professionals that dozens of persons had sought emergency department (ED) care for severe eye pain after attending a party the previous evening. Syndromic surveillance was used to identify persons who had sought ED care with a chief complaint of eye injury.

The case definition was an eye injury in a person who had attended the party and who was symptomatic within a 24-hour window. ED records were reviewed and abstracted, and neighboring ophthalmology clinics, urgent care centers, and hospitals were contacted. Patients were interviewed using an event-specific questionnaire. Social media was used to reach out-of-area partygoers. This outreach provided an additional 26 cases; a total of 56 cases were identified of an estimated 350 partygoers. Eye injuries were moderate to severe; corneal abrasions occurred in half of all cases diagnosed.

TAKE-HOME POINTS

Use of syndromic surveillance to identify increases in symptoms is a useful component in environmental investigations. Additional follow-up with all sources of data, including social media, can result in a more complete case ascertainment.

Source: Reference 22.

BOX 20.6
OUTBREAK OF PESTICIDE POISONING FROM CONTAMINATED WATERMELONS

PUBLIC HEALTH PROBLEM

During the summer of 1985, state health departments in three states received reports by alert clinicians of illness suggestive of pesticide poisoning. Symptoms were gastrointestinal (nausea, vomiting, and diarrhea), neurologic (blurred vision, salivation), and muscular (weakness, twitching) consistent with exposure to organophosphate or carbamate insecticides.

PUBLIC HEALTH RESPONSE

Watermelons were suspected on the basis of food consumption information from initial case-patients. Officials issued advisories to avoid eating watermelons, which were subsequently embargoed. Health investigators developed a case definition based on symptoms and contacted poison control centers and emergency departments to conduct thorough case ascertainment. Approximately 1,000 cases of pesticide poisoning, some severe, were ultimately reported. Tests on watermelons indicated contamination with aldicarb, an acutely toxic carbamate insecticide not registered for use on this crop. Unfortunately, watermelons could not be traced to a specific source.

TAKE-HOME POINT

Public health notifications of an exposure event often rely on alert clinicians. Cooperation of local health departments and laboratories, poison information control, emergency departments, and others is important, particularly given the widespread nature of food contamination.

Source: Reference 23,24.

(Box 20.6), inpatient hospitalization records, and self-reports or interview responses. When most of the instances of exposure have occurred at an event or exposure is widely dispersed (such as product contamination or chemical release in a public place), locating potentially exposed persons might require other methods. Use of conventional print and broadcast media, social media, blasts to providers and facilities, email listings, and other methods might help capture as many cases as possible.

CHARACTERIZING THE DISEASE CLUSTER

Summarize case information, paying attention to basic demographics, place, and time. Constructing and examining the classic epidemiologic curve (the histogram of the number

---

BOX 20.7
ACUTE SELENIUM TOXICITY WITH DIETARY SUPPLEMENT

PUBLIC HEALTH PROBLEM

In March 2008, an unusual clustering of symptoms was reported to public health officials among persons taking a dietary supplement. Symptoms worsened when supplement dosage was doubled. Product tampering or manufacturing contamination was considered, and selenium was suspected based on symptoms reported.

PUBLIC HEALTH RESPONSE

Multiple states worked with the US Food and Drug Administration to investigate. Product testing of suspected lots revealed 200 times the labeled concentration of selenium present. A case was defined as hair loss, nail discoloration or brittleness, or two or more of certain symptoms (muscle or joint pain, headache, foul breath, fatigue and weakness, gastrointestinal symptoms, or cutaneous eruption) in supplement users with onset within 2 weeks after supplement ingestion. Symptoms of 201 persons met the case definition.

The Food and Drug Administration initiated a product recall; implicated lots were identified as having been distributed beginning in January 2008. The epidemic curve indicated cases dropped off after product recall, corroborating the source of illness. Employee error at an ingredients plant was traced as the source of contamination. Despite widespread publicity and outreach, cases were thought to be undercounted.

TAKE-HOME POINTS

Production of an epidemic curve can illustrate and corroborate successful mitigation efforts, including a decrease in cases after product recall of a widely distributed product.

Source: Reference 25.

---

of new-onset cases by date or time) is just as useful in environmental investigations as in field investigations of infectious sources (Box 20.7). The epidemiologic curve can be considered in conjunction with such events as dates of product use, chemical release, and probable exposure, and with knowledge of the lag time between exposure and measured health effect (that is, latency).

Dates, times, and circumstances of symptom *resolution* can also be important. For example, affected persons might report symptom exacerbation when they are in specific locations, possibly pointing to locations or exposures of specific concern. Symptom abatement when absent from a location (work or school) also is an important detail.

Mapping the locations of cases during symptom onset can yield important clues and suggest hypotheses about exposure and symptoms or disease and actions to be undertaken to prevent disease.

DEVELOPING PRELIMINARY HYPOTHESES AND ANALYZING HEALTH AND EXPOSURE DATA

On the basis of data collected, investigators should develop preliminary hypotheses about the relationship between the exposure and symptoms, taking into consideration the following questions:

- Are the symptoms or illnesses that define the cases biologically plausible on the basis of what is known or suspected about the nature and magnitude of exposure?
- Were symptom onset times congruent with the timing of exposure and what is known about the latency of effect?
- Does the epidemiologic curve suggest a discrete event, multiple episodes of exposure, or continuous exposure?
- Does a map of the locations of cases (at time of exposure or disease onset) suggest something about the nature of the source (e.g., localized or widespread, through air or water)?

At this point, ask whether the illness or disease cluster could be associated with an exposure or multiple exposures. Comprehensive resources on toxicologic effects of chemicals are readily available for consultation on exposure–symptom relationships (26–29).

Depending on how the hypothesis is framed, consider testing differences in the proportion of persons with symptoms or disease by varying levels of measured or estimated exposure. The exposure measure to be tested might be physical proximity to a suspected exposure source, environmental measures or modeled values, or biological metrics. Also, ask whether mean levels of exposure differ by varying severity of specific health outcomes. Consult textbooks on standard statistical methods (e.g., 30).

Preliminary analyses might point to the need for more sophisticated methods to better understand the data gathered. Similarly, a systematic epidemiologic investigation might be needed to link exposure and illness in at-risk populations, although this link might be difficult to confirm. In this stage of the investigation, engaging subject matter experts is especially relevant.

DETERMINING THE NEED FOR FURTHER SYSTEMATIC STUDY

The primary goal of any public health investigation is to prevent further disease or death. In an environmental investigation, mitigation efforts might achieve this goal without benefit of detailed environmental or biological information. However, a public health agency can consider a number of next steps, particularly when working with subject matter experts, to refine the investigation. These steps can include exposure modeling (such as air dispersion modeling) to refine exposure estimates. Other classic next steps include a case–control study, a retrospective cohort study, or other relevant study design. Sometimes more extensive use of existing information, including vital statistics, registry data, or hospitalization data, can provide appropriate information. Use of cluster detection methods to refine spatial and temporal bounds of a cluster or to locate other possible clustering of disease also is possible. Most of these next steps are resource intensive and might not lead to confirmation of the association between exposure and cases. Consider the resources available to public health, community needs, and expectations and scientific soundness of any approach.

SUMMARIZING FINDINGS AND DEVELOPING CONCLUSIONS AND RECOMMENDATIONS

Communicate about the status of the investigation to the community and other stakeholders as work proceeds, and prepare a written summary report of methods and findings at investigation end. In the final report, include clearly articulated conclusions that are supported directly by the findings and recommendations to the community and other stakeholders.

Present the summary investigation report to the community and other stakeholders in settings, places, and times convenient for the community. Tailor findings and prevention messages to different audiences, taking into account literacy level and language barriers that might impact the effectiveness of written and spoken communication.

IMPLEMENTING PREVENTION AND CONTROL MEASURES TO REDUCE EXPOSURE AND ILLNESS

Consider prevention and control interventions throughout each step of the investigation. These interventions will usually involve work with environmental regulatory and emergency response partners to take actions to prevent further human exposure. In emergent situations, especially early on, interventions will have to be undertaken in the face of

---

BOX 20.8
CARBON MONOXIDE POISONING AT AN INDOOR ICE RINK

PUBLIC HEALTH PROBLEM

A male hockey player lost consciousness after participating in an indoor hockey event that included a large number of players and spectators. The fire department detected elevated levels of carbon monoxide (CO) inside the arena.

PUBLIC HEALTH RESPONSE

Emergency responders encouraged all attendees to be medically assessed for CO poisoning. Health department staff abstracted local emergency department records for persons who sought care for CO exposure on dates surrounding the event. After additional follow-up, illnesses of 74 persons met the case definition for CO poisoning, including 32 of 50 hockey players and 42 other attendees. Two persons were hospitalized and treated, including a pregnant attendee. Blood carboxyhemoglobin levels among case-patients ranged from 5.1% to 21.7% and were highest among hockey players.

Informant interviews revealed that CO measurements that night ranged from 45 ppm to 165 ppm; acceptable air quality standards for CO levels at an ice arena are 20 ppm or lower. Emissions from the ice resurfacer were determined to be the source of CO.

TAKE-HOME POINT

CO is colorless, odorless, and tasteless and can impact a large gathering. Mitigation steps can include installation of CO detectors, requirements for scheduled maintenance on ice resurfacers, and CO monitoring requirements at indoor ice arenas.

Source: Reference 31.

---

substantial uncertainty. For example, steps should be taken immediately to stop exposure to an elemental mercury spill or release in a residential or school setting. Evacuation of building occupants might need to be considered as soon as possible, followed by appropriate site cleanup steps (Box 20.8).

Other examples of public health actions that can mitigate exposure include

- Providing bottled water to private well water owners after discovery of high levels of contamination.
- Public messaging on prevention of carbon monoxide poisoning before, during, and after power outages related to storms or other disasters.
- Warnings or recalls related to contaminated consumer or food products.

Sometimes an investigation calls attention to the need for larger, more proactive primary prevention efforts that are not necessarily community-specific, such as new legislation (e.g., requiring carbon monoxide detectors in new residences or rental properties), increasing training (e.g., tailored training for emergency response personnel on chemical release), setting new standards (e.g., establishing buffer areas for facilities that handle flammable or toxic chemicals in large quantities), or increased outreach and education (e.g., providing brochures for private well owners on proper well maintenance and testing). Similarly, investigators should take the time to consider lessons learned from the incident response and make recommendations regarding agency best practices for improving the effectiveness of responses to future events.

Field investigations of exposures and diseases of environmental origin require unique partnerships and expertise that might be outside of traditional public health. Effective risk communication is a critical component of response in an environmental investigation. Public expectations of clean food, water, and living areas place increased expectations on public health during these investigations. Public health needs to maintain expertise in environmental issues, maintain strong partnerships with state and federal environmental partners and be skilled at risk communication to successfully complete environmental investigations.

REFERENCES

1. Etzel RA. Field investigations of environmental epidemics. In: Gregg MB, editor. *Field epidemiology*. 3rd ed. New York: Oxford University Press; 2002:355–75.
2. Harada M. Congenital Minamata disease: intrauterine methylmercury poisoning. *Teratology.* 1978;18:285–8.
3. Bertazzi PA, Bernucci I, Brambilla G, Consonni D, Pesatori AC. The Seveso studies on early and long-term effects of dioxin exposure: a review. *Environ Health Perspect*. 1998;106(Suppl 2):625–33.
4. Centers for Disease Control and Prevention. Investigating suspected cancer clusters and responding to community concerns. Guidelines from CDC and the Council of State and Territorial Epidemiologists. *MMWR*. 2013;62(RR-8):1–24.
5. Williams LJ, Honein MA, Rasmussen SA. Methods for a public health response to birth defects clusters. *Teratology*. 2002;66(Suppl 1):S50–8.
6. Henning KJ. Overview of syndromic surveillance: what is syndromic surveillance? In: Syndromic surveillance: reports from a national conference, 2003. *MMWR*. 2004;53(Suppl);5–11.
7. Agency for Toxic Substances and Disease Registry. Health consultation: medical exposure investigation using serial urine testing and medical records review, Kiddie Kollege, Franklinville, Gloucester County, New Jersey. EPA Facility ID: NJN000206028. June 13, 2007. http://www.atsdr.cdc.gov/HAC/pha/KiddieKollege/KiddieKollegeHC061307.pdf
8. Kulkarni PA, Duncan MA, Watters MT, et al. Severe illness from methyl bromide exposure at a condominium resort—U.S. Virgin Islands, March 2015. *MMWR*. 2015;64:763–6.
9. Centers for Disease Control and Prevention. Crisis and emergency risk communication (2014 edition). https://emergency.cdc.gov/cerc/resources/pdf/cerc_2014edition.pdf

10. US Environmental Protection Agency. *Seven Cardinal Rules of Risk Communication.* Washington, DC: US Environmental Protection Agency; 1988.

11. Bellinger DC. Lead contamination in Flint—an abject failure to protect public health. *N Engl J Med.* 2016;374:1101–3.

12. Hanna-Attisha M, LaChance J, Sadler RC, Schnepp AC. Elevated blood lead levels in children associated with the Flint drinking water crisis: a spatial analysis of risk and public health response. *Am J Public Health.* 2016;106:283–90.

13. Kennedy C, Yard E, Dignam T, et al. Blood lead levels among children aged <6 years—Flint, Michigan, 2013–2016. *MMWR.* 2016;65:650–54.

14. New Jersey Department of Health. Surveys of residents of Paulsboro, New Jersey following a train derailment and vinyl chloride gas release. Trenton, New Jersey, September 5, 2014. https://www.state.nj.us/health/ceohs/documents/eohap/haz_sites/gloucester/train_derail/survey_report.pdf

15. New Jersey Department of Health. Air quality in Paulsboro, New Jersey following a train derailment and vinyl chloride gas release. Trenton, New Jersey, September 5, 2014. https://www.state.nj.us/health/ceohs/documents/eohap/haz_sites/gloucester/train_derail/air_quality_report.pdf

16. National Transportation Safety Board. *Conrail Freight Train Derailment with Vinyl Chloride Release, Paulsboro, New Jersey, November 30, 2012.* Accident report NTSB/RAR-14/01. Washington, DC: National Transportation Safety Board; July 29, 2014.

17. Centers for Disease Control and Prevention. National Notifiable Diseases Surveillance System: current and historical conditions. https://wwwn.cdc.gov/nndss/conditions/

18. Council of State and Territorial Epidemiologists. Position statement archive. http://www.cste.org/?page=PositionStatements

19. Council of State and Territorial Epidemiologists. Biomonitoring in public health: epidemiologic guidance for state, local and tribal public health agencies. http://c.ymcdn.com/sites/www.cste.org/resource/resmgr/OccupationalHealth/2012CSTEBiomonitoringFINAL.pdf

20. National Research Council, National Academies of Science. *Human Biomonitoring for Environmental Chemicals.* Washington, DC: National Academies Press; 2006.

21. Centers for Disease Control and Prevention. National report on human exposure to environmental chemicals. https://www.cdc.gov/exposurereport/index.html

22. Cavicchia PP, Watkins S, Blackmore C, Matthias J. Notes from the field: eye injuries sustained at a foam party—Collier County, Florida, 2012. *MMWR.* 2013;62:667–8.

23. Goldman LR, Smith DF, Neutra RR, et al. Pesticide food poisoning from contaminated watermelons in California, 1985. *Arch Environ Health.* 1990;45:229–36.

24. Green MA, Heumann MA, Wehr, HM, et al. An outbreak of watermelon-borne pesticide toxicity. *Am J Public Health.* 1987;77:1431–4.

25. MacFarquhar JK, Broussard D, Melstrom P, et al. Acute selenium toxicity associated with a dietary supplement. *Arch Intern Med.* 2010;170:256–61.

26. US Environmental Protection Agency. Integrated Risk Information System. https://www.epa.gov/iris

27. Agency for Toxic Substances and Disease Registry. Toxic substances portal: toxicological profiles. http://www.atsdr.cdc.gov/toxprofiles/index.asp

28. US Environmental Protection Agency. Acute exposure guideline levels for airborne chemicals. https://www.epa.gov/aegl

29. Klaassen CD, editor. *Casarett & Doull's Toxicology: The Basic Science of Poisons.* 8th ed. New York: McGraw Hill Education; 2013.

30. Armitage P, Berry G, Matthews JNS. *Statistical Methods in Medical Research.* 4th ed. Malden, MA: Blackwell Science, Ltd.;2002.

31. Creswell PD, Meiman JG, Nehls-Lowe H, et al. Exposure to elevated carbon monoxide levels at an indoor ice arena—Wisconsin, 2014. *MMWR.* 2015;64:1267–70.

/// 21 /// OCCUPATIONAL DISEASE AND INJURY

KATHLEEN KREISS
AND KRISTIN J. CUMMINGS

INTRODUCTION

For most adults and some teenagers, work accounts for at least one-third of the work week and half of waking hours. Work stress and work hazards constitute a public health burden that differs substantially from many public health responsibilities in the location of expertise and practice and in societal stakeholders. Even three centuries ago, Ramazzini described the maladies of particular occupations and called on physicians to always inquire about the nature of work in persons who consulted them for illness (1).

Miners developed phthisis, now attributed to silicosis and mycobacterial disease to which they are rendered susceptible by silica dust's toxicity to macrophages. Weavers developed asthma, now attributed to organic dusts contaminated with endotoxin. Mercury-exposed workers developed neurologic sequelae. Most public health workers believe that these workplace toxins are long-controlled, but old diseases crop up again in new industries, as a result of new technologies, or in the absence of regulation or enforcement. In addition, with the introduction of new exposures, new diseases are identified.

IDENTIFYING AND ENGAGING STAKEHOLDERS

One of the first and most critical steps in conducting a field investigation of illness or injury in a workplace is identifying and engaging the stakeholders. The three basic stakeholder groups are workplace management, labor, and government.

Management

- *Small workplace.* In a small workplace, the owner of the business may be the main contact for operations, health and safety issues, and human resources. Thus, this one person may be able to provide field epidemiologists with key information pertinent to the investigation, such as
  - A description of work processes.
  - Safety data sheets.
  - Recorded injury and illness data.
  - Employee rosters that include names, hire dates, departments, and job titles.
- *Workplaces operated by large companies.* In contrast to small workplaces, workplaces operated by large regional or multinational companies may have entire departments dedicated to each function and personnel at the local, national, and international levels. In such situations, the epidemiologist needs to establish early in the investigation who will represent the management and serve as the main contact for investigators. Local-level managers are generally best informed about the workplace, and advocating for their involvement may be worthwhile. However, particularly in contentious situations (e.g., a worker death or severe illness or injury), local management may not be empowered to provide information or make decisions related to the investigation. It is not unusual for larger employers to refer public health investigators to an attorney.
- *Accessing workplaces and worker populations,* and recognizing management concerns.

- Management controls access to workplaces and on-site worker populations. Even with regulatory or statutory access for public health concerns, field epidemiologists benefit by developing trust with sensitivity to management concerns and clarity about public health procedures.

- Economic concerns may derive from workers' compensation claims or insurance rates. If a field investigation demonstrates product hazards, employers may encounter third-party lawsuits from workers in companies downstream that purchase a product. Even consumers of downstream company products may bring suit against the upstream manufacturer of a hazardous ingredient, as occurred in the manufacture of microwave popcorn with the butter flavoring diacetyl, which causes obliterative bronchiolitis (2).

- Management may fear increased labor unrest and poor publicity.

- Management also may be concerned about disclosure of proprietary business information and trade secrets, which can have economic ramifications.

Labor

- *Employees.* Employees frequently are the stakeholder that brings concerns about workplace health and injury risks to public health attention. They might do this through consultation with physicians, who subsequently alert public health agencies, or through direct request. Confidentiality is important to most employees, who want to avoid being fired or disciplined for reporting to government authorities. Although legal protections exist for whistleblowers, access to legal representation may be limited by lack of familiarity and by economic constraints.

- *Labor unions.* Historically, labor unions have been important stakeholders in requesting public health investigations. In 2017, just 6.5% of the US private sector workforce was represented by a labor union (3). When they represent employees, labor unions' involvement in public health investigations is critical. They can provide an overview of the workplace and labor relations. International unions can leverage findings from an investigation across an industry by notifying local unions in other companies and by contract negotiations to include health and safety provisions, such as biological monitoring.

- *Contract labor.* The use of contract labor has been growing for years. Employment arrangements, such as those involving both a contracting agency employer and a worksite employer, can complicate field investigations by introducing ambiguity about responsibility for workplace health and safety and workplace access. The National Institute for Occupational Safety and Health (NIOSH) of the Centers for Disease Control and Prevention has had experience with contracting agencies not allowing their employees to participate in public health investigations of the worksite employer. On the other hand, the California Department of Public Health required flavor manufacturers to include contract employees in monitoring for possible flavoring-related pulmonary function abnormalities (4). The field epidemiologist should explore the complexities of employment because contract employees may be at the highest risk for workplace injury and illness (5). The likelihood of success in an occupational investigation might increase if the public health investigator anticipates participation anxieties by labor stakeholders who might perceive their employment as increasingly precarious and fear plant closure or loss of a contingent labor contract.

Government

Government is a third stakeholder in occupational health and safety. The stake of government can be viewed as advancing the social contract that maintains a cohesive and productive society and enforcing laws and regulations. Occupational laws and regulations are national in scope and set by the federal government. The federal government delegates responsibility for their enforcement to some state agencies, which then have overlapping responsibilities in occupational health. At the federal level, relevant government roles are separated into two different departments: regulation/enforcement and research consultations/service.

- *Regulatory*. In the US Department of Labor, the Occupational Safety and Health Administration (OSHA) and Mine Safety and Health Administration (MSHA) set and enforce workplace standards for exposures and safety in most workplaces. Under the General Duty Clause of the Occupational and Safety Health Act of 1970 (6), employers are required to provide their employees with a place of employment that "is free from recognizable hazards that are causing or likely to cause death or serious harm to employees." In addition, these agencies have permissible exposure limits on a chemical-by-chemical basis. Permissible exposure limits exist for only a fraction of all potential workplace hazards and do not typically account for potential additive or synergistic properties of mixtures that might be present in workplaces. Thus, regulation has not eliminated many opportunities for hazardous exposures in the workplace (7).
- *Research and service*. The primary federal government stakeholder pertinent to public health research and service investigation is NIOSH. NIOSH responsibilities

encompass research to make recommendations for standards to guide OSHA and MSHA in setting regulations; investigative service to employees, industry, and state and local health departments; and education in occupational safety and health. In making recommended exposure limits to protect health, NIOSH is not required to consider cost or feasibility, but the regulatory agencies in the Department of Labor must consider those factors in setting permissible exposure limits. NIOSH's role in recommending health-protective guidance for regulations makes NIOSH particularly interested in emerging, unregulated problems that warrant further investigation in workplaces or throughout an industry. In addition, NIOSH funds many state and local health departments to conduct surveillance of selected occupational health indicators, diseases, and injuries that are commonly reported without identifiers for national-level estimates of the burden of work-related disease.

BASIC OPERATIONAL CONSIDERATIONS IN RECOGNIZING AND INVESTIGATING OCCUPATIONAL DISEASES, INJURIES, AND OTHER CONDITIONS

Approaches to recognizing and investigating occupational conditions can be readily distinguished from approaches to infectious disease. These differences especially pertain to initial recognition of the problem; types and availability of resources for investigations; need for quantitative exposure assessment; approaches to surveillance; and characterization and implications of differences in settings of exposure and occurrence.

Recognition

Public health agencies at local, state, and federal levels have mandated responsibilities and authorities to control both communicable and noncommunicable infections, and physicians are accustomed to regulations requiring reporting of many infections to state public health departments. In contrast, few physicians are trained to recognize work-related diseases, apart from infections. When state health departments have implemented reporting requirements for special surveillance efforts in occupational diseases or injuries, few physicians report (8). Nevertheless, occupational health has benefited from many astute physicians who have recognized or suspected new occupational diseases, such as bladder neuropathy resulting from a new catalyst in polyurethane foam manufacture (9), interstitial lung disease in nylon flock workers making upholstery (10), indium lung disease in workers making sputtering tiles for touch-sensitive screens (11), and obliterative bronchiolitis in microwave popcorn (12), flavoring (13), and coffee processing workers

(14). When clinicians recognize possible occupational disease or injury, they commonly contact state or local public health agencies.

For many occupational diseases, physicians can treat patients without considering an occupational cause. For example, occupational asthma, which accounts for at least 15% of adult-onset asthma (15), could respond to pharmacologic treatment even though removal from the inciting workplace exposure early in the clinical course can result in permanent cure. Patients with carpal tunnel neuropathy may undergo surgery, when eliminating occupational repetitive motion of the wrist in nonneutral positions can relieve symptoms and progression. Such individual patients may be sentinels that co-workers sharing common exposures or physical stresses have similar health outcomes. Public health investigation of sentinel cases of suspected work-related injury or disease can result in remediation of causal factors and prevention of other cases.

Employees often recognize that a cluster of illness or injury exists among co-workers. Unless a physician serves a small geographic area or population, he or she is unlikely to suspect an association between several cases of a disease or chronic injury and a particular workplace.

Resources for Investigation

Upon receiving physician or employee reports of suspected work-related health outcomes, the field epidemiologist can try to ascertain whether the health problem results from a regulated exposure or work circumstance or from unregulated or unrecognized exposure or circumstances. For regulated exposures, OSHA or MSHA are appropriate resources. The regulatory agency can inspect the workplace to measure exposures and assess safety measures to prevent other cases by ensuring that standards are enforced. For example, lead poisoning in a lead-exposed worker can elicit corrective action from OSHA. Twenty-one states and one US territory have OSHA-approved state plans for enforcement that cover both private and local government workplaces, and five states and one territory cover only local government workers. In all other states, federal OSHA is responsible for investigation and enforcement. The potentially overlapping responsibility for occupational health and safety of state and federal government contrasts with most other public health responsibilities, which are state and local in authority, rather than federal.

Where standards for exposures do not exist, OSHA's regulatory enforcement role is limited to the General Duty Clause (6). Examples of an unregulated hazard are repetitive motion injuries, frequently associated with force and rates of repetition, and indoor

BOX 21.1
DEATHS IN FRACKING AND OIL WORKERS

PUBLIC HEALTH PROBLEM
In 2010 and 2012, young workers in Montana and North Dakota died on catwalks while gauging fluid levels of crude oil and gas storage tanks.

PUBLIC HEALTH RESPONSE
These possible sentinel events triggered review of media reports, OSHA case-fatality investigations, and the NIOSH Fatalities in Oil and Gas database. Seven similar nontraumatic deaths occurred during January 2010–March 2015 in three other states. Workers died while gauging or sampling tanks associated with concentrated sources of hydrocarbon gases and vapors in open air. Exposure assessment documented very low oxygen concentrations over open hatches and elevated hydrocarbon gas and vapor concentrations, which can cause acute central nervous system symptoms.

TAKE-HOME POINT
Sentinel event investigation can document new occupational hazards that can be prevented with alternative fluid sample collection points, remote monitoring of fluid levels, proper use of gas monitoring, and worker training.

Source: Reference 16.

air–related complaints in damp buildings in which bioaerosol measurements that predict adverse health outcomes, such as asthma and hypersensitivity pneumonitis, do not exist. Obviously, emerging problems in the process of being recognized and investigated have no applicable regulations. An important responsibility of field epidemiologists is to investigate emerging occupational health problems and formulate exposure-control guidance. Investigation of known occupational diseases and other conditions in new settings also can have public health ramifications (Box 21.1) (16). Consultation with NIOSH or with academic centers that have occupational health expertise might be an efficient first step in contributing to the knowledge base of public health prevention of occupational diseases and injuries.

Quantitative Exposure Assessment

In contrast to most infectious disease investigations, quantitative exposure assessment is a priority in occupational health investigations. In attributing health outcome to working conditions, the level of exposure determines both the plausibility of an adverse health

---

BOX 21.2
OBLITERATIVE BRONCHIOLITIS IN FLAVORING-EXPOSED MICROWAVE POPCORN WORKERS

PUBLIC HEALTH PROBLEM

Eight former microwave popcorn workers had severe lung disease; four were listed for lung transplantation.

PUBLIC HEALTH RESPONSE

Review of medical records established a cluster of cases of fixed obstructive lung disease of unknown origin. The Missouri Department of Health and Social Services and NIOSH conducted a cross-sectional study of current workers, which demonstrated that 25% had spirometric abnormalities related in an exposure–response manner to exposure to diacetyl, the principal ingredient of artificial butter flavorings. Subsequent investigation of five other microwave popcorn workforces found cases consistent with obliterative bronchiolitis in four other factories.

TAKE-HOME POINT

An industrywide risk existed from diacetyl exposure, later implicated in cases in flavoring, cookie, and coffee production. Animal toxicology experiments provided biologic plausibility for risk assessment and recommended exposure limits.

Source: References 2, 12–14, 17.

---

outcome and guidance for its control. Most epidemiologists will need to seek expert assistance from environmental scientists or industrial hygienists who have the training to determine levels of exposure in the workplace. Guidance for control of exposure depends on the exposure level and may include exhaust ventilation, other engineering controls, administrative controls, or personal protective equipment.

Field investigation of new occupational diseases or injuries often requires a cluster of cases that can be addressed in a workplace population–based manner. Exceptions are a work-related fatality and uncommon conditions known to have environmental causes, such as hypersensitivity pneumonitis. In most instances of a new disease, a single case cannot result in attribution to the workplace in the absence of an epidemiologic (population-based) approach to risk factors. Most emerging occupational diseases cannot be identified with a causal biomarker, such as blood lead level. For an actionable preventive outcome of investigating an emerging disease, clusters are usually necessary (Box 21.2) (2,12–14,17).

Surveillance

Surveillance is a long-standing public health tool to trigger field investigation. However, occupational disease and injury surveillance is rudimentary in comparison with infectious disease surveillance. In 1983, pioneers in occupational health surveillance (18) described 50 sentinel occupational health events that represented failures in prevention that should trigger public health action. The authors lamented that death certificates in many states did not have industry and occupation codes; although this remains true, some uniquely occupational diseases (e.g., pneumoconiosis) can be studied with death certificate surveillance. Many state health departments lack staffing to follow up on reported occupational diseases. Several states participating in NIOSH-funded sentinel event notification have contributed greatly to understanding certain conditions, including occupational asthma, silicosis, lead poisoning, and pesticide poisoning. In addition, the Council of State and Territorial Epidemiologists has developed recommendations for occupational health and injury surveillance (19), which many state health departments have adopted.

Other efforts involving occupational health surveillance are examination of workers' compensation claims, which exist in each state; federally mandated surveillance of coal miners through submission of chest radiographs to NIOSH by physicians or clinics hired by coal mine operators; and supplemental federal surveillance of coal miners by NIOSH mobile teams visiting individual mines or regions to take chest radiographs and conduct pulmonary function tests. However, these unique programs for health surveillance of coal miners are not duplicated for other occupations and industries, for which health surveillance remains uncharacterized.

States with considerable initiatives in occupational health, such as California, Massachusetts, and Wisconsin, recently have contributed substantially to understanding new occupational health conditions. For example, the California Department of Public Health approached the emerging issue of flavoring-related obliterative bronchiolitis by partnering with California OSHA (CalOSHA) in a preventive program called the Flavoring Industry Safety and Health Evaluation Program. It required flavor manufacturers to report medical screening questionnaire and spirometry data on their employees to identify presumptive cases of flavoring-related lung disease (4). Employers were motivated to participate by assurance that CalOSHA would provide preventive consultation and not issue citations. Linking questionnaire and medical surveillance data on flavoring-exposed workforces also enabled characterization of risk factors (13,20). These risk factors, such as the annual amount of diacetyl used in production, reinforced the exposure–response relations found in a previous NIOSH investigation in Missouri (12).

CalOSHA worked with the riskiest flavor workplaces to monitor implementation of respiratory protection and engineering controls.

Workplace Investigation

Clusters of suspected work-related disease and injury usually require access to employees in workplaces to conduct population-based epidemiology investigations. To identify risk factors that can guide preventive measures, field epidemiologists must establish common ground with employers, their lawyers, employees, and sometimes their union representatives. Usually the common ground is the desire to avoid harm to employees.

On-worksite collaboration with industrial hygienists or environmental scientists is nearly always required to plan and execute successful field investigations that examine the relation between environmental characteristics and evidence of ill health. Such collaboration is usually important in designing questionnaires for employees about job titles, work areas and practices, and potential work exposures by specific processes. Industrial hygienists measure exposure levels and observe work practices that allow estimation of exposure characteristics, such as average, peak, or episodic exposures. Such quantitative and qualitative evaluation is critical to investigating whether there are exposure–response relationships for adverse health effects found in questionnaire responses, biological indices, and physiologic tests administered by the health team. Thus, a workplace investigation usually involves a multidisciplinary team that requires space for confidential interviews and medical tests, requests for employees to wear personal exposure monitoring devices, and accommodation to production schedules. Good communication among team members and with management and workers is necessary for success in determining whether a workplace is safe for workers and what preventive interventions might be appropriate.

Part of communication with workplace stakeholders is the limits of any proposed investigation. For emerging occupational health problems, epidemiologic associations alone seldom establish the etiology. Newly recognized diseases or injuries trigger expectations that work-related health conditions should be compensated, exposures regulated, and surveillance instituted. These outcomes seldom result from field investigations alone. The contribution of field studies is to establish burden of health outcomes, exposure–response relations, temporality (e.g., by follow-up showing that exposure cessation interrupts the outbreak), and replicability among investigators and populations. Carefully designed field studies can contribute to the accumulation of evidence that workplace exposures are causally related to a new health problem. Effective field studies motivate experiments in laboratory settings to establish biologic plausibility of suspected causal agents, guidance for controlling exposures with engineering interventions and personal protective equipment, and medical and exposure surveillance to establish the effectiveness of interventions. Ultimately, these collective investigative efforts underlie the proposal of regulations to protect employees in diverse settings (2,21).

CHALLENGES AND OPPORTUNITIES

Challenges

Occupational health poses several challenges for field epidemiology.

- *Exposure range and assessment.* When a range of exposure does not exist, use of standardized questions can facilitate external comparisons to population-based data, such as the National Health and Nutrition Examination Survey or the Behavioral Risk Factor Surveillance System. Exposure assessment usually requires multidisciplinary access to a workplace with observational and measurement components. These aid in developing a workplace-specific questionnaire that includes information about tenure, job category, tasks or processes suspected to be risk factors, area or department of the workplace, and spills or mishaps. Exposure assessment usually is best informed by interdisciplinary collaboration regarding sentinel cases (including exploratory interviews) and review of company or OSHA exposure data before designing strategies for environmental sampling.
- *Misclassification of health outcome.* New diseases found in a workforce may be misclassified as other diseases. For example, in the investigation of obliterative bronchiolitis associated with diacetyl exposure in a microwave popcorn factory, sentinel cases were diagnosed with asthma, emphysema, and bronchitis. Although field investigators found these sentinel cases more likely to have obliterative bronchiolitis, they did not consider current workers with abnormal restrictive spirometry to potentially have this occupational lung disease, another example of misclassification (2).
- *Healthy worker effect.* Workers who become too ill to work or who recognize temporal relations of symptoms to aspects of the work environment might not stay in such work environments, as commonly is the case in occupational asthma clusters. This "healthy worker survivor effect" can result in underestimation of work-related disease when only the current workforce is studied, or it might obscure

the exposures associated with disease onset when only current job is considered and miss persons who have transferred to another area to diminish work-related symptoms.

- *Management resistance.* Management resistance to worker requests for public health assistance and access to workplaces for investigation can present additional challenges. Management might designate needed information as trade secret, might request investigators to sign confidentiality contracts, and might resist protection of worker confidentiality. Employers have considerable information about their employees, which enables presumptive identification of persons when aggregate results are stratified by race, sex, age group, tenure, or job category. NIOSH guidance for its field studies (called Health Hazard Evaluations) might be of interest to all field epidemiologists encountering workplace complaints (22).

Opportunities

Recognition and solving of occupational health concerns are underresourced (https://www.cdc.gov/niosh/oshworkforce/pdfs/NASHW_Final_Report-508.pdf). Moreover, protective regulations about exposures and safety, even when they exist, may not be enforced because fewer than 1% of workplaces are inspected in a calendar year (7). Under these circumstances, field epidemiologists can play a critical role. Table 21.1 documents examples of past contributions of field epidemiologists to prevention and knowledge of new occupational risks (2,9–14,20,23–30).

- *Identification of regulated hazards can trigger enforcement and follow-up by OSHA or MSHA.* Beneficial effects can be immediate when causality is unquestioned or when lowering of exposure can be implemented by working with medical care providers and employers on appropriate restrictions of duty and guidance for intervention in workplaces.
- *Prevention of newly discovered disease associations across an industry usually depends on motivating others beyond the epidemiologic team to address causality.* Guidance for interpreting epidemiologic associations as causal may depend on laboratory animal studies, replication in other workplaces and by other investigators, longitudinal follow-up to establish temporality, and establishment of exposure–response relations. These iterative efforts for emerging issues require other stakeholders to contribute to evidence that can be used in risk assessment to establish recommended or permissible exposure limits. Successful public health field investigations motivate efforts by other disciplines, agencies, and stakeholders and stimulate professional

TABLE 21.1 Selected occupational conditions identified by field epidemiologists

Condition	Industry/activity	Agent, when known
Occupational asthma	Pesticide manufacture	3-amino-5-mercapto-1, 2, 4-triazole (23)
Hypersensitivity pneumonitis	Leisure pool lifeguards	Unspecified bioaerosols (24)
Obliterative bronchiolitis	Microwave popcorn, flavoring, and cookie dough manufacture and processing of roasted and flavored coffee	Diacetyl (2,3-butanedione) and related alpha diketones (2,12–14,20)
Pulmonary alveolar proteinosis, fibrosis, and emphysema	Indium-tin oxide manufacture	Indium, particularly sintered indium-tin oxide aerosols (11)
Obliterative bonchiolitis	Fiberglass boat building and water tank manufacture	Ingredients of plastic-coated resins, possibly styrene (25)
Lymphocytic bronchiolitis and peribronchiolitis	Flocking of upholstery, greeting cards	Nylon, rayon, and other synthetic respirable particles (10)
Asthma and hypersensitivity pneumonitis	Damp indoor environments from structural water damage, contaminated air conditioning systems	Bioaerosols (26)
Bladder neuropathy	Polyurethane automobile seat manufacture	Dimethylaminopropionitrile catalyst (9)
Color vision loss	Windblade manufacture	Styrene (27)
Tuberculosis	Zoo with infected elephants	*Mycobacterium tuberculosis* (28)
Carpal tunnel syndrome	Poultry processing	Repetitive motion (29)
Carbon monoxide poisoning	Swimming around houseboats	Carbon monoxide from generators (30)

growth. Investigation involving industry partners can sometimes proceed to regulation proposed jointly by industry and labor.

• *Work-related public health opportunities might be more easily met with consultation from persons experienced in occupational health field investigations.* Many NIOSH divisions have such expertise. Access is perhaps easiest by calling on those who conduct NIOSH Health Hazard Evaluations in the Respiratory Health Division or the Division of Hazard Evaluations, Surveillance, and Field Studies (https://www.cdc.gov/niosh/contact/officers.html). Those personnel can guide field epidemiologists through available resources, such as Safety Data Sheets for hazardous chemical products, known hazards associated with specific industries and occupations, and potential emerging problems that may benefit from collaborative investigation to leverage efforts in an understaffed public health agency.

CONCLUSION

Epidemiologists called on to conduct field investigations of occupational health and safety concerns have stimulating opportunities to explore associations of work conditions with adverse health outcomes, to intervene in preventing well-recognized occupational hazards, and to obtain expert consultation as needed. The challenges arising from diverse stakeholder interests at the heart of economic activity, from the need for environmental scientist involvement, and from deficits in surveillance and medical provider familiarity with occupational health concerns are at the forefront of public health development. Occupational health field epidemiology contributes to public health's full potential in protecting our communities from the hazards of working life.

REFERENCES

1. Ramazzini, B. *De Morbis Artificum Diatriba* (Diseases of Workers, from the Latin text of 1713, revised with translation and notes by Wilmer Cave Wright). Chicago: University of Chicago Press; 1940.
2. Kreiss K. Recognizing occupational effects of diacetyl: what can we learn from this history? *Toxicology.* 2017;388:48–54.
3. Bureau of Labor Statistics. News release. For release 10:00 a.m. (EST) Friday, January 19, 2018. Union members—2017. https://www.bls.gov/news.release/pdf/union2.pdf
4. Centers for Disease Control and Prevention. Fixed obstructive lung disease among workers in the flavoring manufacturing industry—California, 2004–2007. *MMWR.* 2007;56:389–93.
5. Cummings KJ, Kreiss K. Contingent workers and contingent health: risks of a modern economy. *JAMA.* 2008;299:448–50.
6. Occupational Safety and Health Administration. OSH Act of 1970. https://www.osha.gov/laws-regs/oshact/section5-duties
7. Silverstein M. Getting home safe and sound: Occupational Safety and Health Administration at 38. *Am J Public Health.* 2008;98:416–23.
8. Rosenman KD, Reilly MJ, Henneberger PK. Estimating the total number of newly-recognized silicosis cases in the United States. *Am J Ind Med.* 2003;44:141–7.
9. Kreiss K, Wegman DH, Niles CA, Siroky MB, Krane RJ, Feldman RG. Neurological dysfunction of the bladder in workers exposed to dimethylaminopropionitrile. *JAMA.* 1980;243:741–5.
10. Eschenbacher WL, Kreiss K, Lougheed D, Pransky GS, Day B, Castellan RM. Nylon flock-associated interstitial lung disease: clinical pathology workshop summary. *Am J Respir Crit Care Med.* 1999;159:2003–8.
11. Cummings KJ, Donat WE, Ettensohn DB, Roggli VL, Ingram P, Kreiss K. Pulmonary alveolar proteinosis in indium workers. *Am J Respir Crit Care Med.* 2010;181:458–64.
12. Kreiss K, Gomaa A, Kullman G, Fedan K, Simoes EJ, Enright PL. Clinical bronchiolitis obliterans in workers at a microwave-popcorn plant. *N Engl J Med.* 2002;347:330–8.

13. Kim T, Materna B, Prudhomme J, et al. Industry-wide medical surveillance of California flavor manufacturing workers: cross-sectional results. *Am J Ind Med.* 2010;63:857–65.

14. Bailey RL, Cox-Ganser JM, Piacitelli C, et al. Respiratory morbidity in a coffee processing plant with sentinel obliterative bronchiolitis cases. *Am J Ind Med.* 2015;58:1235–45.

15. Balmes J, Becklake M, Blanc P, et al. Occupational contribution to the burden of obstructive airway disease. *Am J Respir Crit Care Med.* 2003;167:787–97.

16. Harrison RJ, Retzer K, Kosnett MJ, et al. Sudden deaths among oil and gas extraction workers resulting from oxygen deficiency and inhalation of hydrocarbon gases and vapors—United States, January 2010–March 2015. *MMWR.* 2016;65:6–9.

17. Centers for Disease Control and Prevention. Fixed obstructive lung disease among former workers at a microwave popcorn factory—Missouri, 2000–2002. *MMWR.* 2002;51:345–7.

18. Rutstein DD, Mullan RJ, Frazier TM, Halperin WE, Melius JM, Sestito JP. Sentinel health events (occupational): a basis for physician recognition and public health surveillance. *Am J Public Health.* 1983;73:1054–62.

19. Council of State and Territorial Epidemiologists. Occupational health indicators. http://www.cste.org/group/OHIndicators

20. Kreiss K, Fedan K, Nasrullah M, et al. Longitudinal lung function declines among California flavoring manufacturing workers. *Am J Ind Med.* 2012;55:657–68.

21. McKernan LT, Niemeier RT, Kreiss K, et al. *Criteria for a Recommended Standard: Occupational Exposure to Diacetyl and 2,3-Pentanedione.* Cincinnati, OH: US Department of Health and Human Services, Centers for Disease Control and Prevention, National Institute for Occupational Safety and Health; 2016.

22. National Institute for Occupational Safety and Health. Health hazard evaluation program. http://www.cdc.gov/niosh/docs/2009-167/

23. Hnizdo E, Sylvain D, Lewis DM, Pechter E, Kreiss K. New-onset asthma associated with exposure to 3-amino-5-mercapto-1, 2, 4-triazole. *J Occup Environ Med.* 2004;46:1246–52.

24. Rose CS, Martyny JW, Newman LS, et al. "Lifeguard lung: endemic granulomatous pneumonitis in an indoor swimming pool. *Am J Public Health.* 1998;88:1795–800.

25. Cullinan P, McGavin C, Kreiss K, et al. Obliterative bronchiolitis in fiberglass workers: a new occupational disease? *Occup Environ Med.* 2013;70:357–9.

26. Cox-Ganser JM, White SK, Jones R, et al. Respiratory morbidity in office workers in a water-damaged building. *Environ Health Perspect.* 2005;113:485–90.

27. McCague AB, Cox-Ganser JM, Harney JM, et al. Styrene-associated health outcomes at a windblade manufacturing plant. *Am J Indust Med.* 2015;58:1150–9.

28. Zlot A, Vines J, Nystrom L, et al. Diagnosis of tuberculosis in three zoo elephants and a human contact—Oregon, 2013. *MMWR.* 2016;64:1398–402.

29. Musolin K, Ramsey JG, Wassell JT, Hard DL. Prevalence of carpal tunnel syndrome among employees at a poultry processing plant. *Appl Ergon.* 2014;45:1377–83.

30. Centers for Disease Control and Prevention. Houseboat-associated carbon monoxide poisonings on Lake Powell—Arizona and Utah, 2000. *MMWR.* 2000:29:1105–8.

/// 22 /// NATURAL AND HUMAN-MADE DISASTERS

RONALD WALDMAN

INTRODUCTION

Every year, approximately 400 natural disasters occur worldwide. Added to these are 30–40 armed conflicts (1). Together, these and other emergencies imperil the health of hundreds of millions of people and substantially increase levels of morbidity and mortality. The future may bring more calamity to more places around the world; climate change is a scientific certainty, and with it comes an increased level of dangerous weather events in all coastal areas around the globe.

Natural events and human-made emergencies (e.g., armed conflict; climate change; and "development disasters," such as those ensuing from flooding upstream of dam construction or excessive damage from earthquakes where structures have not been built to code) frequently occur in relatively remote, difficult-to-reach locations, often in the poorer countries of the world that are least able to cope. The tasks of field epidemiologists who participate in response efforts include (1) accurately determining the number of people affected, (2) calculating rates of morbidity and mortality, (3) assessing the health-related needs of the population, (4) establishing priorities for providing health services, (5) monitoring progress toward rehabilitation and recovery, (6) evaluating the results of emergency interventions, and (7) improving future responses by communicating the consequences of these emergencies.

HISTORICAL HIGHLIGHTS OF THE USE OF FIELD EPIDEMIOLOGY IN HUMANITARIAN EMERGENCIES

The approach to the way supplies and services are delivered to emergency-affected populations has changed radically during the past 50 years. The application of epidemiologic principles to emergency response is generally considered to have begun during the massive international relief effort mounted during the civil war in Nigeria during the late 1960s. During that war, which resulted in widespread starvation, massive internal displacement, and high rates of mortality, epidemiologists developed methods to help determine the health status of the affected populations so that appropriate assistance could be delivered (2). Nutritional surveillance evolved over subsequent years, and, by the late 1970s, internationally approved guidelines for measuring nutritional status had been developed (3).

Toward the end of the 1970s, the genocidal practices of the Khmer Rouge regime in Cambodia resulted in a massive exodus of survivors to Thailand, where hundreds of thousands of people were given refuge in several large camps. These so-called "death camps" quickly became the sites of numerous outbreaks of disease, but the extent and principal causes of morbidity and mortality were measured in quantifiable terms only when epidemiologists from the Center for Disease Control (later Centers for Disease Control and Prevention), working together with colleagues from the International Committee of the Red Cross and a group of nongovernmental organizations (NGOs), instituted a formal disease surveillance system and conducted methodologically sound surveys (4).

Before the regular use of field epidemiology techniques, emergency response was guided mainly by the best intentions of relatively inexperienced medical and surgical teams with inappropriate skills and inadequate logistical support. Doctors would build makeshift clinics, throw open the doors, and provide services to people who were able to access them—in most instances, only a small proportion of the affected population. Available services frequently did not match the public health needs of the population.

Planners and managers were in the unenviable position of directing major relief operations with little information to guide their efforts (5). However, as sound epidemiologic practices emerged and were more regularly applied, reasonably accurate denominators on which to calculate rates of illness and death were generated and a more disciplined approach to the delivery of humanitarian assistance in the health sector evolved.

Unfortunately, disasters that have needed more honed epidemiologic approaches have continued to occur regularly. Examples include repeated famines and conflicts (the two are not unrelated) in the Horn of Africa; cyclones and tsunamis leading to massive flooding in countries bordering the Bay of Bengal and elsewhere in the Indian Ocean; earthquakes and hurricanes in the Caribbean and Central America; and wars in the Balkans, the Middle East, and Central Africa. All of these required distinct responses, but eventually, because of the development and application of epidemiologic techniques, including more formal approaches to rapid assessment, surveillance, and impact evaluation, patterns of morbidity and mortality emerged. In addition, training programs were established that resulted in an emergency response workforce that was more knowledgeable, more sophisticated, and more capable of reducing illness and saving more lives in less time (Box 22.1) (6).

BOX 22.1

GOMA: THE ORIGINS OF THE SPHERE PROJECT

One notable watershed occurred in the wake of the Rwanda genocide of 1994, when more than 500,000 refugees fled that country to then-Zaire, with many settling in a few camps near the northern tip of Lake Kivu. Within weeks, an estimated 45,000 refugees had died of cholera, despite the presence of hundreds of nongovernmental organizations, United Nations agencies, military medical contingents from at least nine Western countries, and many other public health officials (7). The collective failure to respond effectively to this situation clearly underscored the need for the emergency relief community to develop indicators for a successful intervention and to work to achieve those indicators in every emergency. This need led to development of the Sphere Project and its accompanying Handbook (*Humanitarian Charter and Minimum Standards in Humanitarian Response*) that remains obligatory reading for persons working in this field (8). In addition to establishing standards in key areas (shelter, food security, food aid and nutrition, water and sanitation, and health services, and the cross-cutting areas of gender and protection), the Sphere Project has provided opportunities for epidemiologists and other public health experts to agree on a relatively standardized approach to emergency relief. A fourth edition of this essential Handbook will be published in Fall, 2018.

More recently, notable humanitarian crises resulting from natural disasters have included a massive earthquake in Haiti (2010); flooding that displaced 20 million people in Pakistan (2010); several typhoons in the Philippines, including Typhoon Haiyan/Yolanda in 2013; and the ongoing (2017) severe drought in the Horn of Africa. Human-made emergencies commanding the attention of the international humanitarian community have included ongoing conflicts in South Sudan, Central African Republic, and throughout the Middle East. Although the peer-reviewed literature addressing responses to such disasters remains relatively sparse, field epidemiologists preparing to respond to future crises should be encouraged to learn from these case studies.

ROLE OF FIELD EPIDEMIOLOGISTS IN HUMANITARIAN EMERGENCY RESPONSE

The principal objectives of epidemiologic field investigations and response in emergency settings are to

- Establish the magnitude and distribution of the public health consequences of the event.
- Assess the size and health needs of the affected population.
- Help provide and promote epidemiologically derived data as the principal basis for resource allocation.
- Help guide implementation of public health programs to minimize postemergency morbidity and mortality.
- Monitor progress of the relief effort.
- Evaluate the effectiveness of the relief effort.

The field epidemiologist is a core member of the emergency response team. Increasingly, the international response to emergencies is organized in a command-and-control manner, in accordance with the Incident Command System (see Chapter 16) or similar systems approaches (9). Knowledge of the organizational structure of the relief effort and identification of the decision-makers is important, as are being a team player and understanding the roles of other team members. In the face of tragedy, many unseasoned hands will adopt an "act first–think later" approach and view the methodical collection and analysis of data as a frivolous, time-wasting activity. In these instances, the field epidemiologist must be an affirmative voice of reason—strongly advancing an evidence-based approach to health interventions that maximizes benefit to the affected population.

Although no cookbook approach exists to emergency response, flexibility and sound judgment are hallmarks for the successful use of field epidemiology. Accordingly, a flexible framework of steps for the epidemiologist includes

- Determining the impact of the event on the public's health by establishing rates of illness and death with an optimal attainable level of accuracy (note: "the perfect should not be the enemy of the good"). In doing so, it is, of course, essential to focus on the determinations of both numerators (cases and deaths) and denominators (total population and, wherever possible, age and sex breakdowns).
- Initiating disease surveillance as quickly as possible, beginning with a minimum amount of data to collect and augmenting as deemed appropriate and feasible.
- Identifying personal, household, and environmental risk factors for elevated rates of illness and death.
- Advocating for the early initiation of essential public health interventions and disease-control programs on the basis of knowledge of the actual and potential distribution of diseases in the population.
- Arguing forcefully that health actions of lesser priority be deferred.
- Becoming an essential member of the health response team by attending appropriate meetings; working with public health officials and other responders from different organizations, including government officials; and providing frequently updated reports about the situation to those who have a need to know.

This last point (i.e., providing situation reports) is critical; in emergency response, "consequential epidemiology" needs to be practiced (10). The contribution of epidemiologists reflects their ability to provide timely and accurate data in a way that decision-makers can easily understand, analyze, and use for action. The use of those data should enable effective implementation of appropriate public health measures. Conversely, collecting and providing potentially useful information that decision-makers do not act on might be viewed, in part, as a failure of field epidemiology, as is the implementation of health interventions that relevant data do not support. Thus, epidemiologic skills are necessary but not sufficient: equally critical are the abilities to communicate effectively, advocate successfully, and provide strong leadership in support of the policymakers directly responsible for consequential actions.

COMMON ISSUES

Logistics

In its early stages, the emergency relief environment is always chaotic. However, every responder has the same essential needs: food, water, shelter, transportation, communication, and a place to sleep. Thus, the field epidemiologist's first priority is to arrange to meet these basic needs. This is important because the more independent one can be, the less others will have to divert attention from their work to provide assistance.

Hiring staff is another early priority, especially in international emergency relief. Because field epidemiology is a population-based discipline, the epidemiology team should include members who know the local language, geography, and customs. Therefore, recruiting and retaining people who can be relied on to be effective liaisons with the local communities is a high priority. Although English-speaking translators are highly valued, because they do not always represent the community and are unlikely to be professionally trained, information they provide should be carefully assessed and verified.

Establishing Rates of Illness, Injury, and Death

In most emergency relief settings, accurate measurement of the size of the affected population and its current health status is missing and difficult to establish. For the field epidemiologist, though, it is critical to determine a reasonably precise denominator on which to base the calculation of rates, such as crude, age-, sex-, and disease-specific death; prevalence of moderate, severe, and global acute malnutrition in the affected community; incidence of high-priority conditions; and access to use of health services. Determining rates is essential for comparing population groups and prioritizing public health interventions. A variety of methodologic options can be used to calculate population size, ranging from the more basic, such as extrapolating from the number of people in a sample of dwelling units, to the more sophisticated, such as using aerial photography and/or satellite imagery. The field epidemiologist needs to consider the context in which the relief effort is occurring to select the best method—one that provides reasonably accurate numbers in a culturally and contextually sensitive way.

Rapid Assessment

Field epidemiologists play a key role in the earliest stages of any relief effort. In addition to an appreciation for quantifiable data and for how and when to collect it, the "shoe leather" component of epidemiology is valuable in and of itself for conducting an initial rapid assessment. A wealth of information can be gleaned from observation during a walk-through of the affected area if one knows what to look for and how to employ basic qualitative techniques.

- If commodities are being sold or traded in the marketplace, then their price, compared with preemergency prices, indicates their availability or scarcity.
- Black markets spring up quickly in postdisaster settings, and the willingness of people to make major sacrifices to pay for essential commodities indicates dire need.
- Indicators such as the amount of and type of jewelry being worn can be meaningful (Box 22.2). The absence of traditional adornment in a society in which it is customary might signify food insecurity and that everything of value already has been sold.

Interviews with community leaders, transect walks through affected areas, and results from a constellation of methods that frequently are grouped as participatory rapid appraisals can be useful even before the analysis of survey data that might provide more accurate information but at the cost of timeliness. Of paramount importance for the field epidemiologist is reaching the disaster location as quickly as possible, visiting all affected

---

BOX 22.2
PRIORITIZATION BY OBSERVATION

In 1980, in one of the many emergencies on the Horn of Africa, women were observed to be wearing no jewelry, a sign that all valuables had been sold to purchase food that had become available at exorbitant prices. There was one exception, however: almost all women wore a thin string around their necks with a small, spoon-shaped pendant attached to it. The significance of this oddity eluded field epidemiologists assessing the health status of the population until a visiting ophthalmologist mentioned that this population suffered from an unusually high prevalence of trachoma. The spoon-shaped device, it was learned, was used to remove inverted eyelashes, an action that helped relieve the irritation and pain associated with the scratched and ulcerated cornea that are a feature of this disease. Their ubiquity was a testament to the importance of the disease—and keen observation was the key to diagnosing this public health problem.

Source: R. Waldman, unpublished data.

areas and population groups, and helping the relief community gather, collate, and assess the value of all information. Postemergency settings are dynamic, but ultimately decisions about public health and health service delivery must be made from day 1 on the basis of existing evidence (11).

Surveys

As valuable as nonquantitative data might be, the lack of routinely collected health information means that, as soon as is feasible, surveys will need to be conducted. A precise sampling frame will be difficult to establish at first, and careful judgment is needed to ensure that samples drawn from the population are representative. However, in most circumstances, a less than optimally representative systematically chosen sample will be superior to a convenience sample, especially if the results are to guide the equitable distribution of commodities and services.

A commonly used survey method is *two-stage cluster sampling*, first developed by the World Health Organization to measure vaccination coverage rates (12). The logistical demands of this method are far less than for either simple random sampling or systematic random sampling because relatively few clusters need to be visited to obtain statistically valid results with a reasonable degree of precision. Although sample sizes can be relatively large, the advantages of using this method usually outweigh the disadvantages. Nonetheless, two distinct disadvantages should be noted:

- Cluster sampling is not well suited for measuring characteristics that are not homogenously distributed in the population. For example, if malnutrition is clumped in certain areas, then cluster sampling might miss it entirely or, conversely, overidentify it, resulting in skewed, nonrepresentative values for the population as a whole.
- Cluster sampling can be difficult to explain to decision-makers.

Finally, a frequently overlooked problem with surveys is that nonsampling error is likely to be more important than the disadvantages of any sampling method. Surveyors need to be carefully trained to understand the objectives of the survey and the importance of collecting accurate and unbiased information. When people affected by an emergency have lost their possessions or suffered other shocks, they can be eager to please those they perceive to be in a position to help them by providing answers they think the surveyors want to hear, resulting in a sincere, but inaccurate, picture of reality. For example, people might not report household deaths because they fear having their rations decreased. Therefore, the field epidemiologist needs to be aware of the many real and potential biases in obtaining accurate information from an emergency-affected population and must take steps to ensure that none of the epidemiologic activities inadvertently contributes to further deterioration of the situation. For epidemiologists, as for clinicians, "do no harm" is an important rule.

Organizing Priority Interventions

The main goals of emergency relief are to save lives and restore individuals and communities to their preemergency conditions. Although individual- and population-directed health interventions are important in many settings, other types of interventions might take precedence. In the book, *Refugee Health*, the medical relief organization Doctors Without Borders suggested 10 top priorities in disaster response (13). Of the top five, only one—measles vaccination—is a health-specific intervention, and its importance might have diminished since publication of that book as more countries have achieved high measles vaccine coverage rates through routine health services. (In situations of protracted conflict, however, where primary healthcare services have been unavailable to the population for some time, vaccination coverage levels can fall dramatically. As a result, measles outbreaks have occurred increasingly throughout the Middle East and in migrant populations in Europe.) The other priorities are initial assessment; water and sanitation; food and nutrition; and shelter and site planning. Although these are clearly related to public health, in most international emergency responses they are considered to be distinct from the health sector.

Some humanitarian interventions address basic needs of the emergency-affected population slowly and even inadequately. For example, in the area of nutrition, field epidemiologists have been called on to identify, diagnose, and design appropriate interventions for rare conditions (e.g., scurvy, pellagra, and beriberi) while simultaneously implementing surveillance for acute moderate and severe malnutrition. Although relief team members who are experts on specific problems understandably will focus on those problems, the field epidemiologist needs to address the overall spectrum of the relief effort and promote the most appropriate interventions, regardless of the sectors to which the interventions might belong.

Public health surveillance is a critical element of disaster response, and its establishment usually becomes the responsibility of the on-site epidemiology team. In humanitarian settings, epidemiologists attempting to implement effective surveillance might have to address several challenges, including

- Balancing speed *and* accuracy in adverse conditions.
- Integrating multiple sources of sometimes conflicting data while determining which are credible and which are not.
- Soliciting others to participate in the surveillance effort when they might not assign it the same priority the epidemiologist does.
- Assisting decision-makers in using surveillance data to take action.

Rapidly established, well-monitored, and widely used surveillance systems have been instrumental in preventing deaths as, for example, in the aftermath of the Asian tsunami of December 1994, when on-scene, experienced epidemiologists helped conduct effective surveillance.

Conditions targeted for surveillance vary in relation to specifics of the setting. In most developing countries, at the start it may be sufficient to target a simple surveillance system toward syndromic presentations and easily recognizable conditions, such as acute lower respiratory illness (a proxy for pneumonia), acute watery or bloody diarrhea (cholera, dysentery), fever with or without stiff neck (malaria, meningitis), and measles. In other settings—especially in middle- and higher income countries—the focus might be on measuring the needs of chronically ill persons who might be cut off from their medications or procedures; in these situations, such conditions might be more prevalent than common acute communicable diseases. In all settings, surveillance should focus on the most vulnerable segments of the population (e.g., infants, children, older persons, women, destitute and underserved persons, and persons with special needs). To ensure they are not neglected, epidemiologists should disaggregate data to facilitate identification of health problems in these groups.

Coordination

Emergency relief almost always occurs in emotionally charged environments. Although the need for highly coordinated action is universally recognized (some have suggested that "poor coordination" should be recorded as a cause of death on death certificates), many responders might want to coordinate but not "be coordinated." The most common scenario is for a health cluster to be established at the onset of the relief effort. Government officials, representatives of the World Health Organization, and a designated person from a nongovernment organization usually are assigned joint responsibility for chairing cluster meetings and overseeing their functioning. In large disasters, such as the Haiti earthquake of 2010, several hundred responders regularly attended health cluster meetings, many seeking guidance on how to respond effectively (14).

The epidemiologist, for better or for worse, frequently is thrust into a position of responsibility and authority because most responders will not be familiar with the published medical and/or public health literature and few will be able to view the chaos through the objective lens of unbiased data. Epidemiologists responding to an emergency for the first time might be unfamiliar and even uncomfortable with the amount of respect they are accorded.

CONCLUSION

Humanitarian response settings are the emergency rooms of public health. Lifesaving, irreversible decisions frequently are made in the early phases of the relief effort. A fundamental task of the field epidemiologist is collection and circulation of essential data on the health and nutritional status of the affected population as accurately as possible in the shortest possible time. The purpose of these data is to help first responders prioritize the interventions most likely to limit excess preventable death. The environment is often chaotic, uncoordinated, and characterized by logistical and resource constraints, but the epidemiologist needs to be calm, assertive, and able to convey the power of accurately collected and analyzed data. Ultimately, however, successful contribution to a disaster response will be measured not on the basis of the elegance of the epidemiologic investigations, but rather as a function of how many lives are saved (15).

REFERENCES

1. Centre for Research on the Epidemiology of Disasters. http://www.cred.be
2. Brown RE, Mayer J. Famine and disease in Biafra: an assessment. *Trop Geogr Med*. 1969;21:348–52.
3. De Ville de Goyet C, Seaman J, Geijer U. *The Management of Nutritional Emergencies in Large Populations*. Geneva: World Health Organization; 1978.
4. Glass RI, Cates W Jr, Nieburg P, et al. Rapid assessment of health status and preventive-medicine needs of newly arrived Kampuchean refuges, Sakeo, Thailand. *Lancet*. 1980;1:868–72.
5. Sommer A, Mosley WH. East Bengal cyclone of November, 1970. Epidemiological approach to disaster assessment. *Lancet*. 1972;1:1029–36.
6. Toole MJ, Waldman RJ. Prevention of excess mortality in refugee and displaced populations in developing countries. *JAMA*. 1990;263:3296–302.
7. Goma Epidemiology Group. What happened in Goma, Zaire, in July 1994? *Lancet*. 1995;345:339–44.
8. The Sphere Project. *Humanitarian Charter and Minimum Standards in Disaster Response*. 3rd ed. Geneva: The Sphere Project; 2011.

9. Southeast Alaska Petroleum Response Organization. What is the incident command system? http://www.seapro.org/pdf_docs/ICS.Overview.pdf

10. Field Epidemiology Manual Wiki. Field epidemiology manual. https://wiki.ecdc.europa.eu/fem/w/wiki/field-epidemiology

11. Checchi F, Warsame A, Treacy-Wong V et al. Public health information in crisis-affected populations: a review of methods and their use for advocacy and action. *Lancet.* 2017;390:2297–313.

12. Henderson RH, Sundaresan T. Cluster sampling to assess immunization coverage: a review of experience with a simplified sampling method. *Bull World Health Org.* 1982;60:253–60.

13. Médecins Sans Frontières. *Refugee Health—An Approach to Emergency Situations.* London: Macmillan; 1997.

14. World Health Organization. Global health cluster guide. http://www.who.int/hac/global_health_cluster/guide_glossary_of_key_terms/en/

15. Waldman RJ, Toole MJ. Where is the science in humanitarian health? *Lancet.* 2017;390:2224–6.

/// 23 /// ACUTE ENTERIC DISEASE OUTBREAKS

IAN T. WILLIAMS, LAURA WHITLOCK, AND MATTHEW E. WISE

STEPS IN INVESTIGATING ACUTE ENTERIC DISEASE OUTBREAKS

Public health officials investigate outbreaks to identify the source, prevent additional illnesses, and learn how to prevent similar future outbreaks. This chapter provides an overview of how the public health community detects, investigates, and controls outbreaks of foodborne, waterborne, and other enteric (intestinal) disease and emphasizes multijurisdictional foodborne illness investigations in the United States.

An investigation of an outbreak of enteric disease involves certain procedural steps (Figure 23.1) (1). They are described here in sequence, but in reality and as explained in previous chapters, investigations are dynamic, resulting in multiple steps

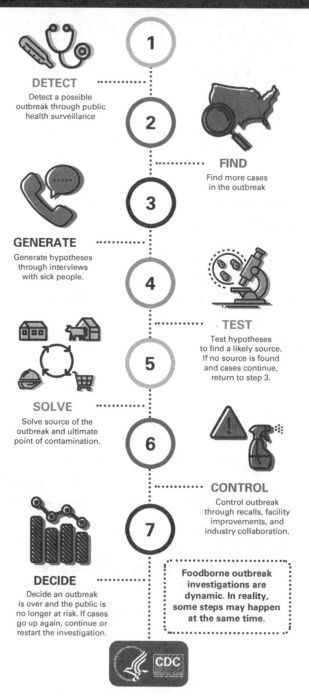

STEPS IN A FOODBORNE
OUTBREAK INVESTIGATION

1

DETECT
Detect a possible
outbreak through public
health surveillance

2

FIND
Find more cases
in the outbreak

3

GENERATE
Generate hypotheses
through interviews
with sick people.

4

TEST
Test hypotheses
to find a likely source.
If no source is found
and cases continue,
return to step 3.

5

SOLVE
Solve source of the
outbreak and ultimate
point of contamination.

6

CONTROL
Control outbreak
through recalls, facility
improvements, and
industry collaboration.

7

DECIDE
Decide an outbreak
is over and the public is
no longer at risk. If cases
go up again, continue or
restart the investigation.

Foodborne outbreak
investigations are
dynamic. In reality,
some steps may happen
at the same time.

CDC

FIGURE 23.1 Steps in an outbreak investigation. *Source*: Reference 1.

occurring simultaneously. Typically, enteric disease outbreak investigations involve the following steps:

- Detecting a possible outbreak.
- Defining and finding cases.
- Generating hypotheses about likely sources.
- Testing the hypotheses and evaluating evidence.
- Finding contamination sources.
- Controlling the outbreak.
- Determining when the outbreak is over.

Detecting a Possible Outbreak

Detecting a cluster or possible outbreak of enteric illnesses can occur in different ways. One way health officials find outbreaks is through public health surveillance. By systematically gathering reports of illnesses occurring over time, they know approximately how many illnesses to expect in a given period in a given area. A *cluster* occurs when a higher number of persons than expected appear to have the same illness in a given period and area. When an investigation reveals that ill persons in a cluster have something in common to explain why they all acquired the same illness, the group of illnesses is called an *outbreak.*

Informal reports occur when members of a community call the local or state health department to report a group of suspected enteric disease–related illnesses. This might happen, for example, if several persons became sick after eating at a group dinner. Health departments often maintain a system to monitor these reports. Sometimes a clinician (e.g., an emergency department physician) realizes that he or she is encountering more cases of an illness than would be expected and calls the health department directly to discuss it with the epidemiologists there.

Formal pathogen-specific reporting systems also play a vital role in outbreak detection, particularly for multijurisdictional outbreaks. Clinicians and microbiologists in each state must report infections that are on a list of notifiable diseases when they diagnose them among their patients. This list includes many foodborne and other enteric illnesses. As public health officials review disease reports, they might notice that the number of persons with a particular illness is higher than expected.

For certain enteric pathogens (e.g., *Listeria monocytogenes, Salmonella enterica,* and Shiga toxin–producing *Escherichia coli*), public health laboratories perform specific tests to help detect clusters that might otherwise be missed. When a clinician suspects that a patient has a foodborne illness, he or she might ask the patient to submit a fecal or other type of sample, depending on the clinical presentation of the illness or the suspected pathogen causing illness. The clinician sends the patient's sample to a clinical laboratory, where bacteria can be isolated and identified as, for example, *Salmonella* or Shiga toxin–producing *E. coli* O157. The clinical laboratory informs the clinician of the diagnosis so that this information can be used to determine whether and how to treat the illness. A sample of the bacteria also might be sent from the clinical laboratory to the state public health laboratory for further characterization.

When a culture is available, the state laboratory might conduct subtyping tests on the bacteria, including serogrouping, serotyping, or DNA *fingerprinting*, which can include pulse-field gel electrophoresis (2), multilocus variable-number tandem repeats analysis (3), or whole-genome sequencing (4). Serogrouping and serotyping categorize bacteria on the basis of certain markers on the surface of the bacteria. Although serogroup or serotype information often can provide enough information to identify a possible outbreak, especially when the cluster is localized, further subtyping is often needed to separate background illnesses, unrelated to an outbreak, from those connected to a common source. DNA fingerprinting methods are more specific than serogrouping or serotyping, and bacteria that share the same DNA fingerprint are more likely to share a common source: the more rare the fingerprint, the higher the likelihood that the illnesses are connected in some way. For bacterial enteric pathogens, state laboratories, as well as some local and federal laboratories, submit subtyping information to the Centers for Disease Control and Prevention's PulseNet system (5).

PulseNet is a national molecular subtyping network of public health and food regulatory agency laboratories. By reviewing the PulseNet database, health officials can identify clusters of illnesses caused by bacteria with the same DNA fingerprint at the same time, even if the ill persons are spread across many different health jurisdictions. This is especially useful when the number of illnesses in any one county or state is not large enough by itself to signal a possible outbreak (5).

Defining and Finding Cases

Often, the initially recognized illnesses reflect only a small part of the total outbreak. Finding additional ill persons is key to helping understand the size, timing, severity, and possible sources of the outbreak.

Early in an investigation, health officials usually develop a *case definition* to help determine which ill persons will be included as part of the outbreak. Case definitions may include details about the

- Pathogen or toxin, if known;
- Certain signs or symptoms typical for that pathogen or toxin;
- Time range for when the illnesses occurred;
- Geographic range (e.g., residency in a state or region); and
- Other criteria (e.g., the pathogen's DNA fingerprint).

Multiple case definitions might be used in an outbreak investigation, each with a different purpose. For example, one case definition might be for confirmed illnesses and another for probable or suspected illnesses. Generally, case definitions start more broadly and are updated and refined over the course of an investigation as new information becomes available. The number of illnesses that meet the case definition is called the *case count*.

Using the case definition, investigators search for more illnesses related to the outbreak. They do this by

- Reviewing local disease surveillance reports;
- Reviewing reports to laboratory surveillance systems (e.g., PulseNet);
- Asking local clinical and laboratory professionals to report cases of the particular illness more quickly (i.e., as soon as they suspect the diagnosis);
- Reviewing emergency department records for similar illnesses;
- Surveying groups or interviewing persons who might have been exposed to the suspected outbreak source (e.g., attended a common meal or event); and
- Asking health officials in surrounding areas to watch for illnesses that might be related (e.g., through *Epi-X* [6]).

Health officials monitor the progression of an outbreak by keeping track of who became ill, when they became ill, and where they live. Investigators use a graph called an *epidemic curve* or *epi curve* that displays the distribution of the number of illnesses occurring across a selected period (7). The pattern of the epidemic curve can help investigators determine whether ill persons were most likely exposed to the same contaminated source during a short period (e.g., at a single meal) or whether the exposure occurred over a longer period (e.g., several weeks or months). Investigators also use maps to denote where ill persons live so that they can see whether and how the outbreak is spreading within an area or community.

Generating Hypotheses About Likely Sources

A hypothesis is a reasonable suspicion of a vehicle as the contamination source for an outbreak and is based on specific facts and circumstances. Health officials use a process for developing and then testing a hypothesis to identify the source of the outbreak. The number of possible outbreak vehicles and the number of potential points of contamination can be enormous, especially for enteric pathogens transmitted through foods or ingredients. Hypothesis generation is an iterative process in which possible explanations are continually refined or refuted.

Pathogens that cause acute enteric disease outbreaks can spread by contaminated food or water, direct contact with an ill person, or direct or indirect contact with an infected animal or its environment. When investigating the illness source, health officials first need to decide on the likely mode(s) of transmission. The pathogen causing illness, the historical sources of illness with that pathogen, where ill persons live, the ill persons' demographic characteristics (e.g., age, sex, and race/ethnicity), and the shape of the epidemic curve can all provide clues about the source.

When exposure to a contaminated food is suspected, health officials must consider the considerable number of foods and ingredients that might be the source or vehicle of infection. They may also need to consider the ingredients used in the foods that ill persons report eating. Health officials interview the ill persons to find out where and what they had eaten and other exposures during the days or weeks before they became sick. The focus of the investigation is then further narrowed to the specific foods or other exposures reported by many of the ill persons. Sometimes health officials also interview ill persons' family members or other persons with similar exposures but who did not become ill. These interviews are called *hypothesis-generating interviews*.

The period interviewers focus on depends on the pathogen's incubation period—the time between becoming ill and the likely exposure that made the person ill (e.g., eating the contaminated food, drinking contaminated water or a beverage, having direct contact with an ill person, or direct or indirect contact with an infected animal). This period varies by pathogen. Which foods or other exposures they ask about depends on what health officials have learned so far in the investigation. If several ill persons had attended a single restaurant, hotel, or catered event, for instance, interviews will focus on the menu items prepared, served, or sold there. If no obvious place of exposure is identified, investigators might use a standardized questionnaire, also known as a *shotgun questionnaire*. This type of hypothesis-generating questionnaire includes questions about a long list of food items or open-ended questions that review each meal a person ate during the days before illness began (8). It typically also includes questions about grocery shopping locations, restaurant dining or attendance at events where food was served, dietary restrictions and use of dietary supplements, travel history, animal contact, and recreational water exposures.

From the interviews, health officials create a short list of the foods, drinks, or other exposures that many of the ill persons had in common. Exposures that none or few ill persons reported are considered less likely to be the source. Health officials then look at other information (e.g., population-based surveys of food consumption) to help determine whether exposure frequencies from ill persons are higher than would be expected among the general population (9). On the basis of the information they gather, health officials develop a hypothesis about the likely outbreak source. However, shotgun interviews can only identify potential vehicles that are included on the questionnaire. If this approach does not lead to any testable hypotheses about the outbreak source, intensive open-ended interviews might be better suited to elucidating hypotheses that are not included in structured questionnaires.

A *dynamic cluster investigation* process can help to quickly identify a hypothesis. In this process, initial ill persons in the cluster are interviewed by using a detailed exposure history questionnaire. As new exposures of interest are indicated during interviews, the initial ill persons are systematically reinterviewed to assess these new exposures uniformly. Newly identified ill persons also will be uniformly asked about these exposures. This approach is particularly helpful in identifying new or unusual exposures not listed on standard shotgun questionnaires.

Investigating illness subclusters can provide crucial clues about an outbreak source. If multiple unrelated ill persons ate at the same location of a restaurant or purchased food or groceries from the same store location within days of each other, it suggests that the contaminated food item most likely was served or sold there. A useful method for generating hypotheses in multistate outbreaks includes rapid and thorough investigation of restaurant or store clusters. Subcluster investigations can identify specific food vehicles and provide detailed information about such items for *trace-back investigations*. A trace-back determines and documents the producer, manufacturer, supplier, and distribution pathway(s) for the food item(s) of interest. A key goal in a trace-back is to determine whether there is a supplier or other point in the distribution chain in common.

Generating a plausible hypothesis is often challenging and can take substantial time for several reasons. First, interviews of ill persons highly depend on their ability to recall events. The time from illness onset to knowing the ill person was part of an outbreak is typically 2–4 weeks for outbreaks that rely on DNA fingerprinting (10). Ill persons might not remember in detail what they ate that long ago. Also, if the contaminated food is an ingredient, the task becomes even more difficult. Ill persons often do not remember or know the ingredients of their meals. These challenges can delay or prevent development of a plausible hypothesis. In certain situations, ill persons might be interviewed multiple times as new ideas arise about possible sources. Visiting someone's home and examining the foods in their pantry and refrigerator or obtaining permission to review information from purchase receipts, shopper cards, or food journals can be helpful.

Testing Hypotheses and Evaluating Evidence

Three types of evidence, or pillars, are used when evaluating hypotheses about the contamination source(s) in an enteric disease outbreak (Figure 23.2) (11).

- *Epidemiologic evidence* (e.g., data from interviews of ill persons; distribution of cases by person, place, and time; results of analytic epidemiologic studies; and the history of the suspected pathogen and the past outbreaks it has caused);
- *Evidence from a trace-back* of a suspected vehicle linked with ill persons to identify a common point where contamination might have occurred and an assessment of the production facility at that common point; and
- *Laboratory results* from testing a suspected vehicle or the production facility where contamination might have occurred.

Evidence from each of these pillars is evaluated in concert to determine whether the data support the conclusion that a suspected food or other exposure is the outbreak cause. Investigators typically determine they have identified the likely source of the outbreak when they have clear and convincing evidence from two pillars. In rare instances, data from one pillar alone might be sufficient to determine the likely source of an outbreak (e.g., point source clusters linked to a meal or single event). In investigations of products with a short shelf life (e.g., unpasteurized milk or leafy greens), conducting testing on products during the likely period of contamination might be impossible, and investigators must rely on evidence from the other pillars to determine the likely source of the outbreak.

A hypothesis should be tested to determine whether the source has been identified correctly. Epidemiologic analytic studies are often used to test hypotheses. Case–control studies or cohort studies are the most common types of analytic study conducted. Health

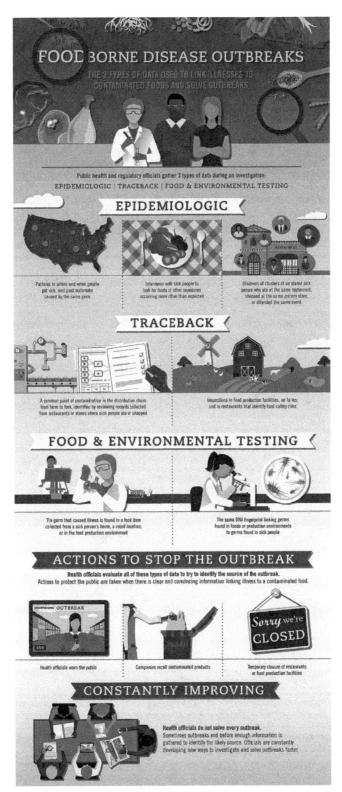

FIGURE 23.2 Evidence used to link illnesses to contaminated foods during outbreak investigations.
Source: Reference 11.

officials analyze information collected from ill persons and comparable well persons to determine whether ill persons are more likely than well persons to have eaten a certain food or to report a particular exposure. These types of analytic studies are often done for outbreaks associated with a single event or restaurant.

If ingestion of a particular food or some other exposure is reported more often by sick persons than by well persons, that food or exposure might be causing the outbreak. By using statistical tests, health officials can determine the strength of the association (i.e., how likely it is to have occurred by chance alone) and whether more than one food or other exposure might be involved. Investigators analyze many factors when interpreting results from these studies, including the frequencies of exposure(s) of interest; strength of the statistical association; dose-response associations; and the production, preparation, and distribution of the product.

If an outbreak is linked to a food that was prepared in different kitchens or to a food that was purchased from different stores and consumed without further preparation, the contamination event probably happened during the production and before preparation in the kitchen. In that situation, investigators perform a trace-back investigation to determine where the contamination occurred (Figure 23.3) (12).

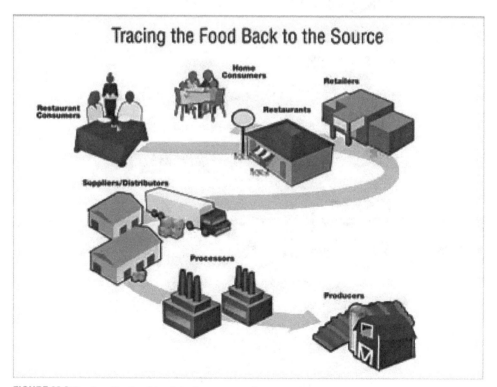

FIGURE 23.3 Tracing the food back to the source. *Source*: Reference 12.

Formal trace-back investigations are conducted by regulatory agencies at the state or federal level. These agencies rely on collecting records and documents to support possible product actions, such as a food recall. Trace-backs typically begin by identifying suspected food item(s) reported by ill persons or identifying restaurants or store locations where ill persons dined or shopped. The next step is to determine whether the production chain of the suspected food item(s) converges to a common point. Finding this point helps to define where contamination occurred and to support the hypothesis. Officials review purchase and shipment information from suppliers of the suspected item for the stores, restaurants, or cafeterias where they believe the item was bought or eaten. They then ask suppliers where they received the suspected item, and so forth, back to the point of production. Trace-back investigations can be resource-intensive and challenging, especially when the distribution pathway is complex or when detailed records are lacking at producers, suppliers, stores, or restaurants in the distribution chain.

During investigations where an ingredient is the cause of the outbreak, identifying the culprit can be more difficult because the contaminated ingredient might have been consumed as part of many different foods. In these situations, epidemiologic product tracing can be an important part of the process for identifying a foodborne outbreak vehicle (13). The overall goal of product tracing to aid an epidemiologic investigation is to determine whether a food item or items eaten by multiple ill persons in subclusters have a source or distribution point in common. Product distribution patterns can add specificity to exposures and assess the plausibility of one or more vehicles.

Testing of food, the environment, or water can provide useful information and support a hypothesis. Finding bacteria in an unopened container of food or in a food production facility with the same DNA fingerprint as clinical samples from ill persons in the outbreak can be convincing evidence of an illness source. However, investigators might not be able to identify a pathogen in the contaminated item for multiple reasons.

- Food items with a short shelf life (e.g., contaminated milk or produce) might be unavailable by the time the outbreak is identified and therefore cannot be tested.
- Even if the suspected food or water source is available, the pathogen might be difficult to detect because it might have decreased in number since the outbreak or other organisms might have overgrown the pathogen as the food started to spoil.
- The pathogen might have been in only one portion of the food. A sample taken from a portion that was uncontaminated will have a negative test result. Therefore, a negative result does not rule out this food as an illness source or outbreak cause.

- Leftover items or items in open containers might have been cross-contaminated from contact with an ill person or a meal preparation item or from contact with the item that actually caused the outbreak.
- Certain pathogens cannot be detected in food or water sources because no established test exists that can detect that pathogen in the suspected food or water.

Not finding a link between a specific item or other exposure and illness can happen for different reasons.

- When a restaurant serves meals containing multiple ingredients that are mixed or cooked together or used in multiple menu items, conducting epidemiologic studies to identify the specific contaminated ingredient can be difficult because of collinearity among exposures.
- Health officials might have recognized the outbreak so long after it occurred that they could not fully investigate it (e.g., food items might be unavailable for testing, ill persons might be unable to recall food histories accurately).
- An initial investigation might not have led to a specific, testable hypothesis; therefore, no analytic study was performed. Alternately, the initial hypothesis might have been wrong, making the results of any analytic study inaccurate or misleading.
- An analytic study might have been performed but did not find a specific exposure because the number of illnesses to analyze was limited, multiple food items were contaminated, or the contaminated item was a food that persons might have eaten but are unlikely to remember (e.g., ice in drinks, garnishes, condiments, or ingredients that are part of a food item).

If the outbreak has ended without the source being identified, the source is declared unknown. If the outbreak has not ended, health officials must keep gathering information and studying results to try to find the food or other source that is causing the illnesses. In these situations, the hypothesis generation process might have to be repeated as the investigation continues.

Finding Contamination Sources

If a likely source is identified, officials might perform an *environmental assessment* to determine the root cause and contributing factors for the outbreak (14). In foodborne illness outbreaks, this assessment might involve one or several facilities along the path from farm to fork. Illness in persons who had eaten food prepared in only one kitchen indicates that the contamination might have occurred in that kitchen. Health officials interview the persons who prepared the food to determine the ingredients used, the steps followed in preparing the food, and the temperatures used to prepare and hold the food. They review employees' health practices and training and the kitchen's cleanliness. They also check the health status of the workers at the time the exposures occurred. In a commercial or institutional kitchen or primary food production farm or facility, officials review past inspection reports for history of problems. Information from the environmental assessment can indicate ways to control the outbreak and prevent future similar outbreaks.

Controlling an Outbreak

After the likely source of illness is identified, immediate control measures might be needed. If a contaminated food stays on store shelves, in restaurant kitchens, or in home pantries or refrigerators, more persons might become sick. Outbreak control measures might include requiring specific measures to clean and disinfect meal preparation facilities, temporarily closing a restaurant or processing plant, recalling food items, informing the public about how to make the food safe, or telling consumers to check their homes and discard the suspected item. As health officials learn more during the investigation, they might modify, focus, or expand control measures and advice to the public.

Determining When an Outbreak Is Over

Not all outbreaks are solved. Investigators should continue to develop and test hypotheses if cases continue to be identified. An outbreak ends when the number of new illnesses reported returns to the number health officials normally expect. The epidemic curve helps health officials determine whether illnesses are declining. However, if illnesses begin to increase again after a noted decline, health officials will reopen the investigation. An increase in illnesses might indicate that the source was not completely controlled or that another unknown source of contamination is involved.

CONCLUSION

Investigating acute enteric disease outbreaks can be a dynamic and complex undertaking, often involving multiple public health and regulatory partners in different jurisdictions. Certain aspects of how the public health community detects, investigates, and controls foodborne and other enteric disease outbreaks are beyond the scope of this chapter. A more comprehensive review of outbreak detection and investigation methods for foodborne disease outbreaks is available in the Council to Improve Foodborne Outbreak Response's *Guidelines for Foodborne Disease Outbreak Response* (15).

ACKNOWLEDGMENTS

This work is based in part on "Multistate and Nationwide Foodborne Outbreak Investigations: A Step-by-Step Guide" (available at http://www.cdc.gov/foodsafety/outbreaks/investigating-outbreaks/investigations/index.html). The authors gratefully acknowledge the many staff at the Centers for Disease Control and Prevention who have helped contribute to developing these ideas and content, especially Robert Tauxe, MD, MPH, and Patricia Griffin, MD.

REFERENCES

1. Centers for Disease Control and Prevention. Steps in outbreak investigation. https://www.cdc.gov/foodsafety/outbreaks/pdfs/steps-in-oubreak-investigation-508c.pdf.
2. Centers for Disease Control and Prevention. Pulsed-field gel electrophoresis (PFGE). http://www.cdc.gov/pulsenet/pathogens/pfge.html
3. Centers for Disease Control and Prevention. Multiple locus variable-number tandem repeat analysis (MLVA). https://www.cdc.gov/pulsenet/pathogens/mlva.html
4. Centers for Disease Control and Prevention. Whole genome sequencing (WGS). http://www.cdc.gov/pulsenet/pathogens/wgs.html
5. Centers for Disease Control and Prevention. PulseNet. https://www.cdc.gov/pulsenet/
6. Centers for Disease Control and Prevention. Epi-X: building a network to save lives. https://www.cdc.gov/about/24-7/savinglives/epi-x/index.html
7. Centers for Disease Control and Prevention. Interpretation of epidemic (epi) curves during ongoing outbreak investigations. http://www.cdc.gov/foodsafety/outbreaks/investigating-outbreaks/epi-curves.html
8. Centers for Disease Control and Prevention. Foodborne disease outbreak investigation and surveillance tools. http://www.cdc.gov/foodsafety/outbreaks/surveillance-reporting/investigation-toolkit.html
9. Centers for Disease Control and Prevention. Foodborne diseases active surveillance network (FoodNet). http://www.cdc.gov/foodnet/surveys/population.html
10. Centers for Disease Control and Prevention. Timeline for reporting cases of *Salmonella* infection. http://www.cdc.gov/salmonella/reporting-timeline.html
11. Centers for Disease Control and Prevention. Foodborne disease outbreaks. https://www.cdc.gov/foodsafety/outbreaks/pdfs/outbreak-infographic.pdf
12. Centers for Disease Control and Prevention. Finding the point of contamination and source of the food. https://www.cdc.gov/foodsafety/outbreaks/investigating-outbreaks/investigations/contamination.html
13. Council to Improve Foodborne Outbreak Response. *Product Tracing in Epidemiologic Investigations of Outbreaks Due to Commercially Distributed Food Items*. Atlanta, GA: Council of State and Territorial Epidemiologists; 2015. http://cifor.us/news/new-white-paper-product-tracing-in-epidemiologic-investigations-of-outbreaks-due-to-commercially-distributed-food-items

14. Centers for Disease Control and Prevention. e-Learning on environmental assessment of foodborne illness outbreaks. http://www.cdc.gov/nceh/ehs/elearn/ea_fio/index.htm

15. Council to Improve Foodborne Outbreak Response. *CIFOR Guidelines for Foodborne Disease Outbreak Response*. 2nd ed. Atlanta: Council of State and Territorial Epidemiologists; 2014:153–4. http://cifor.us/clearinghouse/cifor-guidelines-for-foodborne-disease-outbreak-response

/// 24 /// SUSPECTED INTENTIONAL USE OF BIOLOGIC AND TOXIC AGENTS

STEPHEN PAPAGIOTAS AND KELLY SHANNON

INTRODUCTION

Most of the chapters in this manual focus on the epidemiologic investigation of exposures, illnesses, or outbreaks that have an unintentional or naturally occurring cause. For these events, epidemiologists and public health, in general, work with traditional health-sector partners who have similar professional cultures and expertise, familiarity with relevant laws, and use of investigative methods. In contrast, events involving the suspected intentional use of a biological or toxic agent require epidemiologists to work with nontraditional partners, specifically law enforcement. Cross-sector collaboration is necessary to prevent loss of life, protect public safety, and minimize adverse outcomes for both public health (e.g., increased morbidity and mortality) and law enforcement (e.g., inability to apprehend and/or convict the perpetrator).

Because most epidemiologic field investigations do not involve collaboration with law enforcement, interactions among the sectors during an investigation involving the malicious use of a biological or toxic agent can be challenging. To ensure successful outcomes of such investigations, public health and law enforcement can develop and implement processes to improve coordination and collaboration. This chapter provides a general guide for building relationships between public health and law enforcement that will facilitate timely identification, assessment, and investigation during outbreaks suspected of being intentionally caused.

EVENTS INVOLVING INTENTIONAL RELEASE OF BIOLOGICAL OR TOXIC AGENTS

The deliberate or intentional use of biological and toxic agents to harm populations is not new. Throughout history, governments, organizations, and individuals have used biological and toxic agents for malicious purposes, including as weapons of war (biowarfare), a form of terrorism (bioterrorism), or criminal acts (biocrime) (Table 24.1).

Because of the potential for many countries and nongovernment actors to be well funded and have the scientific and technical expertise to develop and intentionally use a biological or toxic agent, intentional events by these actors present substantial risks for public health and national security; however, the likelihood of occurrence is low (4). In an intentional situation, an epidemiologist is most likely to encounter an exposure or illness associated with a criminal act (i.e., biocrime) rather than an act of bioterrorism or biowarfare.

TABLE 24.1 Selected examples of biological or toxic agents used for intentional purposes

Agent	Perpetrator	Location	Year	Category
Pancuronium bromide (1)	Individual	Michigan	1975	Criminal
Salmonella typhimurium (2–4)	Organization	Oregon	1984	Terrorism
Bacillus anthracis (5)	Organization	Japan	1993	Terrorism
Shigella dysenteriae type 2 (6)	Individual	Texas	1997	Criminal
Bacillus anthracis (7)	Individual	Multiple US locations	2001	Terrorism
Nicotine (8)	Individual	Michigan	2003	Criminal
Tetrodotoxin (9)	Individual	Illinois	2008	Criminal
Ricin (10)	Individual	Texas	2013	Criminal
Ricin (11)	Individual	Mississippi	2013	Criminal

A *biocrime* involves the threatened or actual use of a biological or toxic agent for the sole intent of causing harm to another individual or group of individuals; in contrast, *bioterrorism* includes motivation to achieve a political or social objective. Because biocrimes usually target an individual or a group of people, public health consequences typically are limited. Although biocrimes can involve sophisticated production and use of biological or toxic agents commonly associated with bioterrorism, most events involve crude production or dissemination techniques and use biological or toxic agents that might not be commonly associated with bioterrorism (12). Additionally, a biocrime can occur even without the use of a biological agent. Many biocrimes result from the threatened use of a biological agent, which can involve the use of a suspicious or unknown substance (e.g., "white powder letter"). Although these "hoax" incidents do not involve the actual use of a biological agent, the threatened use is unlawful and is considered a crime (13). In the United States, most biocrimes are hoaxes or involve the production, acquisition, or use of a toxin, and the Federal Bureau of Investigation (FBI) responds to such incidents almost daily (John Woodill and Kelly Shannon, personal communication, January 27, 2017).

Although intentional events involving the actual use of biological or toxic material—compared with hoaxes—have occurred rarely in the United States, the accelerated pace of scientific advancement, availability of materials, and accessibility of information through the Internet have increased risks and vulnerabilities (14). Therefore, the potential use of biological and toxic agents by individuals and groups is likely to pose a long-term threat.

BUILDING RELATIONSHIPS

Because the response to an intentional event requires combined epidemiologic and law enforcement subject matter expertise, epidemiologists need to be versed in how to work with law enforcement. The first step is to identify the appropriate point of contact in law enforcement and establish a working relationship. An ongoing relationship will improve understanding of respective roles and responsibilities, informational needs, and investigational sensitivities during responses to biological and toxic events, whether intentional or unintentional. Improved understanding also fosters development of strong personal ties and trust that in turn facilitates information sharing and collaboration. Because roles and responsibilities differ among federal, state, and local law enforcement, contacts should be identified and relationships established at all jurisdictional levels.

In the United States, organizational structure and responsibilities for law enforcement differ across jurisdictional levels. For example, certain crimes are subject only or principally to federal jurisdiction; others are addressed primarily at the state or local level. As indicated by law (15), Homeland Security Presidential Directive 5 (16), and the National Response Framework (17), the FBI is the lead agency for criminal investigations of terrorist acts or terrorist threats, which includes weapons of mass destruction (WMD) incidents. As defined by law (18), a WMD is

- Any explosive or incendiary device: bomb, grenade, rocket, missile, mine, or other device with a charge of more than 4 ounces;
- Any weapon designed or intended to cause death or serious bodily injury through the release, dissemination, or impact of toxic or poisonous chemicals or their precursors;
- Any weapon involving a disease organism; or
- Any weapon designed to release radiation or radioactivity at a level dangerous to human life.

In addition to responsibilities specified by federal statutes or other legal authorities, an intentional biological incident might be investigated by state and/or local law enforcement and prosecuted under state criminal codes.

Because most intentional events involving biological or toxic agents are subject to federal statutes or other legal authorities, within a given jurisdiction the primary contact for public health will be the FBI WMD Coordinator at the local FBI field office. The WMD Coordinator, a designated Special Agent at each of the 56 FBI Field Offices, is responsible for federal-level prevention, response, and investigations related to WMD, including biological or toxic events. In addition to investigating WMD-related crimes and acts of terrorism, the WMD Coordinators conduct outreach with federal, state, and local stakeholders; industry; academia; and the scientific community. Through this outreach, the WMD Coordinator builds relationships and trust with partners, which facilitates the timely notification of incidents.

In addition, each FBI Field Office maintains a Joint Terrorism Task Force (JTTF) comprising Special Agents and Task Force Officers who represent a multitude of federal, state, and local law enforcement agencies that might have jurisdiction over other criminal activities identified and/or initially investigated by the FBI. The Field Office WMD Coordinator can be a conduit for communications with the JTTF in the event that public health needs an appropriate point of contact with a state or county police department.

Because of the benefits of established, ongoing relationships between public health and law enforcement entities, some jurisdictions have implemented official protocols or Memoranda of Understanding that outline practices for collaboration before and during events. The purpose for creating a formal document is that it extends the collaboration beyond a personal relationship and instills it as part of the agency culture and operations. Although these agreements are recommended and highly beneficial, the steps outlined within this chapter are relevant regardless of whether a Memorandum of Understanding is in place.

NOTIFICATION

Because most epidemiologic investigations do not involve a criminal act or malicious intent, determining when law enforcement should be notified can be difficult. Public health might be reluctant to share information with law enforcement before an outbreak has been confirmed and intentional exposure is suspected, but delaying notification while awaiting confirmation can hamper the timely exchange of information necessary to contain the outbreak, preserve evidence, conduct an investigation, and apprehend the perpetrators.

Establishing public health triggers for notifying law enforcement contacts can facilitate information sharing. The public health triggers (Box 24.1) are not intended as definitive criteria for notification but rather as a starting point to improve information sharing (19). Public health, with input from law enforcement, bases the triggers on the specific needs and circumstances of each sector and jurisdiction. A communications protocol that identifies an intended recipient, timeline (e.g., 30 minutes, 60 minutes), and a means (e.g., email, phone) for notification should be linked to the triggers. As public health becomes familiar with the process for sharing information with law enforcement,

---

BOX 24.1
SELECTED PUBLIC HEALTH TRIGGERS
FOR NOTIFYING LAW ENFORCEMENT

- A specimen (clinical) or samples (environmental) submitted to public health for analysis that tests positive for a biological or toxic agent.
- Large number of unexplained symptoms, illnesses, or deaths.
- Unusual disease presentation (e.g., inhalation vs. cutaneous anthrax).
- Endemic disease with unexplained increase in incidence (e.g., tularemia, plague).
- Higher than expected morbidity and mortality associated with a common disease and/or failure of patients to respond to traditional therapy.
- Death or illness in humans preceded or accompanied by death or illness in animals that is unexplained or attributed to a zoonotic biological agent.

notifications are anticipated to occur in a timely manner for events of mutual interest, even if they are not specifically identified by a trigger.

Legal Restrictions on Information Sharing

Barriers to sharing information between public health and law enforcement can remain, despite the establishment of relationships and public health triggers. One barrier to sharing information with law enforcement is the legal restriction placed on public health about information disclosure. At both federal and state levels, privacy statutes prevent the release of individually identifiable health information. Public health and other healthcare entities (e.g., healthcare providers, health maintenance organizations, healthcare clearinghouses) can use these statutes as justification for not providing information to law enforcement. However, exceptions exist that allow law enforcement access to protected health information provided certain requirements are met. For example, the Health Insurance Portability and Accountability Act of 1996 (HIPAA) (20) and corresponding HIPAA Privacy Rule (21) allow for disclosure of individually identifiable health information, without an individual's authorization or permission for national priority purposes. During a suspicious biological or toxic event, a likely exemption that law enforcement can use to request patient information from a healthcare entity is the "imminent threat exemption" (Box 24.2) (19).

States' laws governing privacy and information disclosure vary among states. Some states have stringent rules; others have higher standards or elaborate processes regulating information disclosure, such that invoking an exception to the HIPAA Privacy Rule might not be sufficient. Thus, public health should first review federal and state privacy laws to clarify the rules and regulations governing disclosure of protected patient information and then develop approaches with law enforcement to facilitate information

---

BOX 24.2
HIPAA/IMMINENT THREAT EXEMPTION

"A covered entity may, consistent with applicable law and standards of ethical conduct, use or disclose protected health information, if the covered entity, in good faith, believes the use or disclosure is necessary to prevent or lessen a serious and imminent threat to the health or safety of a person or the public and the disclosure is made to a person reasonably able to prevent or lessen the threat." See 45 CFR 164.512 (j)(1)(i).

sharing in accordance with those regulations. Awareness of all laws governing information sharing will facilitate timely identification and investigation of a suspected or actual intentional event.

Breach of the Public's Trust

Perceptions grounded in ethics and trust also can constrain information sharing and notification. Patients routinely provide personal information to physicians and public health with the understanding that their information will not be disclosed. The perception that public health is "informing" on individuals to law enforcement is an important concern, especially when the information might be associated with evidence of a crime (e.g., illicit drug use, prostitution). Infringements on the bond of trust might constrain a patient's willingness to provide information that could be critical to identifying an outbreak source or implementing effective control measures (22). Fortunately, such concerns can be addressed to enable the exchange of information between public health and law enforcement. Public health and medical providers routinely work with law enforcement to share patient information that might be associated with a criminal investigation (i.e., abuse/neglect) or public health intervention (i.e., quarantine), so this process is not uncommon. For a suspected or confirmed intentional event, a primary focus of the investigation is stopping the outbreak. To preserve the trust between public health and the individual, information related to minor or petty crimes, which is not associated with the investigation, is typically not prioritized by law enforcement. However, law enforcement may use this information to seek prosecution at a later date (19).

ASSESSMENT

Because many microbial pathogens are endemic or occur naturally in the environment, the intentional use of a biological agent initially might be difficult to discern from an unintentional outbreak (23). Public health generally considers that the source of a case or an outbreak is an unintentional exposure until proven otherwise. Even when the nature of an exposure has not yet been defined, many public health officials will indicate the illness is "not the result of bioterrorism" or "not bioterrorism." However, determining whether an exposure or illness is intentional is the responsibility of law enforcement (i.e., the FBI), not public health, because the scope of an epidemiologic investigation does not fully encompass determination of intent. The ability to determine intentionality relies on attribution of the act to a specific person or group of persons. The data sources and investigational methods used by law enforcement have been developed and implemented for this specific purpose. Conversely, the purview of law enforcement does not encompass a determination of whether an exposure is "not a health risk" because that determination is a public health responsibility. Therefore, any assessment needs to be conducted jointly, involving both law enforcement and public health (19).

The goal of a joint threat assessment is to determine the nature of the threat (i.e., credible or not credible) and identify potential health risk associated with the event. It can be initiated when either public health or law enforcement identifies a defined trigger for information sharing.

Typically, law enforcement and public health will participate in the joint threat assessment of a suspicious exposure, illness, or outbreak involving a biological or toxic agent; other federal, state, and local partners and subject matter experts also might be included, depending on event-specific circumstances. As part of the threat assessment, public health shares any critical or relevant information so that participants can make an informed decision about the nature (i.e., intentional or unintentional) of the event and appropriate follow-up activities. Specifically, public health should be ready to provide or discuss information related to case reports, laboratory results, exposure source, interventions, and overall health risk to the community and responders. Similarly, law enforcement will provide information relevant to assessing the threat, such as intelligence, criminal records checks, national-level trends, and other investigative data, as appropriate.

Once all available information has been shared, the event is classified into one of three risk categories (19):

- *No Threat*: No indication of a criminal act
- *Possible Threat*: Information suggests the event might be a result of a criminal act.
- *Likely Threat*: There is a reasonable belief the event was caused by a criminal act.

If "No Threat" exists, public health can manage the response. If a "Possible Threat" or "Likely Threat" exists, public health should implement a joint investigation with law enforcement.

JOINT INVESTIGATIONS

The scope of an epidemiologic investigation is similar for unintentional and intentional events—for both situations, epidemiologists will apply the traditional steps for an epidemiologic investigation (24). The distinction is that during a potential intentional event, epidemiologists will investigate jointly with law enforcement, referred to as a *criminal–epidemiologic (crim–epi)* investigation. The goals of crim–epi investigations are to

- Identify the disease- or illness-causing agent;
- Identify the source and location of the exposure;
- Determine the mode(s) of spread or transmission of the biological or toxic agent;
- Identify who might have been exposed;
- Direct interventions to reduce morbidity and mortality;
- Identify possible perpetrators; and
- Collect evidence for prosecution (19).

For public health, the crim–epi investigation does not replace the traditional epidemiologic investigation. Instead, it complements both the epidemiologic and law enforcement investigative processes by increasing the efficiency of the investigation through the exchange of real-time information. When implementing a crim–epi investigation, public health should consider several factors.

Information Sharing and Dissemination

A crim–epi investigation does not allow public health and law enforcement full access to each other's information and data sources. When conducting a crim–epi investigation, both public health and law enforcement will still abide by all applicable laws and regulations that govern their routine activities. For example, patient medical information that is not relevant to the investigation is not shared with law enforcement. Similarly, public health does not have access to law enforcement–sensitive information (e.g., informants, intelligence, and undercover operations) that is not relevant to the epidemiologic investigation.

Public health should continually review pertinent investigative information with law enforcement to ensure the accuracy of the information and avoid inconsistencies in reporting. The investigative information should be maintained in a manner consistent with established requirements to prevent unauthorized release (25). In the event that information is requested by entities other than the principal public health and law enforcement agencies—for example, another investigative party, media, or the public—the originating agency should be contacted and consulted before any information is released (25).

Evidence

The goal of a law enforcement investigation is identification, apprehension, and prosecution of the person(s) who committed the crime. Therefore, any information or materials collected by law enforcement during a criminal investigation is handled as potential evidence. For an intentional event involving a biological or toxic agent, evidence might include dissemination devices, clothing of victims or suspects, clinical specimens (e.g., blood, other body fluids or secretions), environmental samples, documents, photographs, and witness statements (19). Evidence must be collected, maintained through chain-of-custody (i.e., the documented accountability at each stage of collecting, handling, testing, storing, and transporting evidence), and analyzed in a manner consistent with evidentiary standards and that will withstand the challenges expected in a legal proceeding (26). Because a suspected or confirmed intentional biological or toxic event is considered a possible criminal or terrorist act until proven otherwise, information and materials collected by public health need to be preserved according to proper evidence collection procedures. Items that are not of central importance from an epidemiologic perspective might have value for the criminal investigation and should not be unilaterally discarded. In addition, public health participants involved in evidence collection or other aspects of the crim–epi investigation might be called as witnesses during the trial of a suspected perpetrator.

Crime Scene Access

A crime scene might not be readily apparent for an intentional biological or toxic exposure. Without the identification of a dissemination device or confession by a perpetrator, the specific location of the intentional exposure might be identified only through the epidemiologic investigation. Because of evidentiary needs of the criminal investigation, law enforcement will consider any location identified by an epidemiologic association as a potential crime scene, until determined otherwise, so public health access to the crime scene location might be limited and delayed because of the need to preserve evidence. If it is a concern that a time-sensitive health investigation could be negatively impacted by the limited and delayed access, then public health can work with law enforcement to address this issue by ensuring that samples or other evidence collected from the location fulfill both epidemiologic and criminal investigative needs.

Joint Interviews

To collect information from case-patients and potential contacts, a crim–epi investigation uses a joint interview by public health and law enforcement, rather than conducting separate public health and law enforcement interviews. Although the presence of law enforcement during a joint interview can provoke anxiety in the patient and public health, one interview with both agencies might be less disruptive to the patient and the investigation than two or more separate interviews. Additionally, separate questioning by law enforcement and public health can produce conflicting statements, which can jeopardize the outcome of the criminal investigation and public health interventions.

CONCLUSION

After the anthrax attack in 2001, it was indicated that public health and law enforcement need to develop working relationships for the response to biological and toxic agents (26). Although public health generally has made progress in developing partnerships with law enforcement, additional work remains. As part of the normal turnover in positions and key contacts, new relationships need to be constantly built and trust established. Additionally, it is essential that the information sharing, threat assessment, and joint investigation processes be constantly practiced and refined. Finally, as scientific knowledge increases and technology advances, the nature of biological and toxic threats will evolve. The mitigation of dynamic biological and toxic threats requires robust relationships between public health and law enforcement partners, as well as with other sectors (e.g., agriculture, veterinary medicine, food safety). Only through productive partnerships can public health and law enforcement be ready to respond to intentional biological or toxic events.

ACKNOWLEDGMENTS

The authors thank Dr. Toby Merlin and Dr. Satish Pillai for their guidance and contributions to the development of this chapter.

REFERENCES

1. Stross JK, Shasby DM, Harlan WR. An epidemic of mysterious cardiopulmonary arrests. *N Engl J Med.* 1976;295:1107–10.
2. Torok TJ, Tauxe RV, Wise RP, et al. A large community outbreak of salmonellosis caused by intentional contamination of restaurant salad bars. *JAMA.* 1997;278:389–95.
3. *US v Sheela et al.,* CR 86-53, Indictment (D Ore 1986), based on 18 USC §1365(a) and 1365(e).
4. Kortepeter, MG, Parker GW. Potential biological weapons threats. *Emerg Infect Dis.* 1999;5:523–7.
5. Takahashi H, Keim P, Kaufmann AF, et al. *Bacillus anthracis* incident, Kameido Tokyo. *Emerg Infect Dis.* 2004;10:117–20. Erratum in: *Emerg Infect Dis.* 2004;10:385.
6. Kolavic SA, Kimura A, Simons SL, Slutsker L, Barth S, Haley CE. An outbreak of *Shigella dysenteriae* type 2 among laboratory workers due to intentional food contamination. *JAMA.* 1997;278:396–8.

7. Jernigan DB, Raghunathan PL, Bell BP, et al. Investigation of bioterrorism-related anthrax, United States, 2001: epidemiologic findings. *Emerg Infect Dis.* 2002;8:1019–28.

8. Centers for Disease Control and Prevention. Nicotine poisoning after ingestion of contaminated ground beef—Michigan. *MMWR.* 2003;52:413–6.

9. US Department of Justice. Lake in the Hills man sentenced to federal prison for acquiring and possessing deadly neurotoxin [press release]. https://www.justice.gov/archive/usao/iln/rockford/2012/pr0924_02.pdf

10. US Department of Justice. New Boston, Texas woman sentenced for ricin letters [press release]. https://www.justice.gov/usao-edtx/pr/new-boston-texas-woman-sentenced-ricin-letters

11. Federal Bureau of Investigation. Mississippi man Sentenced in ricin letter investigation [press release]. https://www.fbi.gov/jackson/press-releases/2014/mississippi-man-sentenced-in-ricin-letter-investigation-1

12. Budowle B, Murch R, Chakraborty R. Microbial forensics: the next forensic challenge. *Int J Legal Med.* 2005;119:317–30.

13. Title 18 U.S.C. §1038.

14. Berger KM, Wolinetz C, McCarron K, You E, So KW, Hunt S. Bridging science and security for biological research: international science and security. Proceedings from the meeting, 2013 Feb 4–5; Washington, DC. https://mcmprodaaas.s3.amazonaws.com/s3fs-public/reports/International%20Science%20and%20Security%20AAAS-AAU-APLU-FBI%20%282013%29%20v%202.pdf

15. Title 18 U.S.C. §2332(f).

16. Homeland Security Presidential Directive 5. https://www.dhs.gov/sites/default/files/publications/Homeland%20Security%20Presidential%20Directive%205.pdf

17. Federal Emergency Management Agency. National Response Framework. https://www.fema.gov/national-response-framework

18. Title 18, U.S.C. §2332(a).

19. Centers for Disease Control and Prevention. Joint criminal and epidemiological investigations handbook. http://www.cdc.gov/phlp/docs/crimepihandbook2015.pdf

20. Pub L No 104-191, 110 Stat. 1936 (1996).

21. 45 CFR §§160, 164.

22. Quinlisk P, Hutin Y, Carter K, Carney T, Teale K. A community outbreak of hepatitis A involving cooperation between public health, the media, and law enforcement, Iowa 1997. In: Vogelstein B, Kinzler KW, editors. *The Genetic Basis of Human Cancer.* New York: McGraw-Hill; 2002:93–113.

23. Treadwell TA, Koo, D, Kuker K, Khan A. Epidemiologic clues to bioterrorism. *Public Health Rep.* 2003;118:92–118.

24. Pavlin JA. Epidemiology of bioterrorism. *Emerg Infect Dis.* 1999;5:528–30.

25. National Association of State EMS Officials. Joint public health–law enforcement investigations: model memorandum of understanding (MOU). http://www.nasemso.org/Projects/DomesticPreparedness/documents/JIMOUFinal.pdf

26. Bulter JC, Cohen ML, Friedman CR, Scripp RM, Watz CG. Collaboration between public health and law enforcement: new paradigms and partnerships for bioterrorism planning and response. *Emerg Infect Dis.* 2002;8:1152–6.

/// 25 /// SUICIDE, VIOLENCE, AND OTHER FORMS OF INJURY

JOSEPH E. LOGAN AND JAMES A. MERCY

INTRODUCTION

Field epidemiology often is not considered applicable to investigations of suicide, homicide, acts of nonfatal violence, or other fatal and nonfatal injuries. Investigations for such injuries and deaths are commonly believed to be the responsibility of law enforcement or the local or state coroner or medical examiners and not of public health officials. In fact, not until the 1970s and early 1980s were suicide and interpersonal violence recognized as public health problems rather than primarily matters for mental health care and law enforcement (1). The late '80s and early '90s continued to mark a wakeful period when local, state, and national leaders recognized increases in adolescent and young adult suicide, adolescent homicide, and homicide inequities disproportionately affecting African Americans over other racial/ethnic groups (1–3). For example, suicide rates for adolescents and young adults almost tripled during 1950–1990, and rates of homicide among youth in their late teenage years increased by 154% during 1985–1991 (1–3). In the realm of unintentional injury, although rates of motor vehicle–related deaths have declined substantially since the 1960s, during the past 15 years, death rates attributed to drug poisoning have tripled in the United States, driven primarily by the use of prescription and illicit opioids (4,5). These trends have generated demand for new thinking on ways to prevent self-directed and interpersonal violent and unintentional injuries. During 1979–1989, multiple reports from the Surgeon General, the Office of the Secretary of Health and Human Services, and the Centers for Disease Control and Prevention (CDC) pushed the national agenda of making suicide, violence, and other injuries public health priorities (2,3,6–8). Collectively, these reports called for the use of multidisciplinary public health strategies that proactively prevented injury. They also stated that effective approaches needed to involve multiple sectors, including healthcare, mental health, education, social services, and criminal justice. During this period, beliefs began to fade about whether mental health, education, and law enforcement initiatives alone were sufficient to handle the national burden of injury (6–8).

Concurrently, as injury prevention efforts incorporated the public health approach, the use of field epidemiology also gained momentum. Field epidemiologists helped discover new patterns or epidemics of injuries, why injuries sometimes clustered, what protected individuals or placed them at risk, and how public health officials can control local and sometimes national epidemics.

Injury-related epidemic investigations can involve intentional or unintentional injuries, and sometimes both. The *intent* of injury often directs which agencies are involved in subsequent investigations and therefore usually establishes the initial scope of an epidemic early in the investigative process. For example, for fatal injury–related cases, the local medical authorities will establish a "manner of death" of either suicide, homicide, accidental (hereafter referred to as "unintentional"), or undetermined (9). This initial classification sometimes directs which agencies should handle succeeding action if an epidemic of fatal injury cases is perceived. For instance, epidemiologic investigations into clusters of homicides might require stronger coordination with law enforcement efforts. Similarly, the intent behind nonfatal injury cases of interest (e.g., assault cases) can also determine whether law enforcement should be involved and therefore direct the initial scope of an epidemic investigation of nonfatal injuries. Sometimes, field investigators might pursue cases across multiple manners of death (e.g., suicide, unintentional, undetermined) or both intentional and unintentional nonfatal injuries (e.g., self-directed violence, unintentional) if they are most interested in a specific mechanism of injury, such as with drug poisonings. This is described later in the chapter.

Field epidemiologists investigate both nonfatal and fatal injuries, and sometimes both simultaneously. For example, field epidemiologists might investigate patterns of nonfatal and fatal suicidal behavior, nonfatal and fatal unintentional drug overdoses, or homicides and nonfatal violent assaults among specific populations of interest if there is reason to believe that both types of injuries are linked to the same risk factors.

Field investigations also can be short-term based on specific public health actions or services (10). For example, some investigations can be descriptive explorations that describe the magnitude, rate, and/or trends of a problem to determine whether an epidemic truly exists. Others might focus on other public health functions, such as determining the etiology of an outbreak, assessing service needs of a specific at-risk population affected by a traumatic event (e.g., a natural disaster) as part of a response effort or evaluating a public health program or policy, strategy, or surveillance system.

This chapter provides a brief overview on determining injury-related outbreaks, key questions to address, common exposures, and case examples of investigations by intent and by public health action. It also provides a brief overview of challenges often faced with injury-related epidemic investigations and examples of short- and long-term strategies used to help contain epidemics.

DETERMINING EPIDEMICS AND FOCUSING INVESTIGATIONS

An early step in an epidemiologic field investigation is to assess whether an epidemic exists (i.e., whether the occurrence of incidents in a community or region of a group of injuries of similar nature is clearly in excess of normal expectancy and derived from a common propagated source[a]). "Outbreaks" are sometimes referred to as epidemics that have "sudden or violent increases" in injuries at specific locations.[b] Field epidemiologists also can view epidemics, or outbreaks, as "clustering" of cases, another term that implies cases are grouped together, beyond an expected number, in a specific space and time period (11). For injury-related field investigations, common data sources for estimating rates and determining epidemics include census data, death certificates, law enforcement reports, emergency medical service records, and coroner/medical examiner reports. To identify epidemics, field epidemiologists first determine a case definition that includes person-, place-, and time-related characteristics. More advanced analytic techniques, such as density-based modeling (12), also can be used to identify local epidemic clusters. However, the application of such techniques in suicide, interpersonal violence, and other injury-related field epidemiology is still in its infancy because such techniques require large databases and a large number of cases (12,13); the number of cases often identified in injury-related epidemic clusters is too small to detect with such methods.

Once field epidemiologists establish an increased trend in rates and/or a clustering pattern, they need to focus the investigation to help address key epidemiologic questions. The questions include the following:

- What large-scale exposure(s) was (were) involved in propagating the outbreak or cluster?
- What individual-level or personal factors increase one's risk for the outcome of interest in the target population?
- Which risk factors in the target population might be more unique than those of other populations?
- Who is at increased risk?
- What factors protect against the outcome of interest, and are these factors unique in the target population?
- What are the possible points of intervention?

INVESTIGATIONS OF INTENTIONAL INJURY-RELATED EPIDEMICS

Epidemics of Suicidal Behavior

Two basic types of epidemics, or clusters, are known to be related to suicidal behavior: (1) point clusters and (2) mass clusters (14). "Point clusters" are a series of suicides or suicide attempts that occur closely in space and time. These clusters are most commonly investigated and often involve the interaction between at-risk persons and an immediate onset of a localized exposure (e.g., layoffs from a plant closing). "Mass clusters" are widespread geographically but grouped closely in time and are believed to be associated with widespread exposures (e.g., media stories, stock market crash).

Clusters of suicidal behavior occur for a variety of reasons, but "social contagion" is often perceived to play a role. Social contagion refers to a social effect of suicide, whereby one person attempts or dies of suicide and then others who felt connected or drawn to the victim, or the act, follow suit (15,16). The essential element of social contagion is that exposure to the suicidal behavior enhances risk for subsequent suicide attempts. Understanding the mechanism of social contagion (or the path of suicide exposure) can help field epidemiologists and other investigators take action (Box 25.1). Persons who

BOX 25.1
SUICIDE CLUSTER IN COMMUNITY A

PUBLIC HEALTH PROBLEM

During January 2004–December 2007, the suicide rate in a rural community increased from 12 to 141 deaths per 100,000 population, and suicide attempts increased from 273 to 967 per 100,000.

PUBLIC HEALTH RESPONSE

CDC's field investigation found that (1) risk factors for suicidal behavior included male sex (deaths only), adolescent/young adult age, gang activity, physical/sexual abuse, mental health problems, substance abuse, and domestic violence; (2) suicide by hanging was overrepresented, and first attempts by persons who recently had a friend die of suicide increased exponentially during this period (both findings suggested that "social contagion" partially precipitated the epidemic); and (3) residents believed the onset of behavior coincided with activities that "glamorized" the suicide deaths (e.g., spray painting verses in memory of victims on water towers).

TAKE-HOME POINT

Suicide can cluster and spread throughout a community through social contagion, and persons with multiple risk factors are particularly vulnerable to this social effect. Field investigators identified the mechanism/venues driving the social contagion and used that information to help stop the spread of suicide. CDC worked with the community to change the messaging about suicide toward how to seek help as a preventive intervention.

Source: Logan J, Halpin J, Diekman S, Vawter L, Crosby, unpublished data, 2009.

attempt suicide after exposure to suicidal behavior usually are those already at risk or "primed" (i.e., have many risk factors) for suicidal behavior (14). The social contagious path between victims might be strong if the two victims had a tight bond (e.g., suicide of one person resulted from him or her being depressed about another person's suicide). Sometimes the path is less direct: at-risk persons might simply become attracted to a community's reaction to a suicide, especially if local residents "glamorized" the victim or the act (Logan J, Halpin J, Diekman S, Vawter L, unpublished data; 15,16); this positive public attention can make suicide appear to be an appealing and honorable option to solving problems. In some clusters related to social contagion, victims even copy specific mechanisms of suicide (Logan et al., unpublished data). For example, cases may replicate a specific method of hanging.

Epidemics of Homicide and Nonfatal Interpersonal Violence

Similar to investigations into suicidal behavior, homicides and nonfatal forms of interpersonal violence can cluster and be linked to exposures that lend to intervention. When field epidemiologists work with law enforcement officials, the role of field epidemiology is to focus on preventing future injuries and deaths by identifying at-risk persons and relevant exposures in need of immediate public health action. For example, identifying and arresting a homicide perpetrator on a killing spree in a community can sometimes be a long process and not a feasible short-term strategy for intervening on the violent outbreak; however, field epidemiologists can use public health methods to identify ways to protect community members from being victimized by the perpetrator (Box 25.2).

BOX 25.2
CHILD MURDERS (ATLANTA, GEORGIA)

PUBLIC HEALTH PROBLEM
During July 1, 1979–March 15, 1981, 22 unsolved child homicides and two child disappearances occurred in Atlanta.

PUBLIC HEALTH RESPONSE
CDC field investigators conducted a case-comparison analysis of the victims and a case–control study comparing victims with other children in the community. Victims shared similar characteristics (e.g., young [children], black, male, overrepresentation of death by asphyxiation) that were distinct from other child homicide victims; these findings suggested the deaths were a discrete cluster. Case-children were more likely than control children to run errands for money and spend time alone on the streets or in shopping centers, which suggested a single perpetrator who was local and knew the children were approachable.

TAKE-HOME POINT
Field epidemiologists helped law enforcement by determining that case-children were part of a unique cluster, the deaths were most likely linked to the same exposure (i.e., same perpetrator), and specific factors placed children at risk for abduction (i.e., being alone, running errands for money). The public health approach also informed local residents about measures for protecting children (e.g., early curfews, parental supervision) until an arrest could be made.

Source: Reference 17.

Homicide and assault outbreaks also can result from gang activity. Gang-related homicides and assaults can spike when rival gangs engage in conflict and retaliation. Although field epidemiologists might not be able to immediately rid a community of gangs, they may be able to identify locales with escalated gang conflict and provide information to public health programs that specialize in stopping retaliatory gang activity in a community. Such programs include those that use the Cure Violence model (initially called CeaseFire) [18]). This model recruits former gang members and other community leaders who are respected among gang members to resolve gang conflicts peacefully, thereby interrupting the sequelae of retaliatory acts of violence. The Cure Violence program members who conduct these actions are called "the interrupters." A future growth area for this program involves leveraging epidemiologic analyses to better inform and target the efforts of Cure Violence interrupters and other staff members who interact with the communities they serve.

INVESTIGATIONS OF UNINTENTIONAL INJURY-RELATED EPIDEMICS

Epidemics or clusters of nonfatal and fatal unintentional injuries also occur. Unintentional injuries are most often investigated in accordance with the mechanism of injury, such as drowning, motor vehicle crash, drug overdose, or natural disaster (e.g., hurricanes, tornados, earthquakes, tsunamis). The subsequent field investigations of such injuries usually focus on understanding the mechanism, intervening on the mechanism, or determining what places individuals at risk of injury by the mechanism. Investigations initially focused on unintentional injury and/or a specific mechanism may eventually broaden the scope of cases to investigate by including multiple manners of death if manner classification is difficult and unreliable. For example, medical authorities sometimes find it difficult to classify poisoning cases as "unintentional" or "suicide" and therefore sometimes misclassify such poisoning cases as one or the other or as having an "undetermined" manner of death (19).

Field epidemiologists frequently investigate ways to reduce injury and death related to drug overdose. During 2000–2014, unintentional drug poisoning deaths and death rates per 100,000 persons tripled in the United States (4,5). This increase in drug-related poisoning mortality has been attributed largely to abuse of prescription and illicit opioids (20). During the 1990s, opioid prescribing became more common for managing chronic noncancer pain, consistent with clinical recommendations at the time based on the evidence available, and the widespread misperception about the low risk for addiction when opioids were prescribed long term (21,22). Over time, the numbers of prescriptions increased, at higher dosages, and for longer durations. In 2015, the amount of opioids prescribed was three times higher than in 1999 (23). Recently, the supply of heroin and illicitly manufactured fentanyl increased throughout parts of the United States, which has been associated with an increase of overdoses involving these drugs (24). In response to the opioid epidemic, field epidemiology has made important contributions to help understand the associated exposures (i.e., drugs involved in overdose deaths), the characteristics of overdose victims and risk factors for death, and the points of intervention (Box 25.3).

The aggregate findings of many epidemiologic field investigations and evaluation studies have also shown substantial decreases in deaths in areas with stricter laws governing opioid supply channels (e.g., pill mill laws) (26,27), which further highlights the importance of understanding the epidemiologic burden of overdoses in relation to key large-scale sources of exposure. Epidemiologic studies have informed other strategies to help reduce the opioid overdose epidemic. Such strategies include

---

BOX 25.3
DRUG OVERDOSE INVESTIGATION (WEST VIRGINIA)

PUBLIC HEALTH PROBLEM

During 1999–2004, West Virginia had the greatest increase (550%) in unintentional poisoning–related deaths in the United States.

PUBLIC HEALTH RESPONSE

Using data sources provided by the state's Office of the Chief Medical Examiner (i.e., autopsy reports, toxicology reports, death-scene investigation reports, death certificates, and copies of the medical records) and records from the state's controlled substance monitoring program, CDC field investigators characterized West Virginia residents who died of drug overdoses in 2006 with regard to potential risk factors and the types of drugs that were associated with their deaths. Most overdose deaths were associated with nonmedical use of pharmaceuticals, primarily opioid analgesics. Drug diversion (i.e., use without a prescription) was identified in 63% of the cases, and 21% of the decedents sought drugs from multiple providers (i.e., showed evidence of "doctor shopping").

TAKE-HOME POINT

This seminal investigation of overdoses helped focus areas for prevention efforts (e.g., safer prescribing of opioids, clinical use of prescription drug monitoring programs that can identify persons seeking multiple prescriptions).

Source: Reference 25.

- Promoting safe opioid-prescribing practices through guidelines to help reduce future risk for addiction.
- Enhancing clinician use of prescription drug monitoring programs to identify patients who might be seeking prescriptions from multiple providers.
- Implementing naloxone distribution programs (naloxone can inhibit the effects of opioids and immediately prevent death among persons experiencing an overdose).
- Improving access to substance abuse and medication-assisted treatment for persons addicted to opioids (23,28).

EPIDEMIOLOGIC FIELD INVESTIGATIONS BY PUBLIC HEALTH ACTION

As mentioned, field investigations can sometimes focus on public health action or service. For example, investigations can be descriptive in nature, use etiologic inquiries, or be response oriented or evaluation oriented (10). Large epidemics sometime require different agencies taking on different actions. For example, in interagency responses, the local health departments might be tasked with describing the magnitude and timing of an epidemic in their respective geographic areas, whereas a federal agency might conduct the etiologic investigation to help understand why it occurred. This division of labor is sometimes done to help gather resources if the epidemic is believed to be too large for one agency to handle. Field investigators must also focus their investigation based on the needs of the authorities requesting assistance and the communities they represent.

Descriptive Investigations

Description-based epidemiologic field investigations are conducted to help understand the magnitude of a problem and to establish basic epidemiologic patterns (e.g., person, place, time characteristics and recent trends). This type of investigation particularly helps to determine whether there is an epidemic or outbreak and to generate hypotheses. These investigations often use existing data sources or survey data (Box 25.4) or link multiple data sources.

Etiologic Investigations

Etiology-based field investigations examine why an epidemic is occurring, which helps identify appropriate evidence-based practices as prevention strategies. These investigations often assess risk and protective factors in the target population, compare these factors with those of other populations to determine how the target population

---

BOX 25.4
SEXUAL VIOLENCE AGAINST CHILDREN (SWAZILAND, AFRICA)

PUBLIC HEALTH PROBLEM

Concern has increased about sexual violence against children in sub-Saharan Africa.

PUBLIC HEALTH RESPONSE

Using a two-stage cluster design, CDC field investigators and UNICEF surveyed female children to ascertain national estimates of sexual violence among this population, discern characteristics of the sexual violence, and identify who was at highest risk. In addition to determining that one in three women aged 13–24 years experienced sexual violence, investigators learned that the sexual violence largely involved perpetrators who were partners (e.g., husbands, boyfriends) of, or someone well known to, the victims.

TAKE-HOME POINT

Using this information, field investigators provided recommendations to in-country authorities for addressing the problem, including developing programs that improved intimate partner relationships and trained persons in communities to recognize signs of and respond to domestic-related sexual violence incidents.

Source: Reference 29.

---

is unique, determine which factors are associated with the timing and onset of the epidemic, and identify which factors present the best points for interventions. Field investigators might use mixed methods of investigation, including quantitative methods (e.g., case–control, case–cohort or cohort, and cross-sectional study designs) and qualitative methods (e.g., focus group analyses). These investigations sometimes not only identify risk factors but also use advanced analytic models with the etiologic data to refine definition of groups at greatest risk. One example was a field investigation that used predictive analytics with etiologic data to identify youth at greatest risk for firearm violence (Box 25.5).

Response-Oriented Investigations

Epidemiologic field investigations can be conducted after a communitywide traumatic event to identify critical needs and ways to prevent future injuries. Such rapid needs assessments can help local authorities allocate appropriate medical or mental

BOX 25.5

FIREARM VIOLENCE EPIDEMIC (WILMINGTON, DELAWARE)

PUBLIC HEALTH PROBLEM

During 2011–2013, the number of victims of shootings in Wilmington increased from 95 to 154.

PUBLIC HEALTH RESPONSE

Focusing on youth, CDC field investigators identified which groups were at greatest risk for firearm-related crime by analyzing administrative databases across multiple sectors (health, child welfare, juvenile services, labor, and education). They conducted a matched case–control study (case-youths were those who engaged in violent firearm crime and controls were other youth) and compared groups with respect to sentinel life events that were key documented events in these databases that could be risk factors for firearm violence (e.g., having been arrested, having been a victim of violence). Using predictive analytic methods, field investigators determined these linked administrative data sources can identify at-risk persons with great accuracy. Youth involved in firearm crime on average had 13 sentinel events, compared with an average of two for controls.

TAKE-HOME POINT

The key result of this investigation was that cities can merge existing data sources, examine risk factors, and prospectively identify who is at-risk for firearm-associated violence with great precision.

Source: Reference 30.

health services. Examples of response-based investigations are those conducted after Hurricane Andrew in 1993; Hurricane Allison in 2001; the 2002 Washington, DC, sniper shootings (Box 25.6); Hurricanes Rita and Katrina in 2005; the Iowa floods in 2008; the Washington, DC, Metrorail crash in 2009; and tornados in Alabama in 2011. These investigations generally use cross-sectional study designs.

Evaluation-Oriented Investigations

Evaluation-oriented field investigations can provide pilot evaluation findings to inform policy or program efforts, other prevention strategies, public health surveillance systems, or even public health survey instruments. They typically gather pilot data and evaluation results to inform decision-makers on whether they should embark on a larger evaluation

---

BOX 25.6
SNIPER SHOOTINGS (WASHINGTON, DC)

PUBLIC HEALTH PROBLEM

In October 2002, 10 people were shot and killed in public during a 3-week shooting spree in the Washington, DC, metropolitan area. Victims were shot while pumping gas, mowing lawns, walking outdoors, sitting on public benches, and conducting other activities of everyday life. The shootings evoked widespread fear among residents of the affected communities.

PUBLIC HEALTH RESPONSE

CDC launched an epidemiologic field investigation to assess the psychological and behavioral responses to shootings among the local residents. Investigators examined measures of traumatic stress symptoms, perceptions of safety, behavioral responses, and exposures to the shootings. They discovered 45% of residents reported going to public places less frequently, and women who resided within 5 miles of any shooting were more likely than women living farther away to report symptoms consistent with posttraumatic stress disorder.

TAKE-HOME POINT

The findings showed severe violent incidents, such as the sniper shootings, can profoundly affect the psychological well-being of communities. The aftermath of such incidents requires the partnering of clinical and community leaders to address fear and to ensure that residents in close proximity to the violent exposure can access mental health services.

Source: Reference 31.

---

effort. One example is a field investigation that evaluated whether children or parents can validly report on a child's swim skill (Box 25.7). This report greatly enhanced surveillance efforts intended to monitor child swimming ability, a known protective factor against drowning, across different populations.

KEY CHALLENGES

Epidemiologic field investigations of injuries have encountered challenges in common with and different from responses to investigations of infectious disease and other acute outbreaks. Here are three common challenges and strategies for addressing these challenges drawn from experiences in previous investigations:

BOX 25.7

EVALUATION OF SELF AND PARENTAL REPORTS OF SWIM SKILL AMONG CHILDREN (WASHINGTON STATE)

PUBLIC HEALTH PROBLEM

Drowning is the second leading cause of unintentional injury death among children. Although drowning risk is decreased for those who have swimming skills, surveillance data on child swimming ability is normally collected through self- or proxy reports rather than observed in-water performance. The use of validated survey measures of swim skills is essential for public health officials to know the true prevalence and accuracy of this drowning protective factor among youth.

PUBLIC HEALTH RESPONSE

CDC and Seattle Children's Hospital responded to a field epidemiologic aid ("Epi-Aid") request to evaluate the validity of self-reports and parental reports of a child's swim skill. This pilot evaluation also explored which swim skill survey measure(s) best correlated with children's in-water swim performance. A total of 482 parent–child dyads were recruited at three outdoor public pools in Washington state. Parent and child reports of three swim survey measures (i.e., "ever taken swim lessons," "perceived good swim skills," and "comfort in water over head") were compared with the child's in-water swim performance. Only parental reports of "perceived good swim skills" were validated with actual child swim ability.

TAKE-HOME POINT

This field investigation was evaluation-oriented and helped determine how well a public health surveillance system can accurately assess and report on an important protective factor against children's drowning. Parent report of perceived "good swim skills" was a strong survey measure to assess child's swim skill; history of swim lessons was not a useful measure. The findings from this investigation informed a statewide youth health survey on how to accurately measure child swimming skills in a community.

Source: Reference 32.

- Local authorities and stakeholders can exert pressure to influence the investigation and its findings. Sometimes local authorities or stakeholders are motivated to be part of an investigation because of political or even personal reasons (e.g., a family member died by suicide). These stakeholders can set high expectations, demand exploration into personal theories, or simply attempt to derail an investigation to avoid unwelcome consequences. Lead field investigators who briefly explain to requesting parties what an investigation can realistically yield, including that not all questions of interest can be answered because of time and resource constraints and that the findings might not be popular with all stakeholders, will have better outcomes with the community. It would also be beneficial for field investigators to indicate clearly that the investigation will base recommendations on what the findings reveal, even if they are unpopular.

- Sample size constraints can limit the amount of information gleaned from an investigation. Clusters of suicide and homicide in particular can involve a small number of cases. Nevertheless, as the examples in this chapter show, investigators manage to conduct case–control, cross-sectional, and/or other descriptive studies. It is best to be aware of the sample constraints, attempt to focus on the most salient factors, and be cautious about how the findings are generalized to the underlying population when sharing these findings with local authorities. Investigators also should be straightforward with authorities and community stakeholders on the limitations inherent in examining small samples and the possibility that such samples might not provide the statistical power to identify anything beyond what is already known.

- Restrictions on primary data collection can limit access to information. For example, when CDC is sponsoring new data collection in response to a state request for urgent epidemiologic assistance, approval must be sought for the data collection from the US Office of Management and Budget (33). This approval process can last up to a year. Mechanisms exist for rapid approvals, but these mechanisms do not always apply to injury- and violence-related epidemic investigations. Therefore, CDC field investigators often must rely on secondary data, which can greatly restrict the kinds of questions that can be answered and the kinds of analyses that can be undertaken. One way to minimize this potential barrier is to link and analyze existing data sources that capture complementary details on the cases of interest. For example, with regard to homicides and suicides, investigators can link multiple data sources, such as law enforcement, coroner/medical examiner, and toxicology reports, by case incident to review details on each case gathered from multiple perspectives (34).

SHORT-TERM AND LONG-TERM PREVENTION EFFORTS

The essence of epidemiologic field investigations ultimately is to help identify short- and long-term prevention strategies. Short-term interventions are intended to stop the immediate spread of the problem; long-term recommendations are directed at making sustainable communitywide changes. A number of resources on injury-related prevention strategies are available to help take action and save lives. However, a good field investigation is always useful to direct public health officials to the most appropriate ones. Furthermore, field epidemiology will remain a cornerstone for innovation and development of new prevention strategies. Some of the most impactful ideas on preventing injury today were once small ideas generated from field investigations. The frontline work of "shoe-leather epidemiology," a common term for field epidemiology, can change the thinking on injury prevention especially as new problems emerge, technology advances, and the mechanisms for how people interact and communicate evolve. For more details on existing resources useful to field epidemiologists with regard to preventing injury- and injury-related outbreaks, review the following:

- CDC's Striving to Reduce Youth Violence Everywhere (35).
- University of Colorado, Boulder's Blueprints for Healthy Youth Development (36).
- Cure Violence (18).
- Technical packages on the best available evidence for preventing child abuse and neglect (37), sexual violence (38), youth violence (39), suicide (40), and intimate partner violence (41).
- CDC Guideline for Prescribing Opioids for Chronic Pain (42).
- World Health Organization. Global Report on Drowning: Preventing a Leading Killer (43).
- World Health Organization. Save LIVES—A Road Safety Technical Package (44).

NOTES

a. "Epidemic," in Gordis L., ed. *Epidemiology*. 2nd ed. Philadelphia: W. B. Saunders Company; 2000. CDC, the World Health Organizations, and Merriam-Webster all.
b. "Outbreak," Merriam-Webster.com. 2017. https://www.merriam-webster.com/dictionary/outbreak

REFERENCES

1. Dahlberg LL, Mercy JA. The history of violence as a public health issue. *AMA Virtual Mentor.* 2009;11:167–72.
2. Alcohol, Drug Abuse, and Mental Health Administration. Report on the Secretary's Task Force on Youth Suicide. Volume 1: overview and recommendations. https://www.hsdl.org/?view&did=743317
3. CDC. Homicides among 15–19-year-old males—United States, 1963–1991. *MMWR.* 1994;43:725–7.
4. CDC. Web-based Injury Statistics Query and Reporting System (WISQARS). https://www.cdc.gov/injury/wisqars/
5. Rudd RA, Seth P, David F, Scholl L. Increases in drug and opioid-involved overdose deaths—United States, 2010–2015. *MMWR.* 2016;65:1445–52. Erratum in: *MMWR*, 2017;66:35.
6. US Department of Health, Education, and Welfare. Healthy people: the Surgeon General's report on health promotion and disease prevention. Washington, DC: US Department of Health, Education, and Welfare, Public Health Service; 1979. https://profiles.nlm.nih.gov/ps/access/NNBBGK.pdf

7. Institute of Medicine and National Research Council. *Injury in America: A Continuing Public Health Problem.* Washington, DC: National Academies Press; 1985.

8. US Department of Health and Human Services. US Department of Justice. Surgeon General's Workshop on Violence and Public Health Report. Washington, DC: Health Resources and Services Administration; 1986. https://www.nlm.nih.gov/exhibition/confrontingviolence/materials/OB10998.pdf

9. CDC. National Center for Health Statistics. Medical examiners' and coroners' handbook on death registration and fetal death reporting. 2003 revision. Hyattsville, MD: US Department of Health and Human Services; 2003. https://www.cdc.gov/nchs/data/misc/hb_me.pdf

10. Halperin WE. Field investigations of occupational disease and injury. In: Gregg MB, ed. *Field Epidemiology.* 2nd ed. New York: Oxford University Press; 2002:306–23.

11. CDC. Lesson 1: Introduction to epidemiology. Section II: Epidemic disease occurrence. Principles of epidemiology in public health practice, third edition: an introduction to applied epidemiology and biostatistics. https://www.cdc.gov/ophss/csels/dsepd/ss1978/lesson1/section11.html

12. Ester M, Kriegel H, Sander J, Xu X. A density-based algorithm for discovering clusters in large spatial databases with noise. KDD'96 Proceedings of the Second International Conference on Knowledge Discovery and Data Mining. 1996 Aug 2–4; Portland, OR. Palo Alto, CA: AAAI Press; 1996:226–31. http://www.aaai.org/Papers/KDD/1996/KDD96-037.pdf

13. Corcoran JJ, Wilson ID, Ware A. Predicting the geo-temporal variations of crime and disorder. *Int J Forecasting.* 2003;19:623–34.

14. Joiner TE Jr. The clustering and contagion of suicide. *Curr Dir Psychol Sci.* 1999;8:89–92.

15. Ali MM, Dwyer DS, Rizzo JA. The social contagion effect of suicidal behavior in adolescents: does it really exist? *J Ment Health Policy Econ.* 2011;14:3–12.

16. de Leo D, Heller T. Social modeling in the transmission of suicidality. *Crisis.* 2008;29:11–9.

17. Blaser MJ, Jason JM, Weniger BG, et al. Epidemiologic analysis of a cluster of homicides of children in Atlanta. *JAMA.* 1984;251:3255–8.

18. Cure Violence. http://cureviolence.org/

19. Rockett IR, Hobbs G, De Leo D, et al. Suicide and unintentional poisoning mortality trends in the United States, 1987–2006: two unrelated phenomena? *BMC Public Health.* 2010;10:705.

20. Paulozzi LJ, Budnitz DS, Xi Y. Increasing deaths from opioid analgesics in the United States. *Pharmacoepidemiol Drug Saf.* 2006;15:618–27.

21. Leung PTM, Macdonald EM, Stanbrook MB, Dhalia IA, Juurlink DN. A 1980 letter on the risk of opioid addiction. *N Engl J Med.* 2017;376:2194–5.

22. American Academy of Pain Medicine and American Pain Society. The use of opioids for the treatment of chronic pain: a consensus statement from the American Academy of Pain Medicine and the American Pain Society. *Clin J Pain.* 1997;13:6–8.

23. CDC. Vital Signs: Changes in opioid prescribing in the United States, 2006–2015.

24. Gladden RM, Martinez P, Seth P. Fentanyl law enforcement submissions and increases in synthetic opioid–involved overdose deaths—27 states, 2013–2014. *MMWR.* 2016;65:837–43.

25. Hall AJ, Logan JE, Toblin RL, et al. Patterns of abuse among unintentional pharmaceutical overdose fatalities. *JAMA.* 2008;300:2613–20.

26. Rutkow L, Chang HY, Daubresse M, Webster DW, Stuart EA, Alexander GC. Effect of Florida's prescription drug monitoring program and pill mill laws on opioid prescribing and use. *JAMA Intern Med.* 2015;175:1642–9.

27. Kennedy-Hendricks A, Richey M, McGinty EE, Stuart EA, Barry CL, Webster DW. Opioid overdose deaths and Florida's crackdown on pill mills. *Am J Public Health.* 2016;106:291–7.

28. CDC. Injury prevention & control: opioid overdose. https://www.cdc.gov/drugoverdose/index.html

29. Reza A, Breiding MJ, Gulaid J, et al. Sexual violence and its health consequences for female children in Swaziland: a cluster survey study. *Lancet.* 2009;373:1966–72.

30. Sumner S, Maenner M, Socias C, et al. Sentinel events preceding youth firearm violence: an investigation of administrative data in Delaware. *Am J Prev Med.* 2016;51:647–55.

31. Schulden J, Chen J, Kresnow MJ, et al. Psychological responses to the sniper attacks: Washington DC area, October 2002. *Am J Prev Med*. 2006;31:324–7.

32. Mercado MC, Quan L, Bennett E, et al. Can you really swim? Validation of self and parental reports of swim skill with an inwater swim test among children attending community pools in Washington State. *Inj Prev*. 2016;22:253–60.

33. US Environmental Protection Agency. Laws and Regulations. Summary of the Paper Reduction Act. 44 USC §3501 et seq. (1980). https://www.epa.gov/laws-regulations/summary-paperwork-reduction-act

34. Paulozzi LJ, Mercy J, Frazier L, Jr., Annest JL. CDC's National Violent Death Reporting System: background and methodology. *Inj Prev*. 2004;10:47–52.

35. CDC. Striving to Reduce Youth Violence Everywhere. http://vetoviolence.cdc.gov/stryve/

36. Center for the Study and Prevention of Violence, University of Colorado Boulder. Blueprints for healthy youth development. http://www.colorado.edu/cspv/blueprints

37. Fortson BL, Klevens J, Merrick MT, Gilbert LK, Alexander SP. *Preventing Child Abuse and Neglect: A Technical Package for Policy, Norm, and Programmatic Activities*. Atlanta: CDC, National Center for Injury Prevention and Control; 2016.

38. Basile KC, DeGue S, Jones K, et al. *STOP SV: A Technical Package to Prevent Sexual Violence*. Atlanta: CDC, National Center for Injury Prevention and Control; 2016.

39. David-Ferdon C, Vivolo-Kantor AM, Dahlberg LL, Marshall KJ., Rainford N, Hall JE. *A Comprehensive Technical Package for the Prevention of Youth Violence and Associated Risk Behaviors*. Atlanta: CDC, National Center for Injury Prevention and Control; 2016.

40. Stone DM, Holland KM, Bartholow B, Crosby AE, Davis S, Wilkins N. *Preventing Suicide: A Technical Package of Policies, Programs, and Practices*. Atlanta: CDC, National Center for Injury Prevention and Control; 2017.

41. Niolon PH, Kearns M, Dills J, et al. *A Technical Package to Prevent Teen Dating and Intimate Partner Violence*. Atlanta: CDC, National Center for Injury Prevention and Control; 2017.

42. Dowell D, Haegerich TM, Chou R. CDC Guideline for prescribing opioids for chronic pain—United States, 2016. *MMWR*. 2016;65(no. RR-1):1–49.

43. World Health Organization. Global report on drowning: preventing a leading killer. http://apps.who.int/iris/bitstream/10665/143893/1/9789241564786_eng.pdf?ua=1&ua=1

44. World Health Organization. Save LIVES—a road safety technical package. Geneva: World Health Organization; 2017. http://apps.who.int/iris/bitstream/10665/255199/1/9789241511704-eng.pdf?ua=1.

INDEX